RESEARCH IN HEALTH ECONOMICS

A Research Annual

Editor: RICHARD M. SCHEFFLER
Department of Economics
George Washington University

VOLUME 1 • 1979

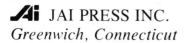 JAI PRESS INC.
Greenwich, Connecticut

CONTENTS

INTRODUCTION

It is my pleasure to introduce the first volume of the annual compilation of research in health economics. Health economics, as a field, has grown and developed at an exponential rate during the last decade. With its growth, the quantity of high-quality research has grown in a corresponding manner.

Some of this research has found its way into the traditional economics journals, while some has appeared in journals oriented toward health services researchers. The research appearing in traditional economics journals, such as the *American Economic Review,* is, for the most part, not policy-oriented or directly relevant to the current problems in the health services industry. On the other hand, the health services research journals are not oriented toward an audience which is trained in economics. Thus most of the research must be softened if it is to appear in these journals. This results in a loss of rigor.

There are also a significant number of high-quality pieces of research which deal with problems and questions in health economics that cannot find a proper publication outlet. They treat a problem in a complete and comprehensive manner. This usually involves the development of an economic model, its empirical testing or estimation, and a discussion of the policy implications. To many health economics, this is the kind of research that is most needed.

It is my hope that this annual series will serve as an outlet for this kind of research. Authors will be given the opportunity to publish their work in health economics in an integrated manner. To facilitate this, manuscripts of 50 to 70 pages will be accepted. However, when warranted, shorter papers, especially those which complement each other, will also be published.

I am fortunate in being able to inaugurate the series with an outstanding set of papers on health manpower. The first paper, by Kenneth Smith, Ralph Andreano, and Uwe Reinhardt, discusses the major analytical problems in making health manpower policy. They discuss manpower substitution, especially as it relates to the physician assistant. Next is a short paper of mine which follows some of their work. In this paper, I present some new production function results for new health practitioners. I also provide examples of how these results may be useful in developing alternative manpower strategies.

The paper by Karen Davis and Ray Marshall concentrates on the the special health manpower problems of rural areas, especially in the South. Davis and Marshall base their findings on data collected via site visits to rural areas. Using a nonmarket approach, they develop a strategy for meeting the health care needs of these areas. A key element in their strategy is the utilization of nurse practitioners.

A crucial issue in health manpower today is the apparent shortage of physicians in primary care. Jack Hadley's analysis is perhaps the most comprehensive piece of work on specialty choice by physicians. With the benefit of a unique set of longitudinal data, he is able to analyze the effect of medical education and training as well as the personnel characteristics of the physicians on their choice of medical specialty.

Another major health manpower problem today is that of distribution. A large volume of research has been done on this subject. However, little, if any, has taken the perspective of the state. Since states have considerable responsibility and influence in health manpower policy, this is an important gap in the litreature. It is partly filled by Gail Wilensky's paper.

Although it is of considerable interest, little is known about the spatial distribution of physicians and their pricing policy or vice versa. Roger Feldman develops a rigorous economic model on this subject and tests the hypothesis he develops from it with data from the periodic survey conducted by the American Medical Association.

Nurses are by far the largest single group of health manpower. Most are women, employed in a hospital setting. Frank Sloan and Richard Elnicki provide an extremely useful and important analysis of the factors that affect wage determination of nurses in hospitals. With an excellent data base, they set hypotheses about monopsony power, the effect of hospital unions, as well as the effect of education and training on nurse wages.

Because of the complexities of the market for nurses, Donald Yett and Robert Deane developed a twenty-five equation simulation model. Although the model's data requirements are beyond those usually available, the model does provide a useful framework to explore the factors that affect aggregate requirement for nurses.

The approach taken by Joseph Lipscomb, Lawrence E. Berg, Virginia L. London, and Paul A. Nutting is unique. It presents a model for allocating health manpower that will maximize the health status of a population. Surely more attention will be paid to models of this type in the near future.

I am really pleased to already have one indicator of the success of this series before its actual publication. It is the outstanding collection of papers that have already been accepted for Volume II of the series. A list of working titles follows:

Volume II: A Theoretical and Empirical Investigation into Hospital Outpatient Measures; Demand for Dental Care; Demand for Medical Care in a Rural Area; Determinants of Children's Health; Economic Incentives in Health Maintenance Organizations; Health Care and Technology; Current Issues in the Economics of Dentistry; The Economics of Community Pharmacies; Physician Reimbursement; Pricing Medical Services: A Segmented Labor Market Approach.

Richard M. Scheffler

PLANNING A NATIONAL HEALTH MANPOWER POLICY: A CRITIQUE AND A STRATEGY

Kenneth R. Smith, NORTHWESTERN UNIVERSITY

Uwe E. Reinhardt, PRINCETON UNIVERSITY

Ralph L. Andreano, UNIVERSITY OF WISCONSIN

I. MANPOWER POLICY AND NATIONAL HEALTH POLICY

Everyone knows that health manpower needs and availabilities at some future date can be substantially affected by public policy. This effect depends on the interaction and independent development of:

1. The internal organization of the manpower resources within the health delivery system; the forces—economic, social, and political—which impinge on the present organization of the system and can, or will, act to change the present structure and performance of the system;

Research in Health Economics, Vol. 1, pp 1–35.

2. What is done in terms of financing consumption of health services on the demand side and what is done to increase or augment the supplies of resources available for providers and producers of health services on the supply side.

Given the critical importance of the government's role in the health manpower arena, the question naturally arises, "What are the ingredients of a rational manpower policy?" This in turn leads to the question, "On what information should such policy be based?"

Forecasts of health manpower have traditionally been based on an independent projection of the aggregate demand for health services, an assumption concerning the productivity of providers and an assumption concerning the relationship between consumption of medical services and the required manpower needs. Aggregate demand projections are typically formulated by applying to independently derived demographic-economic predictions various crude price and income elasticities of demand for a broad range of health services to be consumed from the present delivery system. To determine manpower requirements, some assumption about productivity growth is made, usually just for physicians, seldom for the productivity growth of the entire delivery system and seldom explicitly incorporating substitution effects between the physician and other health manpower. These demand predictions and productivity assumptions are used to derive total manpower requirements which, when compared with an estimate of the supplies, allow shortages and/or surpluses to be assessed at some future date.

In our judgment, and for reasons to be developed further in the next section of this paper, to determine health manpower policy there must be a well-defined and publicly accepted *goal* or *objective* that the Federal government has in health policy. Only in this way will it be possible to predict in advance the unintended, as distinct from the intended, effects of government policies.

What are the implications for national health manpower policy which follow from these observations? First, it simply will not be possible to project needs against availabilities until one has a clear and definite statement of goals from the Federal government. Second, the statement of goals must resolve the differences between consumption of health services through market processes and consumption of health services in terms of *medical* need. Third, no presently existing estimation of future manpower surplus or shortage can have any substantive policy implication. Such estimates have been constructed in too highly an aggregated fashion and with assumptions that are not acceptable. Indeed, the assumption of constant productivity growth, or of assumed price and income elasticities based on historical experience will prove far off the mark unless we know: (a) the internal dynamics of the health delivery system and what forces—internal and external—can move it to a different organization of resources, and (b) the objective function in health which orders national health policy on the part of the Federal government. National health policy then becomes the key link to formulating any sensible and meaningful health manpower policy.

Can one discern from recent government actions the nucleus of a *national health policy?* Three things seem clear: an emphasis on "access" (financial and geographic), on "cost," and on "quality." "Access" is viewed as a surrogate for medical need; increased financial and geographic access is to take place without a deterioration in quality of care. "Cost" is viewed as both private, that is, the net cost of services to the consumer, and public, that is, some balancing of health spending against other federal spending such that the share of the federal budget to health can be set with some predictable accuracy from year to year. "Quality" is often viewed simply as an absolute. Government policies to augment manpower supplies have "access," "cost," and "quality" objectives; government policies to reduce net price to the consumer, or some subset of consumers, have "access" objectives and "cost" implications; government policies to reorganize the delivery system also have these objectives. But the policies adopted often involve a conflict between these objectives in the sense that one policy may increase "access" but also increase "cost" and vice versa. With respect to "quality," if the professed goal of the nation's health system is to provide adequate care to *all* citizens, then any overall index of quality inevitably involves a trade-off between the quality of services *delivered* and the number of persons covered by the system.

The political process in which legislation defining goals of national health takes place inevitably leads to such conflicts and trade-offs. No simple statement would be a meaningful characterization of the goal or goals of the U.S. medical care system. "Better health" is perhaps the highest goal, but the nearer, more direct view of the medical care problem is more difficult to identify. In fact, it is a mistake to talk about "the" problem, to identify "the" goal, for there are many and they are seen differently by different groups of people. Thus, choice among proposals for financing health care producing a different health manpower mix are really not choices among alternative ways of achieving a particular goal: they are choices among the alternative ways of achieving *different* goals! Since there are conflicts between various conceptions of the problem, what is a "solution" for one group becomes a problem for another. The aged, the young, the wealthy, the poor, the government, the hospitals, physicians, other health personnel, to each of these other groups, the "health-care crisis" and its "solution" look different. Physicians see the appropriate health care goal as high standards of patient health care; the Federal government sees the goal as "good health" but at a reasonable cost; the medical research establishment sees the goal as expanded scientific knowledge; and the consumer sees the goal as obtaining the medical services *and knowledge* to which he feels entitled, at "reasonable" cost to him—whatever its total cost may be to society.

At the present time, then, given these conflicts and pressures, what contributions can we make on the manpower side? It is our belief that what can best be accomplished at this point is to identify the key parameters which will affect manpower needs and availabilities in the future and how these parameters can be and/or are being manipulated. The key question is what "state of the world" assumptions can realistically be made; that is, whose health policy goals will dominate?—because manpower demands will differ with different goals that are set. Is the present organization of the delivery system to be assumed? Is universal entitlement the appropriate "state of the world"? If the present delivery system cannot be assumed, how will it be changed, who will change it? How should the system be organized? For the consumer? For the provider? What should the government's role be in influencing whatever "state of the world" is to prevail? What will be its actual role? Is the government's objective to create an efficient delivery system? How can it eliminate present inefficiencies—by a "rewards" or "punishment" approach? What would manpower demands look like in a "state of the world" where government draws a fixed budgetary line, i.e., agrees to spend only a specified fraction of GNP and no more on health? What will closed-end, fixed budgetary commitments imply in terms of alternative manpower combinations? Will they produce surpluses or deficits relative to anticipated, objectively determined, *medical need?*

We cannot hope to provide answers, indeed there may be none, to all these questions. But we insist that all that has been discussed thus far is crucial if any sensible national health manpower policies are ever to be formulated. In the next section we develop these themes by looking explicitly at the usefulness of existing manpower projections. We argue that manpower forecasting, as distinct from manpower policy, has become merely a numerical exercise; the nature of the underlying assumptions on which the forecasts are based are more critical than the numbers themselves.

II. WEAKNESSES INHERENT IN NUMERICAL HEALTH-MANPOWER FORECASTS, OR, THE FUTILITY OF THE NUMBERS GAME

One rather narrow conception of a federal policy for health manpower would be the notion that this policy should essentially be a response to exogenously determined shortages or surpluses of particular types of health manpower. Under that approach, an impending shortage might, for example, trigger Federal health subsidies for the construction of additional manpower training facilities and/or tuition support for potential entrants into the occupation. The policy response to an impending surplus would be to reduce such subsidies to manpower training as have traditionally been given or, if subsidies are not being granted, to maintain a hands-off posture and to let the market take its course.

In view of the often long lead time between policy action and policy impact in the manpower training area, it is clear that the reactive type of policy described above presupposes highly reliable point estimates of future manpower requirements and availability. Since much of past public policy in the manpower area has, in fact, resembled this type of policy, it is not surprising that considerable research energy has been devoted to preparing health-manpower forecasts for up to three decades into the future. Unfortunately, the various forecasts that have been offered in the past have not distinguished themselves by their accuracy and they have therefore left policy makers with a sense of disillusionment. To some extent, the forecasts in question did leave something to be desired from the point of view of methodology or of their empirical foundation. The real problem, however, and one not likely to be overcome even with the best research effort, is the fact that any such forecast must be the product of a complex system of interdependent relationships. In technical parlance, any future manpower estimate is but one variable in a large simultaneous equations system. Within the context of health-manpower forecasting, it is therefore quite legitimate to seek protection behind the well-known caveat that "it is always difficult to predict anything, especially the future."

In this section we shall briefly review the methodology used in traditional forecasts of health manpower and indicate the rather large variance in alternative forecasts made for a given target year. Next, we shall indicate the more important parameters that jointly determine the future demand of a particular type of manpower. The discussion will be followed with an illustration of the sensitivity of future health-manpower requirements to changes in the projected time-path of these underlying parameters. The entire section is intended to highlight the futility of any attempt to structure a Federal health-manpower policy on point estimates of future manpower requirements, for it will become obvious in the course of our discussion that such point estimates inevitably tend to degenerate into a numbers game.

A. Previous Health Manpower Forecasts

Probably the simplest definition of the future requirement of a particular type of health manpower is the algebraic expression

$$R_t = (D_t/Q_t)P_t \tag{1}$$

where R_t denotes the manpower requirement at time t, D_t is the per capita demand for the services produced by that type of manpower, Q_t denotes the average output of such services per unit of that manpower, and P_t is the population to be served at t.

Point estimates of future manpower requirements typically proceed via an equation of this sort. It is assumed that the per capita demand for the service, D_t, is given exogenously and can be predicted for period t. Next, an assumption is made about the average productivity of manpower, Q_t, in period t (also thought to be exogenous) and the resultant ratio D_t/Q_t is multiplied by the projected population for period t. Within the context of the forecasting model described by equation (1), health manpower research is, in the main, an attempt to project reliable values of P_t, D_t, and Q_t under alternative assumptions about the organization of the health care sector.

It is clear that the demand-variable D_t, is a function of an entire array of socioeconomic and demographic variables. In order to predict D_t, one must first of all have empirical knowledge about the precise nature of this function. Next, one must project values for the socioeconomic and demographic determinants of D_t and insert these values into the demand function. To the extent that the empirical per capita demand function has been estimated by relating past, observable *utilization* to the hypothesized determinants of *demand,* one must make allowance for the fact that past utilization patterns will not be a true reflection of past *demand.* In the context of the health care market, any difference between observed utilization and effective demand may have one of two distinct origins. First, it may be the fact that the observed utilization pattern emerged from a system that operated under severe, effective supply constraints so that a part of the effective demand was simply never satisfied. Alternatively, if it is indeed true that, in the health care market, the available supply occasionally generates its own demand, then an observed utilization pattern may contain elements that would not be observed under balanced demand-supply conditions. In short, it should be obvious that any attempt to forecast the future per capita demand for a particular kind of medical service is a hazardous venture and can at best yield point estimates with sizable standard errors of prediction.

Any forecast about the future productivity of any particular type of health manpower is similarly hazardous. At the most general level, the productivity parameter Q_t may be written as a function

$$Q_t = f(L_{1t}, L_{2t}, \ldots, L_{nt}, K_t; A_t) \qquad (2)$$

where L_{jt} denotes units of manpower of type j employed in period t, K_t is an index of the supportive capital available to all employed manpower, and A_t may be taken as a general productivity index whose value may be determined in part by the organizational setup under which health care is delivered and for the remainder by a whole host of quantitative and qualitative factors. The important point to note about equation (2) is the fact that the average productivity of any particular type of health manpower is strongly influenced by the relative amounts of other types of manpower who work either as complements or as partial substitutes along with the type of manpower under consideration. *It is this interdependence among types of health manpower that make the projection of the demand for a particular type of health manpower so enormously difficult.*

In past forecasts, it has generally been assumed that the relative amounts of health manpower would remain more or less unchanged in the future so that the problem of interdependence could simply be forgotten.[1] This approach, however, is in conflict with the historical fact that relative amounts of health manpower have shifted significantly in the past.[2] And, as will be argued later in this paper, it abstracts entirely from the possibility that public policy in the manpower area may be deliberately slanted to produce changes in the overall composition of health manpower.

Once the future variability in the overall composition of health manpower is acknowledged, it becomes clear that any particular point estimate of future manpower requirements is really nothing more than one particular combination from a great variety of alternative manpower combinations technically capable of satisfying a given aggregate demand for medical care. In other words, so long as it is technically feasible to substitute one type of health manpower for another in the production of health services, it will be impossible to translate any given projected demand for health services into a *unique* vector of manpower requirements. Instead, the best that can be achieved in such a forecast is the identification of alternative manpower mixes that can meet the target demand.

While it is true that some of the mixes so identified are more likely to become reality than others, there nevertheless will be sufficient flexibility to permit an entire menu of plausible outcomes. It follows that a narrowly conceived manpower policy which simply seeks to react to predicted shortages is likely to be troubled from the outset. A more fruitful approach is a policy that considers future manpower requirements as a set of endogenous variables that can be influenced by that policy itself. On that view, the policy maker's emphasis should shift away somewhat from the numbers game toward the (often less quantifiable) determinants of variable D_t and particularly of variable Q_t in equation (1). The main objective of the present paper is to identify the logical targets for policy action under this broader conception of federal health manpower policy.

B. Sensitivity of Manpower Forecasts to Productivity Change

It may be well to illustrate the argument presented above at a general level with a concrete numerical example that will underscore the tenuity of point estimates for future health manpower requirements and the futility of a manpower policy heavily dependent upon such forecasts. In presenting the illustration, we shall concentrate on physicians, not only because empirical information is more readily available for that type of manpower but also because physicians have long been of primary concern in health manpower forecasting.

Table 1 below, taken from W. L. Hansen (1970), presents a convenient summary of the physician requirement forecast in a variety of studies for the year 1975. The considerable variance in the projected requirement, and particularly in the projected surplus or deficit, reflects not only the fact that the forecasts were prepared at different points in time, but also differences in the underlying assumptions about the future time path of per capita demand for physician services, physician productivity, and perhaps even about future population growth. It is quite possible that if six completely independent studies were commissioned today, each with the mandate to produce a point estimate of the derived demand for physicians in 1985, a roughly similar variance in projected shortages of surpluses would result. And chances are that the bulk of that variance could be explained by differences in the assumptions (opinions) concerning the future values of the many parameters embedded in the forecasting equation.

Tables 2 and 3 indicate the sensitivity of future physician requirements to one of the parameters alluded to above: the average productivity of practicing physicians. The top rows in Table 2 indicate the projected supply of all physicians (row 1) and of practicing physicians (row 2) in Canada for the years 1961 to 1991 [Reinhardt (1971)]. Rows 3 to 5 indicate the *required* number of physicians in those years on the assumption that the per capita demand for physicians' services will remain a constant 5.37 visits and on the assumption of alternative rate of productivity growth. It is seen that in the absence of productivity growth, a deficit of about 7,000 physicians (about 30 percent of the available supply) is forecast for 1991.

Table 1. Summary of Physician Projections for 1975

Projection study	Requirements (I)	Supplies (II)	(-) Deficit** (+) Surplus (III)
1 Bane Committee Report	330,000 (minimum)	(a) 312,800 (b) 318,400	-17,200 -11,600
2 Bureau of Labor Statistics (1966)	305,000	– –	– –
3 Fein	(a) 340,000 to 350,000 (b) 372,000 to 385,000	361,700	+21,700 to +11,700 -10,300 to -23,300
4 National Advisory Commission on Health Manpower	346,000 (minimum)	360,000	+14,000
5 Bureau of Labor Statistics (1967)	390,000	360,000	-30,000
6 Public Health Service	(a) 400,000 (b) 425,000	360,000	-40,000 -65,000

Note: *Physicians include both M.D.'s and D.O.'s, except for Line 2 which excludes D.O.'s.
**Column (II) minus Column (I). A (-) indicates a deficit; (+) indicates a surplus.

Sources:

Line (1) Surgeon General's Consultant Group on Medical Education. Frank Bane, Chairman. *Physicians for a Growing America.* (Washington: GPO, 1959)
Column (1) Table 2, p. 3.
Column (II) (a) and (b) Table 2, p. 3.
Column (III) Calculated.

Line (2) U.S. Bureau of Labor Statistics. "America's Industrial and Occupational Manpower Requirements, 1964-1975." In: *The Outlook for Technological Change and Employment,* Appendix Volume I to *Technology and the American Economy,* Report of the National Commission on Technology, Automation, and Economic Progress, (February 1966)
Column (I) Page 1-141; obtained by multiplying the number of employed physicians in 1964 (265,000) by the "nearly 15 percent" projected rise in "employment" from 1964 to 1975. A study of this report indicates that the word "employment" is used as a synonym for "requirements."
Column (II) No figure is available.
Column (III) Not calculated.

Line (3) Fein, Rashi, *The Doctor Shortage: An Economic Analysis.* (Washington: The Brookings Institution, 1967)
Column (I) (a) Based on 12-15 percent increase due to population growth above. (b) Based on 22-26 percent increase due to all factors. See pp. 134-135.
Column (II) Table III-9, p. 87.
Column (III) Calculated.

Line (4) National Advisory Commission on Health Manpower. *Report, Vol. II.* (Washington: GPO, 1967)
Column (I) Based on 13.5 percent increase in total visits by 1975. See p. 243.
Column (II) Table 4, p. 235.
Column (III) Calculated.

Line (5) U.S. Bureau of Labor Statistics. *Health Manpower 1966-1975, A Study of Requirements and Supply.* (Washington: GPO, 1967)
Column (I) Page 18.
Column (II) No figure is given. I assume NACHM supply figure of 360,000 is appropriate to use.
Column (III) Calculated.

Line (6) U.S. Public Health Service, *Health Manpower, Perspectives 1967.* (Washington: GPO, 1967)
Column (I) (a) and (b), Table 8, p. 15, and accompanying text.
Column (II) Same as Column II, line 5.
Column (III) Calculated.

Source: W.L. Hansen, (1970).

Table 2. The Effect of Productivity Growth on the
Requirements of Private Medical Practitioners

CANADA, 1961 - 1991

	1961	1971	1981	1991
Expected Total Supply of Physicians	21,290	25,826	29,069	31,410
Expected Number of Physicians in Private Practice[a]	15,450	18,800	21,100	22,800

I. Required Number of Private Practitioners if d = 5.3784 Visits per Capita. Assuming:[b]

	1961	1971	1981	1991
$q_t = 6336$ for all t	15,481	19,174	23,976	29,799
$q_t = 6336 e^{.01 (t-1961)}$	15,481	17,352	19,636	22,073
$q_t = 6336 e^{.02 (t-1961)}$	15,481	15,703	16,070	16,355

II. Required Number of Private Practitioners if d = 6.7320 Visits per Capita. Assuming:[b]

	1961	1971	1981	1991
$q_t = 6336$ for all t	19,352	23,969	29,972	37,251
$q_t = 6336 e^{.01 (t-1961)}$	19,352	21,692	24,547	27,593
$q_t = 6336 e^{.02 (t-1961)}$	19,352	19,631	20,088	20,445

[a] Calculated as 72.5 percent of total supply of physicians.
[b] Zero, 1 percent and 2 percent productivity growth, respectively.

Table 3. Physician-Population Ratios Required to Service a Constant per
Capita Demand for Physician Services

Assumed Annual Rate of Increase in Q_t	Required Physician Population Ratio (Base-Year Ratio set at 100)		
	5 Years Hence	10 Years Hence	20 Years Hence
0%	100	100	100
1%	95	90	82
2%	90	82	67

The shortage all but disappears on the assumption of an annual productivity growth of 1 percent. At a productivity growth of 2 percent per year, the deficit of 7,000 physicians becomes a surplus of about 6,500 physicians (about 28 percent of the available supply). Rows 6 to 8 repeat the experiment for a higher per capita utilization of services. Table 3 illustrates the same phenomenon but more compactly and at a more general level.

The question arises, of course, whether the rates of change in physician productivity suggested in Tables 2 and 3 are at all realistic. For U.S. industry as a whole, the long-run growth rate in output *per manhour* during the postwar period has been on the order of 4 percent per annum, although due to shorter working hours the rate of output *per person employed*—the analogue to parameter Q in equation (1)—has grown at only about 3.3 percent. The corresponding rate in the commercial *services* industries, however, have been only 1.8 and 1.1 percent, respectively. The notion that productivity growth in the professional services industries—such as law, teaching, or medicine—is even more difficult to achieve than in the commercial services sector as a whole has led some students of the health care sector to believe that sustained productivity growth of even as much as 1 percent per annum cannot be expected in medical practice.

Past research on productivity growth in medical practice during the postwar years has suggested that physician productivity in those years did indeed increase by between 2.0 percent and 4.5 percent per year [Klarman (December 1969)]. There is, however, little information about the sources of this productivity growth. It is reasonable to assume that the almost complete shift from relatively time-consuming home visits to less time-intensive office visits has enabled the physician to handle a far greater patient load than was previously possible. The postwar period was also one during which a number of important antibiotics were introduced, and one may suppose that widespread use of these antibiotics had yielded significant economies in the use of the physician's own time. To what extent pharmaceuticals can contribute toward physician productivity in the future is at this time an open question. In fact, those who argue that there is still considerable room for further improvements in physician productivity typically base their case on the following potential developments:

1. The substitution of registered or licensed nurses, medical technicians and clerical personnel for the physician's time (such personnel will hereafter be referred to as "traditional" paramedical personnel).

2. The substitution of more carefully trained *physician extenders* for the physician's time.

3. The potential impact of technological advances on manpower productivity in the health care sector.

4. The introduction of new organization forms (e.g., health maintenance organizations) into the health care delivery system.

The main problem at this stage is that, for the most part, there does not exist sufficient empirical information on the potential impact each of these factors can have on the productivity of health manpower. Although such information is gradually emerging from ongoing research, any health manpower forecast that currently seeks to incorporate these factors must remain something of an educated guess.

B.1. The Potential Role of Traditional Types of Auxiliary Personnel

A rough idea about the potential impact on physician productivity achievable through task delegation from physicians to the *traditional* types of paramedical assistants may be obtained from an evaluation of previous production function research on that problem. One production function that has been proposed and estimated has the general algebraic form [Reinhardt (1972)]:

$$Q_t = A_t H_t^{a-1} K_t^b e_{dL_t - gL_t^2} \tag{3}$$

where Q_t is the rate of patient visits processed by the individual physician (i.e., it *is* parameter Q_t in the forecasting equation (1) above), H_t is the number of physician hours worked per period, K_t is an index of supportive capital and L_t is the number of traditional paramedical assistants supporting the physician. Equation (3) can be used in conjunction with the general manpower forecasting equation (1) above to calculate the following magnitudes:

1. Suppose we postulated a future time path for L_t (e.g., we assumed that the number of traditional aides available to support the physician in period t) and furthermore assumed given time paths for the per capita demand of physician services and the size of the population to be served, what must the time path of the available number of physicians be if we want to see the demand generated by the population met? An illustration of that calculation is shown in Table 4.

2. Given time paths of the per capita demand for physician services, of the number of physicians available, and of the size of the population to be served, what is the time path of the number of aides per physician (L_t) such that at any point in time t, the demand for physician services can, in fact, be met with the number of physicians then available? An illustration of that calculation is shown in Table 5.

In making the calculations shown in Tables 4 and 5, it has been assumed that the number of hours physicians work per week (H_t) will remain constant over time. Furthermore, it has been assumed that the population to be served (P_t) will increase at an average annual rate of 1 percent. The postulated growth of per capita demand (D_t) is based on the assumption that the nation has adopted a comprehensive health insurance plan with relatively modest deductibles and co-insurance rates. Thus, in Table 4 it has been assumed that the insurance plan will, through a gradual learning process, drive the per capita demand for physician services to a level that reaches about 125 percent of the pre-insurance level after about one decade. The time-phased demand increase postulated in Table 5 assumes an even larger price elasticity of the demand for physician services, after about one decade, D_t is assumed to reach a level close to 155 percent of its pre-insurance level. Finally, since our intent here is merely to illustrate the point rather than to generate a concrete forecast, all timepaths have been expressed in the form of index numbers, with base-year values set equal to 1. The only exception is the time series of the number of aides per physician which has been expressed in actual numbers. The calculations are based on an actual production function estimate for a nationwide cross section of self-employed medical practitioners [Reinhardt (1972)].[3]

Tables 4 and 5 bring out a number of important points. First, it is seen from Table 4 that a given increase in the demand for physician services can be met with quite distinct mixes of health manpower. If the number of aides per physician are permitted to increase by only 1 percent per year, then the postulated demand can be met only if, by year 25, the number of physicians has increased by about 59 percent over its base-year level. This corresponds to a physician population level that has increased by about 23 percent over its base-year level. By contrast, if the number of aides per physician is permitted to increase as fast as 5 percent per year, then the same demand profile can be met with far less physician manpower. As is seen from the table, by year 25, the number of physicians would have to be only about 26 percent higher than the base-year value, and the physician-population ratio could actually be permitted to decline somewhat from its base-year value. Given the size of the actual stock of physicians in this country (roughly 350,000) these changes in the index numbers certainly reflect nontrivial differences in medical manpower.[4]

In Table 5, it is assumed that the number of physicians is increasing in step with population growth, so that the physician-population ratio remains at one. The table indicates to what extent the fairly strong demand pressure posited in column 2 can be met by increasing the average productivity of physicians. As mentioned above, this presentation is based upon the assumption that the only potential source of such productivity increases will be increases in the number of traditional auxiliary personnel supporting the physician. The columns headed by the symbol L_t/L_t indicate the annual increase in the number of aides required to meet the

Table 4. Estimated Future Physician Requirements at Given Growth Rates in the Stock of Traditional Paramedical Assistants (Base-Year Values Set Equal to Unity)

Year	Per Capita Demand D_t	Population P_t	Total Demand $D_t P_t$	Time Path of Future Physician Requirements (R_t) if the Number of Aides Increases At					
				1 Percent/Year			5 Percent/Year		
				Number of Aides[a] L_t	Number of MD's R_t	Phys./ Popul. R_t/P_t	Number of Aides[a] L_t	Number of MD's R_t	Phys./ Popul. R_t/P_t
0	1.000	1.000	1.000	1.800	1.000	1.000	1.80	1.000	1.000
1.	1.030	1.010	1.04	1.818	1.037	1.027	1.892	1.021	1.011
2.	1.073	1.020	1.09	1.836	1.086	1.064	1.989	1.052	1.031
3.	1.127	1.030	1.16	1.855	1.149	1.115	2.091	1.095	1.063
4.	1.174	1.041	1.22	1.873	1.203	1.156	2.199	1.128	1.084
5.	1.209	1.051	1.27	1.892	1.247	1.186	2.311	1.150	1.094
6.	1.234	1.062	1.31	1.911	1.280	1.205	2.430	1.161	1.093
7.	1.246	1.073	1.34	1.931	1.301	1.213	2.554	1.160	1.082
8.	1.252	1.083	1.36	1.950	1.315	1.214	2.685	1.154	1.065

9.	1.259	1.094	1.38	1.970	1.330	1.215	2.823	1.148	1.049
10.	1.265	1.105	1.40	1.989	1.345	1.217	2.968	1.142	1.034
11.	1.271	1.116	1.42	2.009	1.360	1.218	3.120	1.137	1.019
12.	1.278	1.127	1.44	2.029	1.375	1.219	3.280	1.133	1.005
13.	1.284	1.139	1.46	2.050	1.390	1.220	3.448	1.130	0.992
14.	1.290	1.150	1.48	2.070	1.405	1.222	3.625	1.129	0.981
15.	1.297	1.162	1.51	2.091	1.421	1.223	3.811	1.129	0.971
16.	1.303	1.173	1.53	2.112	1.436	1.224	4.006	1.131	0.964
17.	1.310	1.185	1.55	2.134	1.452	1.225	4.211	1.135	0.958
18.	1.317	1.197	1.58	2.155	1.468	1.226	4.427	1.143	0.955
19.	1.323	1.209	1.60	2.177	1.484	1.228	4.654	1.154	0.954
20.	1.330	1.221	1.62	2.199	1.501	1.229	4.893	1.169	0.957
21.	1.336	1.234	1.65	2.221	1.517	1.230	5.000[b]	1.187	0.962
22.	1.343	1.246	1.67	2.243	1.534	1.231	5.000	1.205	0.967
23.	1.350	1.259	1.70	2.265	1.551	1.232	5.000	1.223	0.972
24.	1.357	1.271	1.72	2.288	1.568	1.233	5.000	1.242	0.977
25.	1.363	1.284	1.75	2.311	1.585	1.234	5.000	1.260	0.982

[a] In absolute numbers, per physician.
[b] At five aides/physicians, negative marginal returns to aides set in.

15

Table 5. Estimated Required Future Growth in the Number
of Aides per Physician
(Base-Year Values Set Equal to Unity)

Yr t	Total demand for services $D_t P_t$ [a]	Supply of physicians M_t	Phys./ popul. ratio M_t/P_t	Required percentage increase in no. of aides L_t/L_t	Number of aides per physician [b] L_t	Time path of productivity of physicians Q_t
0	1.00	1.00	1.00	– –	1.80	1.00
1	1.04	1.01	1.00	7.6%	1.94	1.03
2	1.09	1.02	1.00	9.9	2.15	1.07
3	1.16	1.03	1.00	12.1	2.42	1.13
4	1.25	1.04	1.00	14.7	2.80	1.20
5	1.32	1.05	1.00	13.1	3.20	1.26
6	1.39	1.06	1.00	12.1	3.61	1.31
7	1.45	1.07	1.00	12.1	4.10	1.35
8	1.49	1.08	1.00	– –	– – [c]	– –
-	1.52					
-	1.54					

[a] Based on the assumption that a national health insurance plan is introduced in year t=o, and that the annual percentage increase in per capita demand for physician services increases rapidly during the initial years of the plan as follows:

Year	Increase in D_t	Year	Increase in D_t
1	3%	6	4%
2	4	7	3
3	5	8	2
4	6	9	1
5	5	10	½

and every year thereafter by ½ percent. The population is assumed to increase by 1 percent per year.

[b] Actual number (not index number) of aides per physician.

[c] In year 8, the required number of aides is not defined, because negative marginal returns to aides are assumed to set in after employment of the 5th aide.

demand for health services. The effect of these increases in auxiliary personnel on the physician's productivity can be read off the last column in the table. It is seen from that column that task delegation to paramedical aides can—according to the underlying production function—increase physician productivity by about 35 percent over the base-year level. Thereafter, however, the employment of additional aides is characterized by negative (or at least nonpositive) marginal returns. A similar effect will be observed in Table 4 (see especially note b to that table).

A second important point to emerge from Tables 4 and 5 is therefore that the substitution of traditional types of paramedical for medical personnel is not an inexhaustible source of increases in physician productivity. For the particular demand profile postulated in Table 5, for example, that source has been fully depleted after about year 7. Thereafter, any increase in the demand for services has to be met by corresponding increases in the number of physicians, or through delegation of higher level medical tasks to specially trained personnel: the so-called *physician extenders*. For situations characterized by less intensive demand pressure, on the other hand, the delegation of tasks to traditional types of auxiliary personnel might well be a sufficient remedy for any impending physician shortage.

B.2   The Potential Role of Physician Extenders

Although the previously cited production function research suggests that considerable increases in physician productivity can be achieved through a judicious use of nurses, medical technicians or even clerical personnel, it is widely suspected that the employment of physician extenders will constitute by far the most important source of such productivity gains during the next few decades. Precisely how important the contribution of this new type of personnel is to the physician's own productivity is as yet an open question, but one on which much research is currently underway. Table 6 below presents a convenient summary of the estimates that have so far emerged from prior research on that issue. As may be seen from the table, the experts on this question are as yet far from agreement. It would be hazardous indeed to base a manpower forecast on any particular of these numbers.

Tables 7 and 8 below—taken directly from the APPLIED MANAGEMENT SCIENCES, November 10, 1972, report on *The Effects of Task Delegation on the Requirements for Selected Health Manpower Categories in 1980, 1985, and 1990*, represents an attempt to use estimates such as those in Table 6 in the prediction of future manpower requirements. The percentage decreases shown in Table 7 are deviations from a baseline forecast. Although the numbers presented in these tables are not implausible, they do in fact reflect a number of quite arbitrary assumptions about (a) the average impact a physician extender can have on the productivity of the employing physician, and (b) the rate at which physician extenders will be accepted by private practitioners at various points in time. Although one has sympathy with the authors of the forecasts in the sense that arbitrary assumptions must occasionally be made in any type of research, it is nevertheless appropriate to point out that the seemingly firm numbers offered in Tables 7 and 8 are very sensitive indeed to

Table 6. Estimates of Increased Physician Productivity
Which can be Obtained Through the Use
of a Physician Extender

Specialty	Source	Type of data upon which estimate was based	Estimated increase	Percent
General Practice	Estes and Howard	Judgmental	30-50%	
	Smith, Miller and Gollady	Mathematical Model	74%	
				40%
	Pondy	Mathematical Model	70%	
	Medex	Experience	40.4%	
	Bergman, et al.; Hessel and Haggarty; Breeze, et al.	Judgmental	100%	
	Silver	Experience	426%	
				25%
	Charney and Kitzman	Judgmental	25%	
	Schiff, Fraser, and Walters	Experience	18.8%	
	Yankauer, et al.	Experience	25%	
Ob/Gyn	Lang	Judgmental	233%	25%
Surgery	– –	– –	25%	25%

Source: Applied Management Sciences, "The Effects of Task Delegation on the Require-ments for Selected Health Manpower Categories in 1980, 1985, and 1990," Report pre-pared under Contract No. NIH 72-4406 with DMI, BHME, NIH, HEW, November 10, 1972, Table 23, P. 3.47.

changes in the underlying assumptions, a fact that is not apparent from the tables. Any policy based on numerical estimates of this sort certainly skates on thin ice.

Table 7. The Decrease in the Model Number of Physicians
Required after Physician's Assistants Are
Introduced into the Health Care System

Physician Category	1980		1985		1990	
	Number	% Decrease	Number	% Decrease	Number	% Decrease
"General"	-22,866	-16.6%	-27,756	-18.9%	-32,411	-20.8%
"Pediatrics"	- 2,334	-11.4%	- 2,881	-12.8%	- 3,398	-14.2%
"Obstetrics/ Gynecology"	- 2,170	- 9.4%	- 3,810	-11.2%	- 3,549	-13.2%
"Surgery"	-10,294	-13.4%	-11,922	-14.6%	-13,426	-15.6%

Source: Applied Management Sciences, "The Effects of Task Delegation on the Requirements for Selected Health Manpower Categories in 1980, 1985, and 1990," Report prepared under Contract No. NIH 72-4406 with DMI, BHME, NIH, HEW, November 10, 1972,
Table 24, p. 3.48.

Table 8. The Projected Number of Physician's Assistants
Required in 1980, 1985, and 1990

		Number of Physician's Assistants Required		
	Speciality	1980	1985	1990
	General Practice	80,031	97,144	113,441
Number of Physician Assistants	Pediatrics	11,678	14,405	15,317
	Ob/Gyn	10,848	14,054	17,747
	Surgery	51,474	59,612	67,131
	Total	154,031	185,215	213,636

Source: Applied Management Sciences, "The Effects of Task Delegation on the Requirements for Selected Health Manpower Categories in 1980, 1985, and 1990," Report prepared under Contract No. NIH 72-4406 with DMI, BHME, NIH, HEW, November 10, 1972,
Table 25, p. 3.48.

B.3 The Potential Role of Technological Advances

Predictions concerning the impact on manpower requirements of potential technological advances in the future are even more difficult and more

tenuous than predictions about the impact of task delegation. There is, first of all, the difficulty of identifying probable direction of future technological advances. But even if these directions were clear, it is not always known whether technological advances in health care delivery are of a manpower-saving or manpower-using nature. The difficulty in this respect is amply illustrated by a report on the topic by GEOMET, Incorporated (1972). Although much of the report stresses that technical advances in medicine are often of the manpower-using type (i.e., of a type that tends to increase the demand for health manpower), the authors go on to present point estimates of the manpower savings due to technological advances by the year 1990. These estimates are presented in Table 9 below. The figures in the table are again reductions from a baseline forecast. Once again, the apparent precision of these figures obscures the fact that these estimates are based upon quite arbitrary assumptions about the future rate of technological advances, about the rate at which these advances will be incorporated into actual medical practice, and about the likely impact of technological advances on the efficiency of health workers. Our intent in citing these figures is not to berate their authors but instead to indicate the inevitable tenuity of any particular forecast in this area. Since the figures themselves raise more questions than they answer, they are best used as a stimulus and guide for future research, and not as a basis for manpower planning.

B.4 *The Role of Changes in the Organization of Provider Facilities*

In addition to significant productivity gains from task delegation within traditional forms of provider facilities—particularly small private medical practices—some students of the health care sector also expect major economies in the use of manpower from a shift towards large-scale group medical practices, preferably of the prepaid variety. Although the idea of large prepaid, fully integrated group practices (PGP) has been with us for

Table 9

Selected Manpower Reductions in 1990

Total Manpower	632,000 persons — 9%
Physicians	101,000 persons — 23%
Registered Nurses	194,000 persons — 21%
Allied Health Manpower	241,000 persons — 5%

Source: GEOMET, Incorporated (1972).

a good many decades—in both theory and practice—the concept has recently been skillfully repackaged and marketed under the new label "Health Maintenance Organization" (HMO).[5] In fact, so successful has been the relabeling of the old PGP concept that, while prepaid group practices of the Kaiser or HIP variety had long been thought to be quite effective where they functioned, the HMO is now viewed as a panacea for the entire American health system. It is a notion based on intense belief and some supporting (though controversial) empirical evidence.

One of the major benefits attributed to the prepaid-group-practice mode or HMO concept is a substantial saving in medical manpower relative to the traditional form of medical practice (solo practices or small partnerships). In an early paper on the subject, Klem and Hollingsworth asserted that PGP promises savings of as much as 30 percent in the physician-population ratio;[6] the National Advisory Commission on Health Manpower of 1967 indicated a saving of 27 percent in the physician-population ratio between California's Kaiser-Permanente program as compared to the state of California as a whole.[7] The Nixon Administration White Paper *Towards a Comprehensive Health Policy for the 1970's: A White Paper* (May 1971) appears to suggest that savings of 40 percent in the physician-population ratio are feasible under the HMO mode. Finally, a study of the impact of a widespread adoption of HMO's on future health manpower requirements,[8] concluded that if, by 1990, 38 percent of the U.S. population were enrolled in HMO's, then total health manpower requirements in that year would be about 90–93 percent of a baseline forecast for an unchanged health care sector and these figures were further reduced to 79 percent from 88 percent if 83 percent of the population were covered by HMO's. The forecast reductions vary considerably by type of manpower. For physicians as a group, the reduction vis-à-vis the baseline was about 12 percent, although there would actually be an increase in the requirements of some physicians (e.g., pediatricians and ophthalmologists). The largest HMO-induced reductions in health manpower requirements are said to occur in registered nurses and other allied health manpower categories: if 83 percent of the population were covered in 1990 by HMO's, then the actual requirement for such personnel was estimated to be only about 59 percent (for nurses) and 78 percent (for other allied health workers) of the baseline forecast. These calculations are based, it may be added, on postulated rates of HMO coverage of the population combined with assumed medical-service/health manpower ratios thought to apply to the HMO production mode.[9]

If the reader is somewhat bewildered by this plethora of statistics he joins the authors. Such studies may have merit in identifying areas that require further research or in highlighting the sensitivity of one's manpower forecasts to even rather innocent assumptions about the growth of HMO's, about manpower productivity in HMO's and traditional forms of provider facilities and, in particular, about the performance of HMO's in regions or localities where operating analogues cannot now be found (e.g., rural localities or any areas with low population densities). However, it is not even clear how the bulk of American physicians—who so far have not been strongly drawn to the HMO concept, and the bulk of American patients, who have also not flocked in large number to PGP's—would behave under any widespread HMO system. Some students of PGP's have cited at least suggestive empirical evidence for the view that, on balance, production of health care in PGP's may well be less efficient than it is under competing modes of health-care delivery.[10] Since the physicians now functioning in HMO-type settings and their patients also may be a rather distinct set of Americans, with a common though particular view toward medicine, it is not at all clear whether any of the medical services/manpower ratios now observed for operating PGP's can be taken as a clue for a situation where 83 percent of the nation is covered by HMO's.

In short, then, the studies cited above *are* useful in terms of their impact on future research in this area and interesting in the diversity of their conclusions. But it is inconceivable how, with the present state of our empirical knowledge about HMO performance, these studies can be used by the policy maker in his or her quest to identify future manpower shortages or surpluses.

C. Summary

As will have become apparent by now, it is in general always possible to prepare at least some kind of numerical health manpower projections for a decade or so hence. What is all too frequently overlooked by the users of such forecasts, however, is that they are at best a very informed guess. The simple truth is that the derived demand for manpower at any future point in time is a function of so many interrelated variables that the most useful kind of forecast will ultimately be a parametric one, i.e., a *model* capable of generating manpower forecasts upon ingesting specific (even if arbitrary) assumptions about the parameters that underlie any manpower forecast. Given such a model, the policy makers in the health area can then concentrate their effort on ways in which the public sector can influence the value of these parameters. And crucial among the latter will be the factors that can make the health-care sector receptive to innovations in the organization of health-care production. It is to a discussion of these factors that we shall now turn.

III. TECHNICAL FEASIBILITY AND MANPOWER GOALS

As has been noted, public policy can, within certain restraints noted below, intervene to alter the manpower mix and the level of supplies in any direction it wishes. Whether or not the manpower mix and aggregate supply will be an efficient one, however, depends on how policies that produce them relate to some clearly enunciated goal. Moreover, efficient use (i.e., accomplishing a stated objective at a minimum of resource costs) does not simply depend on the availability of the manpower supplies: the existence of manpower supplies, even if policy defines these as the appropriate ones, does not guarantee acceptance and use of the supplies within the health system; technical feasibility as a policy concern must be viewed in the context of translating feasibility into actual practice. To formulate manpower policy and goals and translate these goals into actual supplies will be meaningful and will produce efficient results only if there are no obstacles—market, professional, or legal—to the acceptance of technically feasible manpower combinations. To translate technical feasibility into actual practice turns on how decision makers respond and on the motives and incentives they face. It becomes important, therefore, when one is formulating health-manpower policy to confront the obstacles that must be overcome if one is to translate a seemingly legitimate goal into actual practice. That is true not only of health manpower but of any economic policy; just because something is technically feasible does not guarantee that it will happen or that if it happens it will be at the time and pace that is desired. A policy based only on technical feasibility, therefore, if it does not also assess whether or not "things *will* happen" can result in serious miscalculation and, to the extent that public resources are involved, serious misuse of society's resources.

We now turn to an examination of some of the impediments that lie between technical feasibility and actual practice.

1. The impact of national health insurance on utilization depends critically on the (not necessarily constant) price and income elasticities of demand. Historical evidence may be a rather poor guide to actual behavior. In addition, the government must decide whether a large increase in demand, if it occurs, should be honored (and therefore the manpower will be needed) or whether rationing will be considered. Alternatively, the government might consider what it can do to promote "optimal utilization" of the system.

2. A discussion on health-manpower productivity must proceed in terms of a clear distinction between overall gains in manpower productivity and increases in the productivity of a particular type of health manpower, brought on by manpower substitution.

Overall productivity gains are the result of a more effective use of the manpower resources already at a producer's disposition. It is conceivable, for example, that a simple reorganization of a medical practice—involving perhaps a change in the office layout or in the patient flow—can increase the productivity of every person employed by the practice. But even if that reorganization were to enhance the productivity of only some personnel in the practice, one would still speak on an overall productivity gain so long as that gain was not dependent on the employment of additional personnel. In essence, then, one may define gains in overall productivity as those gains that follow from increases in the so-called *technical efficiency* of a provider facility. In general, such productivity gains tend to be costless from society's point of view.

It may be tempting from the policy maker's viewpoint to regard gains in the technical efficiency of health-care production as primarily the result of prayers or manna from heaven. After all, the technical efficiency of a medical practice depends ultimately on the managerial acumen of the individual physician, an attribute that does not seem to offer a ready policy handle. This conclusion overlooks, however, that the typical medical school curriculum tends to neglect completely the mundane though important problem of *managing* a provider faculty. The assumption seems to be that every medical graduate will somehow know how to attend to the business side of his or her practice, just as the education of a college professor is almost invariably based on the notion that every Ph.D. will somehow know how to teach. There is reason to believe that in either case this assumption is invalid. The ability can surely be enhanced through formal instruction.

One way in which the public sector could impact on the curricula of health-manpower training centers would be to make public subsidies to such institutions contingent on the inclusion of appropriate management courses in the institution's curricula. In the case of medical schools, for example, the management course would introduce the student to alternative provider structures, to efficient modes of task delegation and to the cost implications of alternative modes of health-manpower utilization. It would, in short, render the physician literate in the economics of health-care delivery. And one would suppose that, other things being equal, physicians so trained would tend to be more efficient both *technically* and *economically*.

3. The mere fact that manpower substitution in the production of health care is *technically* feasible and that adequate numbers of paramedical assistants have been trained is, of course, no guarantee that the providers of health care will automatically exploit the productivity potential available to them.

If the market for health services were competitive in the classic sense, then one could assume that the discipline of the market would simply force individual health-care providers to adopt the most efficient combination of productive inputs for any rate of output. Unfortunately, the health-care market is a far cry from the competitive norm.

In order to determine the impact of task delegation to the new intermediate-level health worker (the physician extender) on manpower policy, we must know (1) the increase in productivity actually obtained from utilization and (2) the rate at which physicians will hire a physician extender. Both these factors will depend upon the objectives—other than productivity—that the physician wishes to accomplish with a PE, the physician's attitudes, and the ability of his practice to generate additional demand so that a productivity increase can be realized in actual practice. The other objectives which the physician may obtain through the use of a physician extender are (1) more leisure time, (2) a more leisurely working pace, or (3) an upgrading of the quality—completeness or comprehensiveness—of medical care which the physician can provide to his patient. The fact that higher quality of care may be a specific physician objective places in question the notion that all physicians deliver only the highest quality of care. This upgrading of quality may involve either the provision of additional types of medical services (i.e., more preventive care or patient education) or more systematic medical responses for those problems that can benefit from a thoughtful, unhurried diagnostic process. In fact, the ability to undertake a more careful diagnostic effort in some cases may lead to lower hospital utilization rates.

The physician must *perceive* some personal benefit in hiring a health practitioner, either economic (income obtained by expansion of the practice) or noneconomic (leisure, enjoyment from his practice, the quality of care delivered to his community). These benefits, coupled with the knowledge of how physicians can use the physician extender will determine the rate at which the PE concept spreads.

In short, physicians must make the decisions about what quantities of each type of health manpower are to be used and the way in which each is to be utilized in producing a given volume of medical services. Furthermore, the level and composition of demand for the services of the practice place constraints on the economically efficient utilization of health manpower. As noted above, the question of whether there will be sufficient demand for the additional patient visits will influence the physician's decision to hire a health practitioner. To the extent that this additional demand does not exist, the physician will hire a health practitioner only if his objective is more leisure time or higher-quality care. This has crucial implications for manpower projections. If the problem of access to medical care is, as some have suggested, merely geographical, we might have the ironical situation that there is no physician to hire the extenders where they are needed and no need for them where there is a physician to hire them.

It is also imperative that manpower policy come to terms with the important topic of independence from supervision. If physician extenders are expected to work under supervision, then their contribution to the medical care delivery problem may be severely restricted. The evidence seems to suggest that the greatest productivity impact of using a physician extender is obtained when some subset of patients is totally delegated. Furthermore, in small communities it may be optimal and mandatory to have the PE operating under remote supervision. If this is the case, then the role of the PE as a solution to the rural medical problem is dependent upon the development of new medical delivery systems that can better facilitate their use.

There are a number of other reasons why physicians may prefer not to push task delegation to the point that is technically feasible, economically desirable, and legally permissible. One can think here of a number of reasons for such a decision:

a. Physicians themselves may hold to the notion that the quality of their care is more or less proportionate to their own time input into the production of that care.

b. Physicians may fear, rightly or wrongly, that increased task delegation may increase the probability of malpractice suits (and/or higher malpractice insurance premiums).

c. The reimbursement policies adopted by third-party payers (private insurance companies or the public sector) may render increased task delegation unprofitable.

There is little that can be achieved through public policy in connection with point (a) other than, perhaps, the previously suggested reorientation of the medical school curriculum. It might be possible, for example, to emphasize in the clinical part of the medical school program training in the use of ancillary personnel and to impart to the medical school graduate a realistic view of the relationship between task delegation and quality of care.

Whether or not increased task delegation does in fact increase the probability of malpractice suits (point (b) above), or whether it does lead to increases in malpractice insurance premiums, is an empirical question to which a conclusive answer has so far, to the best of our knowledge, not been furnished. If the physician's fear in this respect turns out to be well founded, public policy can nevertheless impact on the issue via consumer education and via legislation that prescribes the capricious resort to malpractice litigation. It is an area that requires more careful analysis in the future.

For reasons that are not entirely clear the emergence of the "physician extender" has led to some controversy concerning the rate at which physicians should be reimbursed for services performed by physician extenders employed by a physician. In this connection the Social Security Administration (SSA) has ruled that, under Title XVIII of the Medicare Act, a noninstitutional medical practice cannot be reimbursed for any services rendered solely by a physician extender even if these services were performed on the premises of the employing physician's practice and under the physician's supervision. Services produced by the traditional types of auxiliary personnel, on the other hand, can be included as part of the physician's fees or charges. This ruling appears to rest on the notion that the traditional types of health manpower render their services "incident to" the physician's own activities, while a physician extender substitutes directly for the physician. The fact is that the current SSA policy cannot but reduce the economic attractiveness of health-manpower substitution from the viewpoint of individual practitioners. The policy contradicts the government's efforts elsewhere to train paramedical aides and to encourage their acceptance by health-care providers. This contradiction led to the development of an experiment, now in progress, designed to explore the relationship between the nature of the SSA reimbursement policy and the impact of the physician extender on practice activity and productivity. Unfortunately, the experiment is not designed to obtain any information on the more important relationship between reimbursement policy and the rate at which the physician extender is introduced into American medical practice.

4. A fourth obstacle to the introduction of new types of health manpower (e.g., physician assistants) or to more extensive delegation of tasks to traditional types of ancillary personnel will undoubtedly be patients' resistance to such changes. There is some evidence that particularly the lower-income groups tend to view group medical practice as "medicine for the poor." Similarly, it is to be expected that these groups are likely to view the emergence of the physician assistant as an attempt to develop a new, low-cost and hence low-quality care for the poor.

A public policy designed to enhance the effectiveness with which health manpower is being used may therefore have to be preceded or at least accompanied by an intensive program of consumer education. It is probably fair to suggest that the medical profession has contributed in no small part to the mystique now surrounding the physician and to some misconception patients may have about the determinants of the quality of health care. Since it is this mystique in part which leads patients to assume that, say, an injection administered by a physician obviously constitutes care of a higher quality than an injection administered by the physician's aide, the medical profession should now lend its authority to any program designed to enlighten patients in this area, and to create patient acceptance of a more extensive use of paramedical professionals.

The SSA reimbursement policy referred to above also impairs the status of physician extenders in the eyes of patients. After all, a policy under which, *for a given service*, a high price is paid when the physician performs it and a lower price if a physician extender performs it may inadvertently communicate to consumers the view that, in the eyes of the SSA, the *quality* of service produced by the physician extender is relatively lower and hence warrants a lower price. This is clearly not the intent of the SSA ruling; the entire idea of using physician extenders is based on the premise that certain tasks can be delegated to such personnel without impairing the quality of medical treatments being dispensed. But it may, in the end, have that effect.

The actual magnitude of the negative effects generated by the current SSA reimbursement policy is, of course, an empirical question that deserves intensive research effort. What is clear is that policy in this area needs to be formulated with extreme caution lest the government frustrate its own efforts to move the health-care sector toward a more efficient production mode in the longer run.

The existing legal barriers to more effective health-manpower utilization are likely to act as a very strong impediment to more extensive task delegation in the future. In the United States, the licensure of physicians is mandatory and persons not licensed as physicians are prohibited by law from performing any of the functions that go into the definition of "medical practice" in the licensure laws of the various states.

Licensure of medical and paramedical personnel is justified primarily as a means of protecting patients from unqualified or unethical practioners and in that justification lies the popular appeal of such laws. Actually, however, there is little empirical evidence that, with respect to the quality of care, licensure always performs its expected function. After all, licensure merely certified that *at the time of completing his or her formal training* the licensee was, indeed, technically competent. At this time of writing, only the State of New Mexico requires periodic relicensing of health personnel. Since the medical field is characterized by unusually rapid scientific progress, it may be surmised that the beneficial effects of licensure wear off soon after the licensees' graduation. Furthermore, if the physician is the only independent practitioner in the medical delivery system, one can argue that he determines the quality of the care performed under his jurisdiction. Thus, there is no need to place constraints on the pattern of delegation that is legally permissible.

While there is some question concerning the existence and/or magnitude of social benefits that may conceivably flow from professional licensure in the health field, there is very little doubt that it entails significant social costs. These costs have two distinct sources: (1) inefficiencies resulting from the constraints imposed upon the allocation of tasks among various types of health manpower, and (2) overall shortages of various types of health manpower resulting indirectly from the restrictiveness of licensure laws.

With respect to the first point, it should be noted that the licensure laws governing various types of health manpower have rarely, if ever, been designed to encourage an optimal (least cost) allocation of tasks among the various health occupations. And even if the laws were originally tailored to such optima, they do not keep in tune with the rapidly changing organizational and technical innovations that are potentially feasible in health-care delivery.

There is convincing empirical evidence that, at the present time, the typical medical practitioner performs many tasks that could safely be delegated to a paraprofessional assistant and that, within hospitals, registered nurses still perform tasks that could just as well be performed by licensed practical nurses or even orderlies. At the present time, however, any bold experimentation with more extended delegation runs the risk of inviting legal action. While we are on the topic of licensure laws, it may be pertinent to mention also that, as far as the paramedical professions are concerned, these laws may act as a two-pronged deterrent to entry into the health labor force. On the one hand, licensure requirements typically increase the cost of entering particular occupations, and some of these entry costs may not be socially necessary. A less direct but equally potent deterrent to entry is that licensure severely restricts upward occupational mobility. One authoritative student of allied health-manpower problems regards this lack of mobility as one of the more significant contributors to the current shortage of paramedical personnel [Greenfield (1969)].

Without further research into the matter it is impossible to ascertain the true social cost of licensure-induced inefficiency in the health-care sector. High priority should be given to such research. It might quite possibly establish that the current and often anachronistic licensure laws in the health field are a major barrier to technical and organizational progress in health-care production. At any rate, it is surely appropriate to conclude that the widespread use of new types of health personnel—such as physician extenders—will remain a dream unless a more flexible legal basis is established for use of such personnel.

IV. THE PROBLEM OF LAGS

Anthropologists and social psychologists have long used the term "cultural lag" to denote a difference between a society's practices and its institutions. The term has little operational significance. But there are lags between a society's institutions and its actions that have operational significance for public policy. National health manpower policy is one such area where this is true. A myriad of public programs are now, and have been, underway to augment and/or to increase the supply of various kinds of health manpower, including physicians. These supplies are being generated, with an appropriate time lag necessary to do so, to levels that will either match or miss the particular parameter values for consumer demand forecasted. Everyone does not accept the point that the demand forecasts are substantially impacted by the level and skill mix of the manpower supplies available now and in the process of moving to some future point in time. Secondly, most people recognize and do not know how to cope with the notion that the manpower training and subsidy programs which are now underway may be inadequate as to level and skill mix if the disjointed and unintegrated structure of the delivery system is reorganized. Third, most authorities do not recognize that what is manpower "now in the pipeline" will not only affect future demand levels but the ability or inability to restructure and rationalize (i.e., get out all the present inefficiencies) the present delivery system. Finally, most informed persons seem to believe that if the manpower "flow and mix in the pipeline" turns out to be incorrect for either forecasted demand or actual restructuring of the delivery system, what's in the pipeline can be instantaneously changed (stopped, increased, etc.). That is where the problem of lags becomes relevant. If the specialty distribution of physicians, for example, now in the pipeline turns out to be "wrong" (either for demand or delivery reorganization reasons) the private and social cost of that miscalculation may be both high and difficult to correct. Public programs are not easily changed in midstream; the longer a program exists, the greater the sphere of vested interest attached to the program and the more difficult it becomes to mobilize support for a change in the existing program or a new program which circumvents the one in which the original policy miscalculation occurred.

There is also a multiplier effect to public programs, especially manpower subsidy and training programs, which can magnify a miscalculation. By highlighting some national need, a public program induces others not directly affected by the training or subsidy program to find alternative ways, usually through private markets, to become qualified to meet a national need. A recent survey of high school graduates showed that about 12 percent anticipated careers in health, exclusive of becoming physicians and nurses. Educational institutions have been quick to respond to the "health crisis" by instituting programs for allied health-manpower occupations. If the forecasted future demands for allied health manpower turn out to be wrong, the adjustment lag will not be instantaneous. Engineers, for example, are today in excess supply and the market adjustment process has been slow. Engineers produced under the "national needs of space and defense" turned out to have minimal skill transfer in other uses. The same may well be true with allied health manpower; if anticipated demand does not materialize, the adjustment lag will not be instantaneous.

The main thrust of some of our earlier discussion was to demonstrate that it is almost always possible to increase the productivity of a particular type of manpower in a technically efficient provider facility through health-manpower substitution even though there are always formidable obstacles to be overcome. In contrast to overall productivity gains, however, productivity gains achieved through factor substitution are not costless; increases in physician productivity that seem technically feasible do presuppose rather substantial additions to the pool of allied health workers. The difficult part of devising a policy in this respect is not to find suitable instruments—the most suitable are probably direct subsidies to students and/or the institutions that train them—but to determine precisely how far the shift in the mix of trained manpower should be pushed and, of course, how large the overall pool of health manpower should be. It is a question that has not so far been answered satisfactorily by the research on health manpower.

A priori it is reasonable to suggest that, whatever health manpower policy is implemented by the public sector, every effort should be made not to err on the upward side of the number of required physicians. There is considerable empirical evidence that, across state or regions, the number of physicians per capita is positively correlated to the average level of physician fees. While this phenomenon may be interpreted as the result of differences in the effective demand for health care—a demand to which physicians have simply responded—it is not implausible to entertain the alternative hypothesis that physicians tend to locate primarily in response to the cultural, climatic, and social characteristics of particular localities and that, within limits, medical fees adjust to a level that affords the physicians living in a region a satisfactory standard of living. And if fees are not the sole adjuster, then any potential surplus of physicians in a region may easily translate itself also into physician-generated demand for medical services. These effects would be a natural consequence of the peculiar role played by physicians in the delivery of health services; they act at once as the patient's agent in determining the latter's demand for physician services and as the providers who meet that demand. In other words, the market for medical services is such that the demand for and supply of services are not fully autonomous.

In obtaining their education, physicians typically bear significant costs both in terms of out-of-pocket expenses and foregone earnings (as do, however, other professionals). These costs must be amortized over the physician's professional life. If the description of the market structure offered in the preceding paragraph is at all near the mark, then one may assume that regardless of the aggregate number of physicians available at any point in time, physicians as a group will always be able to amortize the cost of their education and to earn an adequate living in the process. From this perspective, any large increase in the number of physicians who are graduated is very likely to translate itself into strong inflationary pressure on the cost of medical care. Since other types of health manpower do not enjoy nearly the degree of market power commanded by physicians, any oversupply of these types of manpower will, if anything, tend to translate itself into a deflationary pressure on medical-care costs. One concludes, then, that upward errors in the public support given to training programs for allied health workers are actually not as serious as upward errors in the number of trained physicians.

On the other hand, because there are lags in adjustment in both the public and private sectors, and because what's in the health-manpower pipeline is premised on shaky assumptions, there may well be an element of self-fulfilling prophecy; the level of demand for health services will be heavily shaped and influenced by the level and skill mix of the manpower resources (and other resources, too) that *are available* and/or being produced. What this all boils down to is that manpower forecasts are without real meaning for purposes of policy planning unless we have an explicit health policy goal which specifies what it is we are trying to achieve. The organization of the health delivery system cannot be treated as an exogenous variable; the level of demand cannot be forecast in a useful policy-making sense unless the orgnaization of the delivery system is incorporated as an endogenous factor; a forecast, or policy, for the organization of the delivery system cannot treat the manpower flow and mix in the pipeline as exogenous for not only will it shape the delivery system but it will alter and shape demand. These delicate complexities face planners of health manpower strategy. And there is the problem of lag adjustment and the potential for magnifying correct (and incorrect) manpower plans to further invalidate policy. Therefore, manpower policy formulated around specific numbers on manpower needs and requirements is a chimera: the delicate balance of assumptions and predictions required to produce a numeric forecast does not inspire confidence that the policy required to produce those numbers is the correct one.

V. FORMULATING A NATIONAL MANPOWER POLICY

The purpose of this paper has been to question the reliance of health-manpower policy on forecasts of future manpower requirements. In so doing we have attempted to alert the reader to the vulnerability and naiveté of a policy premised on numbers that people think represent future shortages or surpluses of various types of manpower. Such point estimates will rest on assumptions about the values to be taken by a set of key parameters. Our position is that the policy maker's attention should be focused on these parameters: to understand what factors will affect them and how the government can influence them in a desired way.

The first step in the development of a health-manpower policy will be to determine where and what resources are over- or underutilized. Of course, to answer this question one must immediately address the question of what constitutes optimal utilization. This in turn involves the determination of what substitutions among different inputs into the medical care production process are technically feasible and, based upon that knowledge and the relative costs or scarcities of these inputs, what substitutions are economically justified.

There have been a number of studies in recent years that have addressed these questions. For example, Smith et al. have investigated the optimal staffing of ambulatory medical care practice when various types of physician extenders are included in the set of feasible technologies; Reisman, Gravenstein et al. have studied the design of alternative teams for anesthesia coverage in multiple room surgical suites; Lewit et. al. have examined the utilization of surgical assistants rather than surgeons as first assistants for various types of surgical procedures. And the SSA Study of Physician Extenders Reimbursement, referred to in an earlier section, promises to provide an extensive description of alternative manpower utilizations. The list of possible studies is extensive. Our contention is that manpower policy should start from such micro-studies of optimal utilization.

A second component in a national health manpower policy will be the development of programs which facilitate the optimal utilization of resources. Such programs can include the removal of legal or financial disincentives to the productive use of health manpower, educational efforts to improve the physician's understanding of optimal practice organization, and support systems for practitioners who desire to innovate within their practice setting. In fact, the processes by which change is introduced into medical practice are incompetely documented and understood. Again the content of this suggestion is that much more effort must be placed on an understanding of behavior within a micro-organizational context.

A third component of a national health manpower policy will be concerned with the movement of resources into those situations where they are most needed and away from those situations where they are least needed. Having obtained an understanding of what might constitute over- or underutilization, special programs encouraging movement can be developed.

Finally, the production of various types of manpower (or facilities) can be stepped up or stepped down, according to whether current rates of production appear inadequate or excessive. It is by no means easy to make such determinations. As a guide one can take the somewhat conflicting positions that (a) change requires evidence that the current strategy is quite out of line and (b) given the absence of strong competitive forces in the market for health manpower (especially physicians) and facilities it may be better to err on the side of shortfall rather than excess supply.

Certainly the development of a health policy is a complex undertaking. Given this fact, it should be observed that the first three components of the strategy defined above can be beneficial independently of the difficulties inherent in the final component. It is unfortunate that much of our previous effort has concentrated on this fourth component.

FOOTNOTES

1. The more doctrinaire members of the research establishment may have sought to justify this approach on the notion that the production function for health care is homogeneous and that relative factor prices do not change over time. Such a defense, unless empirically supported, is clearly not very helpful.

2. See, for example, Jeffrey H. Weiss (1966).

3. It should be noted that assuming the base year equal to 1 is equivalent to assuming initial balance between manpower demand and supply. While this is not a particularly defensible assumption, it is one that quite frequently underlies past projections of future shortages and surpluses.

4. The difference would be between producing 8,400 physicians plus replacing those who die versus 3,600 plus replacements.

5. See, for example, Paul M. Ellwood (May 1971).

6. Quoted from H. E. Klarman (1971).

7. Ibid.

8. GEOMET, Incorporated (1962).

9. Ibid.

10. See Newhouse (1973), and Bailey (1970).

REFERENCES

Bailey, Richard M. (1970), "Economies of Scale in Medical Practice," in Herbert E. Klarman, (ed.) *Emperical Studies in Health Economics,* Baltimore: The Johns Hopkins Press.

Ellwood, Paul M. (May 1971), "Restructuring the Health Delivery System—Will the Health Maintenance Strategy Work?" in *Health Maintenance Organizations: A Reconfiguration of the Health Services System,* Center for Health Administration Studies, Graduate School of Business, University of Chicago.

GEOMET, Incorporated (November 1972), *The Impact on Future Health Manpower Requirements and Supply of Increasing Productivity Through Use of Technological Advances,* Report No. R-163 prepared under Contract No. NIH 72-4408 with DMI, BHME, NIH, HEW, Table 5-3, pp. 5–7.

———— (October 1972), *The Impact on Future Health Manpower Requirements of the Spread of Coverage of Health Maintenance Organizations.*

Greenfield, Harry I. (1969), Allied Health Manpower: Trends and Prospects, New York: Columbia University Press.

Hansen, W. L. (March 1970), "An Appraisal of Physician Manpower Projections," *Inquiry.*

Klem, Margaret C., and Helen Hollingsworth (1947), "Medical Care," in J. Frederic Dewhurst and Associates, *America's Needs and Resources,* New York: The Twentieth Century Fund, pp. 236–272.

Klarman, H. E. (1969), "Analysis of the HMO Proposal—Its Assumptions, Implications, and Prospects, in *Health Maintenance Organizations: A Reconfiguration of the Health Services System,* Center for Health Administration Studies, Graduate School of Business, University of Chicago.

———— (December 1969), "Economic Aspects of Projecting Requirements for Health Manpower," *The Journal of Human Resources.*

Lewit, Eugene M., J. D. Bentkover, S. H. Bentkover, R. N. Watkins, E. F. Hughes *(January 1977), "Alternative Uses of Manpower for Surgical Assisting," Office of Primary Health Care Education, College of Medicine and Dentistry of New Jersey, New Jersey Medical School, unpublished.*

Newhouse, Joseph P. (Winter 1973), "The Economies of Group Practice," *The Journal of Human Resources.*

Reinhardt, U. E. (February 1972), "A Production Function for Physician Services," *Review of Economics and Statistics.*

———— (1971), "Physician Productivity: The Supply of Physician Services and the 'Physician Shortage' in Canada," paper read before the Canadian Economic Association, St. John's, Newfoundland.

Reisman, A., J. Gravenstein, et al., "Design of Alternative Teams for Anesthesia Coverage in Multiple Room Surgical Suites: Simulation Study," unpublished.

Smith, K. R., A. M. Over, Jr., M. F. Hansen, F. L. Gollady and E. J. Davenport, (September-October 1976), "An Analytic Framework and Measurement Strategy for Investigating Optimal Staffing in Medical Practice, *Operations Research.*

————, M. Miller, and F. L. Gollady (Spring 1972), "An Analysis of the Optimal Use of Inputs in the Production of Medical Services," *Journal of Human Resources* 7, No. 208.

Weiss, Jeffrey H. (1966), *The Changing Job Structure of Health Manpower,* Ph.D. dissertation, Harvard University.

THE PRODUCTIVITY OF NEW
HEALTH PRACTITIONERS:
PHYSICIAN ASSISTANTS AND
MEDEX*

Richard M. Scheffler,** GEORGE WASHINGTON

UNIVERSITY

Economists working in the health-manpower area have continued to suggest that manpower substitution may be an important solution to alleviating the shortage of health services. Increasing the supply of physicians is a long-term, costly social investment when one considers that it takes an average of seven years to train a physician. An additional problem with this policy is that physicians may have considerable control of the demand for their services. Thus, an increase in the supply of physicians may generate an increase in the demand for medical services. The most important new type of health practitioner, the physician extender (PE), may be the best alternative to increasing the supply of health services

Research in Health Economics, Vol. 1, pp 37–56.
Copyright © 1979 by JAI Press, Inc.
All rights of reproduction in any form reserved.
ISBN 0-89232-042-7.

without training additional physicians. This new category of health manpower is trained for one or two years to perform many of the medical tasks that were previously the exclusive role of the physician.[1]

Previous studies in the productivity of physician extenders, such as those by Smith et al. (Spring 1972) and Galladay et al. (Winter 1974), have used small data sets and simulation techniques to explore the potential productivity of physician extenders.[2] The usefulness of these studies should not be overlooked; however, more accurate and more specific estimates are now required. This paper presents estimates of the realized productivity based on a national sample of data on physician extenders. It is organized as follows: a discussion (primarily for noneconomists) of the production functions used, a description of the data base, and the empirical results followed by policy implications.

THE PRODUCTION FUNCTION

This review of basic production functions is included for noneconomists. Perhaps the most useful production function is the Cobb-Douglas production function. It is described in equation (1)

$$Q = AL^\alpha K^\beta \tag{1}$$

where A, α, β are positive parameters. The marginal product of labor is positive for all finite levels of L and decreases continuously as L increases. The marginal product of capital behaves similarly if $0 < \alpha < 1$.

From equation (1) the technical definition of the measure "returns to scale" is equal to $\alpha + \beta$. "Returns to scale" is the percentage change in output for a simultaneous and equiproportionate change in all inputs. If both labor and capital inputs are increased by 1 percent and output increases by 1 percent, constant returns to scale prevail. If output increases by less than 1 percent, decreasing returns to scale are exhibited, and if output increases by more than 1 percent there are increasing returns to scale.

To utilize this function to study the productivity of medical practice it is respecified in equation (2)

$$V = AH^\alpha L^\beta N^\Delta K^\gamma Z^u \tag{2}$$

where A is a constant, H = hours of physician extenders, L = the number of physicians, N = the number of nonphysician medical personnel excluding PEs, K = a measure of capital, and Z is the stochastic error term. This function is linear in the logarithms as is shown in equation (3)

$$\ln V = \ln A + \alpha \ln H + \beta \ln L + \Delta \ln N + \gamma \ln K + Z \ln u \tag{3}$$

and statistically is relatively simple to estimate. The parameters (α, β, Δ, γ) measure directly the elasticity of output with respect to their input coefficients ("elasticity" is the precentage change in output in response to a 1 percent change in an input). The elasticity of output with respect to P.E. hours is

$$E_{q.h} = \frac{\partial Q}{\partial H} \cdot \frac{H}{Q} = \frac{\partial \ln Q}{\partial \ln H} = \alpha,$$

and similarly, the elasticity of output with respect to physicians and with respect to capital, respectively are

$$E_{q.1} = \beta$$

$$E_{q.k} = \gamma.$$

The output elasticity with respect to all inputs, returns to scale, is the percentage change in output for a simultaneous equiproportionate change in all inputs (i), and in the Cobb-Douglas function is:

$$E_{q.1} = \alpha + \beta + \Delta + \gamma.$$

If: $E_{q.i} = 1$, constant returns to scale prevail,

$E_{q.i} > 1$, increasing returns to scale, and

$E_{q.i} < 1$, decreasing returns to scale.

As a specific functional form, the Cobb-Douglas function has some shortcomings. Given the multiplicative nature of equations (1) and (2), it is necessary that all inputs have positive values in order to have positive output. If the labor input of PEs or physicians were broken down into hours worked by the different skill levels or medical specialties, only those practices which utilized positive input rates of each of the classifications could be used in estimating the production function, and the resulting function would describe only those practices included. In the Cobb-Douglas function, marginal productivities of an input are everywhere declining and positive as that factor is increased, and the elasticity of substitution between factors has a constant value of unity. Also in the Cobb-Douglas function, returns to scale is a constant that is not dependent on the size of the practice. Using the Cobb-Douglas function implicitly assumes that the marginal productivities of inputs, elasticities of substitution between inputs, and returns to scale in medical practice behave as specified. Whether or not these assumptions are true is an empirical question which should be tested with a more general functional form.

Alain de Janvary (1972) has summarized much of the recent theoretical discussion of economic production functions by presenting a production function called the "generalized power production function" which includes as special cases the Cobb-Douglas, the Transcendental, and the Cobb-Douglas with variable returns to scale, and variable production elasticities. The function used by Reinhardt (1972, 1973, 1975) in estimating the production function for physicians' services, and by Boulier (1974) in estimating the function for dentists' services was a form of the Transcendental function that largely overcomes the restrictive shortcomings of the rigid Cobb-Douglas. Most importantly, it permits some of the inputs to be zero (those not required for all production activities) without having the level of output reduced to zero. We utilized this function and the results appear in Appendix A. for the most part, they were inferior to those obtained with the Cobb-Douglas function.

EMPIRICAL SPECIFICATION

The Cobb-Douglas function described in the previous section was estimated with the addition of variables to account for case mix differences, mode of practice differences and individual differences among physician assistants. We now proceed with a discussion of these variables.

In an attempt to standardize for case mix differences (i.e., differences in the type of visit), dummy variables were entered that measured the age and the sex for each patient visit.[3] The percent of patient visits in each of five age groups (PATAGE) and the percent of males treated were included in the specification used. A complete list of variables appears in the Glossary of Variables, below.

The data sample was divided among the PAs (physician assistants) and Medex in private practice (solo, group, partnership) and those in two institutional settings, hospitals and nursing homes. These two types of physician extenders are trained somewh t differently, hence they are analyzed separately [see Scheffler (1974)]. Within these groups dummy variables were included to account for any differences in output due to mode of practice. For example, in the private practice sample, dummy variables for solo, group and partnership were included. In institutions a variable for nursing homes as compared to hospitals was utilized. For the Medex sample, due to a paucity of observations, the data were not split into private and institutional practice. Hence, both sets of dummy variables are included in the estimates for Medex. To account for the different types of visits produced by different medical specialties, a variable was entered to indicate if the visit was in a primary care specialty (Care−, see

GLOSSARY OF VARIABLES

Totpat -	daily average number of patients seen by the PA (Medex), physician(s) and other nonphysican medical personnel with whom the PA (Medex) works
You -	daily average number of patients seen by the PA (Medex)
PAMedhr -	numbers of hours per week the PA (Medex) spends in patient care
Phys# -	number of physicians with whom the PA (Medex) works closely
Totnon -	number of non-physician medical personnel with whom the PA (Medex) works on a daily basis
Solo -	dummy variable equals 1 if the PA (Medex) is employed in solo, private practice
Clinic -	dummy variable equals 1 if the PA (Medex) is employed in a branch or satellite clinic from a private MD practice or a hospital, or a community based public clinic
Hospital -	dummy variable equals 1 if the PA (Medex) is employed in a hospital
Nursing home -	dummy variable equals 1 if the PA (Medex) is employed in a nursing home
Group -	dummy variable equals 1 if the PA (Medex) is employed in a partnership or group practice
Sex -	dummy variable equals 1 if the PA (Medex) is a male
Race -	dummy variable equals 1 if the PA (Medex) is white/Caucasian
Care -	dummy variable equals 1 if the PA (Medex) is employed in primary care
PA age, PA age - squared -	age and age–squared of the PA (Medex)
Patage 1 - Patage 5	percent of patients that the PA (Medex) treats in each of the following following age categories: 0-6, 7-25, 26-44, 45-64, 65+ years
nonfedpop -	number of non-Federal physicians per 100,000 population in county in which the PA (Medex) is employed

Glossary). Although this adjustment is viewed as incomplete, it was the best that the data file allowed.

Finally, a set of variables was included to standardize for a number of personnel characteristics that differed among PAs and Medex. These were the sex and race of the PA or Medex and their age. Sex and race may measure a number of factors that influence patient visits. One such factor may be the existence of discrimination either by the physician or patient. Discrimination by the physician may affect how the PA or Medex is utilized in the practice. Patient discrimination could affect the number of patient contacts. The age of the PA or Medex was included as a proxy measure for experience. Human capital theory suggests that on the job training should be related to the productivity of the worker. To account for the nonlinear pattern that is expected an age-squared term was also included. Previous specifications separated experience into medical experience before and after training as a PA or Medex. However, they were not statistically significant.

DATA

The data were obtained in the spring of 1975 from a mailed national survey of 1,792 formally trained Physicians Assistants and Medex.[4] The overall response rate was 75.6 percent, or 1,355 respondents, and the data collected can be roughly classed into three areas: information pertaining to the mode of practice in which the PA/Medex worked, information relating to their work activities, and data describing the patients who were treated by the practice. In the first of these groups, the PA/Medex was asked to describe his present employer as a private solo practitioner, group, clinic, or a hopsital or nursing home. An estimate of practice size was obtained by asking the number of full-time M.D.'s working in solo, group and clinic practices and the number of beds in nursing homes and hospitals. The PA/Medex was also asked to indicate the number and specialty of physicians with whom he or she worked closely.

Information pertaining to the work activity of the PA/Medex includes data on the hours worked per week as well as how their hours were occupied (i.e., patient care, laboratory work, clerical assignments, teaching, administration, research). Information was also collected on the work experience of the PA/Medex and the number of nonphysician medical personnel with whom the respondent worked on a daily basis. Patient characteristics include breakdowns by sex and the percentage of patients treated in each of five age categories. PAs and Medex were also asked how many patients they treated on a daily basis with (and without) an M.D. being present. From ZIP codes the county of practice was identified, the data on the population, per capita income, hospitals and hospital beds, as well as the number of physicians were added to the file.

Two different output measures were obtained in the study; one was the daily average number of patients seen by the PA/Medex, physician(s) and nonphysician medical personnel with whom the PA/Medex worked, and the other output measure was the number of patients with whom the PA/Medex had direct medical contact. The former output measure is viewed as being more suitable than the latter for the present study for two reasons. First, it more accurately reflects the number of patients seen by the practice as a unit and hence explicitly takes into consideration the different types of manpower that may be employed to produce a visit. Since the PA/Medex must work under the supervision of an M.D. (either directly or indirectly) it is possible that their rate of utilization in the production process may be subordinate or at least related to that of the physician. Therefore, by postulating a production function in which both the physician and the PA/Medex are explicit inputs, more realistic results may be obtained. Second, the a priori specification of a production function in the latter case rests on weaker grounds since it cannot be determined which, if any, other inputs were utilized in the treatment of patients with whom the PA/Medex responded that he had direct medical contact. It is well known that the visit as an output measure has a number of serious analytical drawbacks.[5] Most important is its lack of homogeneity. As will be seen later, a set of variables is used in an attempt to standardize for some of the differences in the types of visits.

EMPIRICAL RESULTS

The means the standard deviations of the dependent and independent variables appear in Table 1.

As would be expected, PAs in institutions have a larger number of patient contact visits than those in private practice. They also work with more physicians and nonphysician medical personnel. Furthermore, they work, on the average, a shorter number of weekly hours, i.e., 40.06 hours in institutions compared to 46.62 hours in private practice. The sex, race and average age of PAs employed in private practice and institutions are quite similar as is the distribution of the ages of patients treated.

Comparing PAs to Medex, we find the most notable difference is the number of non-Federal physicians per 100,000 population in the county in which they practice. The ratio is approximately 141 per 100,000 for all Medex as compared to 188 per 100,000 for PAs in private practice, and 197 per 100,000 for PAs in institutional settings. The remaining variables appear to be quite similar.

Turning to Table 2, we find the estimates of the Cobb-Douglas function for PAs and Medex including the standardizing variables discussed in the previous section.[6] It should be pointed out that this result is the best specification according to R^2 and significant t-values.[7] In addition, we have omitted a measure of capital since it was not statistically significant in the earlier specifications.

The elasticity of output with respect to hours for PAs in private practice is statistically significant at the 5 percent level as are the values for the number of physicians and nonphysician medical personnel. The output elasticity of the PA is 0.175; for the physician, 0.277, and for nonphysician medical personnel, 0.139. These results are appealing, each of the output elasticities is less than one and the relative magnitudes are what one would expect a priori. PA's are approximately 63 percent as productive as physicians and over 35 percent more productive than other nonphysician medical personnel. These results are fairly consistent for PAs in private practice and institutional settings; however, the elasticity of physicians with respect to output increased slightly to 0.425 in institutions. The results for Medex (column 3) were very similar. This result is within

Table 1. Means and Standard Deviations of Variables Used in the Total Patients Treated Equations

Variable	PA Private Practice	PA Institution	Medex
Total patients	69.73 (70.04)	88.03 (84.79)	70.88 (58.61)
PA hourly work week	46.62 (32.44)	40.06 (14.76)	47.33 (15.09)
Number of physicians	2.77 (4.20)	3.25 (2.59)	2.56 (1.90)
Total nonphysician medical personnel	9.93 (14.91)	13.49 (15.02)	9.49 (10.09)
Solo practice*	0.36	+	0.33
Group practice*	0.45	+	0.36
Clinic practice *	0.19	+	0.08
Hospital-based*	+	0.91	0.15
Nursing home*	+	0.09	0.08
Sex* of PA or Medex	0.80	0.88	0.93
Race* of PA or Medex	0.91	0.87	0.86
Primary or non primary care*	0.61	0.55	0.68
Patient age 0-6*	0.14	0.07	0.13
Patient age 7-25*	0.19	0.22	0.21
Patient age 26044	0.25	0.30	0.26
Patient age 45-64*	0.24	0.26	0.22
Patient age 65+*	0.16	0.15	0.18
PA age	31.88 (5.47)	32.89 (5.30)	33.60 (6.70)
PA age squared	1046.07 (411.63)	1109.76 (371.39)	1173.42 (508.36)
Non-federal physicians per 100,000 population	188.66 (218.76)	197.08 (166.83)	141.33 (199.96)

Values in parentheses are standard deviations.
* Variable was entered as a binary variable equal to 1 if the respondent was in the group, zero if he was not. Sample means indicate the percentage or respondents in each group. Standard deviations of such variables have no meaningful interpretation.
+ Indicates no observations were available for this variable.

the range of estimates made by Smith et al. (1974) of a productivity increase of between 40 and 74 percent when introducing a PA into private practice. As expected the actual productivity gain is less than the potential. Reinhardt (1975) found the elasticity of aides to be approximately 0.3; however, his data and specification were quite different and did not include physician extenders. Kimbell and Lorant (December 1973) found physician aide elasticities ranging from positive values of 0.126 to 0.454 as well as negative values depending on the medical specialty and type of practice. The positive values are within the general range of those we have reported.

The other variables in our estimates are also of some interest. According to t-values, the primary care variable, mode of practice variable and some categories of the patient age variable were statistically significant. Primary care practices produce roughly 40 percent more patient visits.[8] Solo and group practices produce more visits than clinics, and nursing homes produce more visits or contacts than hospitals. We found that the sex of the PA was not statistically significant; however, for Medex it was significant. PAs in institutional settings who were white had more visits than did nonwhites. It is interesting to note that the county per capita number of non-federal physicians did not statistically affect the number of visits in private practice. For PAs in institutional settings it approached but did not reach statistical significance and was negative. In the Medex equation, which was not split into private practice and institutions, it was statistically significant and positive.

Table 3 repeats the same regressions, except that the dependent variable is patients with whom the PA/Medex had direct medical contact. These patients represent a subgroup of the total patients seen and being treated by a PA/Medex and does not necessarily preclude treatment of other members of the practice. We found that the number of physicians is significant only for PAs employed in institutions. Since PAs responding to this question were no longer constrained to work in the physical presence of an M.D. but had direct contact with the patient themselves, it is likely that the physician's contribution to output would decline in significance. Physicians are still a significant input in institutions (and this may be due in part to the hierarchical structure described earlier), however both the size of the coefficient and the degree of significance have decreased markedly from the analogous results for total patients treated by the practice. Notice also that while the primary care variable was statistically significant for all cases of the "total patients treated" equations, it is no longer important in "explaining" output. This may be an indication that one's specialty may affect the number of patients one is able to treat or influence the likelihood of treating patients, but once patient contact has been established specialty has little effect on productivity.

Table 2. Cobb-Douglas Results – Total Patients Treated

Variable	PA Private Practice	PA Institution	Medex
Ln (PA hourly work week)	0.175 (2.19)	0.179 (1.50)	0.185 (1.31)
Ln (number of physicians)	0.277 (3.87)	0.425 (5.01)	0.277 (3.00)
Ln (total nonphysician medical personnel)	0.139 (3.45)	0.136 (2.37)	0.138 (2.58)
Solo practice	0.471 (3.78)	+	0.513 (2.69)
Group practice	0.413 (3.79)	+	0.503 (2.88)
Clinic practice	†	+	0.188 (0.83)
Hospital-based	+	+	0.233 (1.11)
Nursing home	+	0.327 (1.78)	+
Non-Federal physicians per 100,000 population	*	-0.0005 (1.45)	0.0004 (1.87)
Primary or non-primary care	0.390 (4.32)	0.481 (4.06)	0.410 (3.62)

46

	(1)	(2)	(3)
Sex of PA or Medex	0.603 (3.42)	-0.144 (0.81)	-0.099 (0.40)
Race of PA or Medex	-0.178 (1.30)	0.358 (2.26)	0.059 (0.43)
PA age	-0.007 (0.09)	0.316 (2.84)	0.003 (0.05)
PA age squared	*	-0.004 (2.59)	*
Patient age 0-6		-0.008 (1.63)	
Patient age 7-25			0.007 (2.52)
Patient age 26-44	0.006 (2.04)		
Patient age 45-64		-0.012 (3.93)	
Constant	1.791	-3.155	2.040
R^2	.236	2.67	.172
Observations	191	246	322

Values in parentheses are t values.
* This value is too small to report and is statistically insignificant.
† Indicates no observations were available for this variable.
‡ Indicated this variable served as the reference group.

47

Table 3. Cobb-Douglas Results — Patients Seen by PA/Medex

Variable	PA Private Practice	PA Institution	Medex
Ln (PA hourly work week)	-0.022 (0.70)	0.300 (3.65)	0.327 (2.94)
Ln (number of physicians)	-0.027 (0.43)	0.105 (2.04)	-0.045 (0.60)
Ln (total nonphysician medical personnel)	0.098 (2.93)	0.060 (1.60)	0.091 (2.32)
Solo practice	0.354 (3.12)	+	0.398 (2.58)
Group practice	0.286 (2.93)	+	0.238 (1.64)
Clinic practice	†	+	0.240 (1.30)
Hospital-based	+	†	0.259 (1.58)
Nursing home	+	0.127 (1.02)	†
Non-Federal physicians per 100,000 population	*	*	*
Primary or non-primary care	-0.002 *	0.054 (0.73)	-0.049 (0.52)

Sex of PA or Medex	0.058 (0.66)	0.129 (1.13)	0.002 *
Race of PA or Medex	0.049 (0.40)	0.188 (1.83)	-0.104 (0.91)
PA age	0.159 (3.56)	0.047 (0.64)	-0.056 (0.81)
PA age squared	-0.002 (3.47)	-0.0003 (0.33)	0.001 (0.79)
Patient age 0-6		-0.007 (2.56)	
Patient age 7-25	0.004 (1.65)		
Patient age 26-44		-0.003 (1.67)	
Patient age 45-64		-0.009 (5.02)	0.004 (1.44)
Constant	-0.259	0.761	2.592
R^2	0.093	0.249	0.069
Observations	309	232	159

Values in parentheses are t values.
* Value is too small to report and is statistically insignificant.
+ Indicates no observations were available for this variable.
† Indicates this variable served as the reference group.

Using the results of this productivity analysis, the Bureau of Health Manpower, DHEW, calculated the number of physicians that would be needed with and without task delegation to NHP. Their analysis for primary care physicians appears in Table 4. For primary care as a whole, they conclude using the low estimate, that 83,000 less doctors (130,890 as compared to 213,510) physicians would be required without task delegation by 1990. These estimates should be viewed only as suggestive.

Table 4. Comparison of Requirements for Primary Care Physicians
With and Without Task Delegation to Physician Extenders,
1975, 1980 and 1990*

Year	With Task Delegation	Without Task Delegation
	Total Primary Care	
1975	107,480 – 131,900	175,110 – 215,010
1980	116,130 – 142,790	189,420 – 232,660
1990	130,890 – 160,950	213,510 – 262,250
	General and Family Practice	
1975	34,400 – 42,240	56,040 – 68,840
1980	35,040 – 43,070	57,100 – 70,170
1990	36,770 – 45,200	59,920 – 73,640
	Pediatrics	
1975	17,760 – 21,590	28,900 – 35,080
1980	17,820 – 21,680	29,060 – 35,920
1990	19,930 – 24,250	32,510 – 39,470
	Internal Medicine	
1975	55,320 – 68,070	90,170 – 111,090
1980	63,270 – 78,040	103,260 – 127,200
1990	74,190 – 91,500	121,080 – 149,140

*Calculations assume a 63 percent gain in physician productivity as measured by visits per week, through task delegation to formally trained physician extenders.
Sources of data on which estimates are based: Scheffler, R.M., "The Productivity of Physician Assistants, Empirical Estimates," presented at the Western Economic Association Meeting, June 1976. American Medical Association, *Profile of Medical Practice, 1975 - 1976,* AMA, Chicago, 1976.

However, their implications seem clear. The utilization of new health practitioners can substantially increase the productivity potential of the existing stock of physicians. Hence, further increases in the supply of physicians may be unwarranted.

POLICY IMPLICATIONS

Perhaps the most important empirical finding of this study is that elasticity with respect to output of a physician assistant or Medex is approximately 63 percent of that of a physician. Although this estimate should not be considered as exact or final, it is probably a reasonable "ball park" estimate. With this estimate as given, it would appear that the training of physician assistants and Medex would be a good investment, given the shorter period (two years) even if the per year cost of training were equivalent to that for physicians. Approximately three PAs could be trained at the social cost of one physician. These three PAs, given our estimates, could produce 1.8 times more visits than one physician. There are many qualifications to be made: PAs and Medex must work with physicians; thus, if physicians do not employ them, additional training will not be productive. The issue of diminishing returns cannot be discussed because so few PAs are employed that estimates diminishing returns cannot be made at this time. Thus, the productivity of the second PA employed by one physician is still unknown. Other issues related to the quality of care and patient acceptance are also of importance.

Given our estimates on the average income of physicians [$41,090 in 1974 (Medical Economics, November 1975, p. 184)], we are able to calculate the imputed wage of PAs and Medex if the physician maximized output or minimizes cost. According to economic theory, the physician should equate the value of the marginal products to the factor input prices. Making this calculation, we find an imputed wage for PAs or Medex of $27,000 ($W/41{,}090 = 0.175/0.277$) when the actual average wage was slightly over $14,000. This suggests, among other things, that the physician shuold be able to profit from the employment of additional physician extenders; whether or not physicians are aware of this is another matter.

Finally, of interest are the projections made for the future supply of new health practitioners. Estimates were based on the known supply in 1975 of formally trained PAs and Medex. The new entrants, i.e., those graduating from approved training, were estimated for each year in the projection. Some of the key assumptions made are that of sex distribution would remain constant, all training programs lasted two years, and attrition rates were assumed to be five percent. The validity of these assumptions are, of

Table 5. Present and Projected Supply of Physician Extenders
(Physician Assistants and Medex) 1975, 1980 and 1990

	1975	1980	1990		
			Basic	Low	High
Total Physician Assistants (PA's)	2,540	7,410	18,520	13,200	27,700
– Physician Assistants	2,100	6,550	16,640	11,790	26,440
– MEDEX	440	860	1,880	1,410	2,860

Source: Physician Assistants: Individual program director's estimates of 1974 – 1980 enrollment. Nurse Practitioners: SUNY. Characteristics of Trainees and Graduates of Nurse Practitioner Programs. Projections made by the Bureau of Health Manpower, DHEW – 1977.
Note: Numbers may not add due to rounding.

course, opened to discussion. In the opinion of the author, the estimates are reasonably "ball park" figures.

Table 5 presents the results of the projections. It is apparent that the supply of PAs and Medex, accouring to these estimates, will increase dramatically in percentage terms. However, the absolute number of these new health practitioners will still be small. A similar projection finds that the supply of physicians will be 559,820 in 1990. Even if we use the high projection of 27,700 PAs and Medex in 1990 there would be about five percent as many PAs as compared to physicians. The number of PAs and Medex does not fully reflect the potential importance of their role in the health care system.

There should continue to be a need for these new health providers. An analysis of the distribution of PAs and Medex (Scheffler 1978) shows that they are locating in rural underserved areas. In addition, they may be helpful in increasing the supply of preventive services to underserved populations.

APPENDIX A

In an attempt to allow for greater flexibility in our model, a translog model was also specified. One of the main attributes of the translog approach is that it allows some of the inputs to have a zero rate of utilization and still obtain output [see Reinhardt (1975)]. Necessary inputs (PA/Medex and physicians) are entered in both log and linear forms in an attempt to get an estimate of decreasing-increasing returns, whereas other inputs are included in nonlog form only. Looking first at the PA results, all of the coefficients for the necessary inputs have the proper sign. However, while the log terms are greatly significant (PA/Medex in institutions are significant only at the 20 percent level), the linear terms are insignificant except for the physicians in institutions. This seems to imply that the model does not need or fully utilize the added flexibility of the translog approach. Due to the constraints and legal barriers under which many PAs are presently employed, this is not a surprising result. The results for the Medex are somewhat disappointing in that only the number of physicians variable attains any statistical significance. However, as in the PA regressions, the Totnum variable retains its significance. The number of nonphysician medical personnel was also entered in squared form to obtain an estimate of the optimal number of aides. The numbers range from 30 to 47, indicating that an increase in aides may be warranted from a productivity point of view.

FOOTNOTES

*This work was supported by funds from DHEW Contract NO1-MB-44184. The author would like to thank Larry Miners, Marilyn Harrington, Elaine Bursic and Roger Feldman for their help on this project

**This paper was written when the author was on leave from the University of North Carolina at the Institute of Medicine, National Academy of Sciences, Washington, D.C.

1. For a discussion of the economics of training these new health practitioners, see Richard Scheffler (February 1975).

2. An earlier study of the earnings of physician assistants is in Richard Scheffler (1974).

3. The sex composition of the patient visits was omitted from the final specification because it was statistically insignificant.

4. A more detailed description of the data base may be obtained from the Project on the Economics of Health Manpower, Department of Economics, University of North Carolina, Chapel Hill. Preliminary analysis suggests that there is not any significant nonresponse bias.

5. Bailey (1970) provides an illuminating discussion of this problem.

6. The empirical results for the translog function are found in Appendix A. In general, they were not as statistically reliable or as plausible as the Cobb-Douglas.

7. The R^2's vary from about 17 percent to over 26 percent. Our concern is primarily with the statistically significant coefficients and not with R^2's.

8. It should be noted that primary care visits are probably less complicated, of shorter duration, and hence easier to provide.

REFERENCES

American Medical Association (1973), *Profiles of Medical Practice:* 199.

Bailey R. M. (1970), "Economies of Scale in Medical Practice," Herbert E. Klarman, ed., *Empirical Studies in Health Economics.* Baltimore: The John Hopkins University Press.

Table A.1. Translog Results — Total Patients Treated

Variable	PA Private Practice	PA Institution	Medex
PA hourly work week	-0.001 (0.74)	-0.005 (0.59)	-0.004 (0.38)
Ln (PA hourly work week)	0.250 (2.28)	0.397 (1.47)	0.323 (0.74)
Number of physicians	-0.007 (0.54)	-0.123 (2.44)	0.183 (2.30)
Ln (number of physicians)	0.329 (3.17)	0.842 (4.52)	-0.208 (0.87)
Total nonphysician medical personnel	0.016 (2.50)	0.015 (1.64)	0.027 (2.32)
Total nonphysician medical personnel squared	-0.00017 (2.40)	-0.00015 (1.42)	-0.00035 (1.44)
Solo practice	0.444 (3.47)	+	0.522 (2.72)
Group practice	0.416 (3.76)	+	0.603 (3.35)
Clinic practice	†	+	0.351 (1.50)
Hospital-based	+	†	0.350 (1.74)
Nursing home	+	0.368 (1.91)	†
Non-Federal physicians per 100,000 population	*	- .00049 (1.54)	*
Primary or non-primary care	0.379 (4.11)	0.444 (3.71)	0.452 (3.95)
Sex	-0.032 (0.32)	-0.174 (0.98)	0.603 (3.42)
Race	0.071 (0.52)	0.308 (1.93)	-0.194 (1.41)
PA age	0.009 (0.19)	0.325 (2.93)	-0.010 (0.13)

Table A.1. (Continued)

PA age squared	-0.00008 (0.13)	-0.004 (2.69)	*
Patient age 0-6		-0.008 (178)	
Patient age 7-25	0.006 (2.33)		
Patient age 26-44			0.005 (1.96)
Patient age 45-64		-0.011 (3.56)	
Constant	1.818	-3.650	1.404
R^2	0.152	0.273	0.239
Observations	322	246	140

Values in parentheses are t values.
* Value is too small to report and is statistically insignificant.
+ Indicates no observations were available for this variable.
† Indicates this group was used as the reference group.

Boulier, Bryan L. (1974), "Two Essays in the Economices of Dentistry: A Production Function for Dental Services and an Examination of the Effects of Licensure. Unpublished Ph.D. dissertation, Princeton University.

De Janvary, Alain (May 1972), "The Class of Generalized Power Production Functions." *American Journal of Agricultural Economics* 54: 234–237.

Golladay, F. L., Mauser, M. E., and Smith, K. E. (Winter 1974), "Scale Economies in the Delivery of Medical Care: A Mixed Integer Programming Analysis of Efficient Manpower Utilization," *Journal of Human Resources:* 50–62.

Kimbell, L. J., and Lorant, J. H. (December 1973), "Physicians' Productivity and Returns to Scale," Econometric Society Meetings, New York.

Kushman, John, and Scheffler, Richard (1978), "Pricing Health Services: Verification of a Monopoly Model for Dentistry," *The Journal of Human Resources.*

—— *(May 1978), "A Manpower Policy for Primary Health Care,"* New England Journal of Medicine 298:1058–1062.

Reinhardt, Uwe E. (1975). *Physician Productivity and the Demand for Health Manpower: An Economic Analysis.* Cambridge, Mass.: Ballinger Publishing Co.

—— (Fall 1973), "Manpower Substitution and Productivity in Medical Practice: Review of Research." *Health Services Research:* 200–227.

—— (February 1973). "A Production Function for Physicians' Services," *Review of Economics and Statistics* 54:55–66.

————. and Smith, Kenneth R. (1974), "Manpower Substitution in Ambulatory Care," *Health, Manpower and Productivity,* John Rafferty, ed., Lexington, Mass.: Lexington Books, pp. 3–33.

Scheffler, Richard M. (February 1975), "Physician Assistants: Is There a Return to Training?" *Industrial Relations* 14: 78–89.

———— (Autumn 1974), "The Market for Paraprofessionals: The Physician Assistant." *The Quarterly Review of Economics and Business* 14, No. 3: 48–60.

———— (Spring 1975), "Further Considerations on the Economics of Group Practice: The Management Input," *The Journal of Human Resources* 10, No. 2: 258–263.

———— (1974), "Production and Economies of Scale in Medical Practice," *Health, Manpower, and Productivity,* John Rafferty, ed., Lexington, Mass.: Lexington Books.

————, and John Kushman (July 1977), "A Production Function for Dental Services: Estimation and Economic Implications," *Southern Economic Journal* 44.

———— (1978), *The Supply of and Demand for New Health Professionals: Physician's Assistants and MEDEX,* Department of Health, Education and Welfare, Contract No. 1-44184, Bureau of Health Manpower.

Smith, K. R., M. Miller, and Golladay F. L. (Spring 1972), "An Analysis of the Optimal Use of Inputs in the Production of Medical Services," *Journal of Human Resources* 7, No. 208.

NEW DEVELOPMENTS IN THE MARKET FOR RURAL HEALTH CARE[1]

Karen Davis,* BROOKINGS INSTITUTION

Ray Marshall,** UNIVERSITY OF TEXAS

In the last decade, health care has received an increasingly important place in Federal and state government budgetary priorities. This growth in public commitment to health care has been paralleled by interest of economists and other researchers in health services research focusing on a wide range of aspects of health-care financing, organization, delivery, and training of health professionals. Little attention, however, has been paid in either the design of public programs or in the conduct of research to the particular needs of rural Americans. This neglect has led to an inequitable distribution of benefits under public programs between urban and rural residents and the implementation of health programs which are not geared toward rural needs.

There are a number of reasons why health research and policy should

Research in Health Economics, Vol. 1, pp 57–110.
Copyright © 1979 by JAI Press, Inc.
All rights of reproduction in any form reserved.
ISBN 0-89232-042-7.

be more sensitive to rural health problems in the coming years. First, neglect of rural health has led to a disproportionately low share of benefits under public programs going to rural residents. A quarter of the nation's population lives in rural areas, nearly half of the nation's poor are rural residents, and 38 percent of elderly people and children live in nonmetropolitan areas. Yet a cursory review of health programs designed to meet the special needs of the poor, elderly, and children indicates limited benefits in rural areas:

- Total expenditures for Medicare in 1976 are expected to be $15 billion. Approximately 29 percent of Part A funds for hospital and posthospital services go to elderly patients in nonmetropolitan areas; about 28 percent of Part B funds for physician and other ambulatory services to the nonmetropolitan residents—but 38 percent of the elderly live outside metropolitan areas.
- Less than 30 percent of Medicaid funds of an estimated $14 billion in 1976 go to nonmetropolitan areas. Average Medicaid payments per poor child were $5 annually for rural children in 1970, compared with $76 for poor children in central cities.
- The Maternal and Child Health program which was explicitly designed to meet rural health problems spends a less than proportionate share in rural areas—23 percent of Federal and state expenditures go to nonmetropolitan areas even though 37 percent of all children and births are in those areas. Over 90 percent of women and children served by comprehensive health centers under this program live in metropolitan areas.
- Seventy-five percent of all neighborhood health centers are in urban areas.
- Those programs which have placed greater emphasis on rural areas have been funded at low levels. Twenty-two out of 39 family health centers have been established in rural areas, but this program has a total annual funding of $13 million. The National Health Service Corps which places physicians and other health professionals in areas of critical shortages also has a budget of $13 million.

A second reason for greater concern with rural health is that some health problems among rural residents tend to be more serious and severe than among urban residents. Low incomes, poor diets, unsafe or deteriorated housing, impure water supplies, poor transportation and communication, and limited medical resources combine to intensify health-care problems. These factors are reflected in such statistics as:

- The rate of deaths from accidents in rural areas is four times the national average.

- Infant mortality rates among the rural poor are 20 percent higher than among the urban poor, and 50 percent higher than the national average. Infant mortality rates among poor rural blacks is double the national average.
- Chronic conditions are much more prevalent among rural residents of all ages. Gallbladder, emphysema, pleurisy, arthritis, rheumatism, hypertensive heart disease, and cerebrovascular disease all afflict rural residents to a greater extent than urban residents.
- Fifty-four percent of all new cases of tuberculosis are in nonmetropolitan areas.
- The life expectancy of migrant farmworkers, 49 years, is 23 years less than the average for U.S. citizens. The infant and maternal mortality is 25 percent greater than the U.S. average. Migrant births occur outside hospitals nine times more frequently than the national average. The death rate from tuberculosis is two and one half times the U.S. average. Death from influenza and pneumonia is three times the national average.

Third, the potential for improvement in health among rural residents may not be realized because of the dominance of urban conditions in health services research and in policy decisions. The latest vogue in health services research is to discount the importance of medical care in improving health. A shift in health care policy appears to be occurring with reduced concern for ensuring access to medical care services and increased concern that many Americans may be "overdoctored, overmedicated, and overhospitalized." High rates of surgery in the United States have been used to bolster the case that most Americans now get "too much" and possible deleterious medical care. Hospitals are accused of acquiring excessive, costly technological innovations. Experts point to the possibility of a physician surplus in the near future. Major new health policy initiatives in the last few years all emphasize *reducing health care* and utilization—including health maintenance organizations, professional standards review organizations, and health planning. This shift in policy and the growing conviction that medical care is not efficacious may be invalid for a number of reasons—our measures of health outcome are crude, improvements may only occur after considerable lag, other factors may be changing to offset improvements in health, our methodological tools may not be sufficiently well developed to detect changes, and so forth. But even if "excessive" medical care is a fact of life for some Americans, it is unlikely to be so universally for all Americans or for all health problems. For those excluded from adequate medical care, serious health problems which could be prevented and ameliorated with modern medical technology may persist. Such is clearly the case among many rural residents for whom additional medical care can be expected to yield quite substantial returns to improved health.

Finally, increased attention to rural health problems is particularly crucial in the next few years because this is an area which appears to be on the threshold of change. Large sums of Federal funds are going for health care so that, if redirected, a substantial impact could be made. State governments are becoming increasingly concerned with rural health problems—passing state rural health acts and establishing rural primary care programs. Private foundations and the Federal government are beginning to experiment with alternative approaches to rural health delivery. New kinds of health professionals, particularly nurse practitioners and physician assistants, are being trained in significant numbers. Family practice residencies are being established. A large influx in the total supply of physicians is expected. Decentralized medical education is being fostered through area health education center programs and the establishment of rural medical school programs. Harnessing these forces to work for better rural health care, however, is unlikely to occur without considerable effort and attention to all aspects of the policy-formulating and policy-implementing process.

I. WHY RURAL HUMAN RESOURCE DEVELOPMENT IS IN THE BEST INTEREST OF URBAN AREAS

Rural health care is important for urban as well as rural people because an effective health-care delivery system is necessary for rural development and rural development could help relieve some of the nation's most pressing urban problems.

- Rural to urban migration transfers rural problems to urban places. If present long-run trends continue, two-thirds of the population of the United States will live in large metropolitan areas with populations of over 30 million by A.D. 2000.
- An effective rural development strategy also might make it possible for rural and urban people to have greater freedom of choice in where they live. People are leaving rural areas not because they want to live in urban places. Opinion polls rather consistently show that most people in the United States prefer to live in small towns and rural areas. The preference of rural people to remain where they are is particularly strong—88 percent of the rural respondents in one national poll preferred to remain in rural areas.
- The main reasons most of these people cannot stay in rural places are economic. Although metropolitan areas also provide advantages of

diversity of economic opportunities and life styles that are not likely
to be available in most small towns or rural areas, the evidence also
shows that many people find the quality of urban life to be negative
and deteriorating.

The preference for rural living undoubtedly accounts for the slight reversal in rural-to-urban migration trends since 1970. For the first time
since 1890, rural areas are gaining population absolutely and relatively.
The rural population was fairly constant absolutely between 1920 and
1970, but was a declining proportion of the total population. However, a
number of developments have made it possible for more people to move
back to rural areas. These include: the rapid expansion of manufacturing
employment in rural areas (manufacturing employment grew faster in
rural than in urban areas during the 1960s); the growth of vacation and
retirement communities in rural places; the growth of rural college communities; and the resurgence of coal-mining areas during the 1970s after a
period of decline.

The main negative aspects of the quality of life in large metropolitan
areas are frequently overlooked until they reach crisis proportions because of the positive market attractions of those places.

The following seem to us to be the most serious of these problems:

(1) There is a positive correlation between population density and vio-
lent crimes. Crime increases in large metropolitan areas because deper-
sonalization and congestion lead to aggressive behavior; moreover, internal social controls tend to break down in those places, requiring the
substitution of external or police controls. This causes the policy problem
to be almost unsolvable.

(2) Population density and size also lead to personal alienation, because of such factors as individual powerlessness in a highly complex and
interdependent society; frustrations caused by congestion and environmental pollution; the boring, menial, repetitive jobs many people hold;
and loss of contact with the natural environment.

(3) Urban congestion also leads to serious *environmental problems,*
which are not counted as economic costs initially but which ultimately
must be considered. These include air, noise, and water pollution and
solid-waste disposal, all of which intensify with the city size, density and
age.

(4) The concentration of people in large metropolitan areas could put
serious strains on the democratic process. Increasingly, metropolitan systems become so complex that only experts can pretend to understand
them. Individual voters in such systems are likely to feel relatively power-
less and apathetic, even if they get sufficient information to understand
the complexities of the issues confronting them. Individual participation

in the democratic process is discouraged by the feeling that one vote has little significance.

Elected officials also have serious problems in governing complex urban systems. They too are likely to rely increasingly on experts, whose value to elected officials is limited because (a) specialists do not have clear-cut answers to problems which are accepted by all or most of the experts and (b) specialists draw narrow limits to their knowledge, making it hard to understand the whole system and put specialized information in a comprehensive perspective.

The problems of large metropolitan areas are compounded by the freedom of movement of people and enterprises. As the quality of urban life deteriorates, those who are able to move tend to do so. These include wealthy people and the more mobile businesses. These movements cause cities to be left with inordinate proportions of poor people and blue-collar workers, whose mobility is limited by economic constraints and who must therefore bear the brunt of the deteriorating quality of life. The cities' financial ability to respond to increasing social problems is weakened by declining tax bases. There are therefore likely to be serious social tensions as the cities attempt to require blue-collar workers to bear increasing tax burdens to help the poor, whose ranks are augmented by people displaced from rural areas. It might be good economics for large metropolitan places to grow, but we think it is a very narrow type of economic analysis that produces this conclusion.

Public policy must therefore be based on a systematic approach which counts nonmarket as well as market costs and benefits. Viewed in this perspective, outmigration from rural to large metropolitan areas is not self-correcting but produces cumulative decline in some rural places and serious problems for larger metropolitan areas. The process of cumulative decline cannot be corrected by market forces alone because those forces tend to be root causes of deterioration. Balanced growth in rural and urban areas will therefore require that market forces be complemented with public policies and nonmarket private activities. A rural development strategy that includes an effective rural health system is therefore in the national interest.

II. CONCEPTUAL FRAMEWORK FOR THE ANALYSIS OF RURAL HEALTH

The basic conceptual approach used in our rural health project focuses on health sytems, and nonmarket as well as market behavior. This systems approach identifies the actors involved in a particular interrelated activity (like the delivery of health care, the practice of a profession like economics or law, agriculture, labor relations, etc.), analyzes the hierarchy of relationships between the actors and their relative power positions, and studies the relationships between the particular system being analyzed and the environmental context within which it operates.

In analyzing health care in the rural South, for example, a systems approach attempts to answer such questions as: What is the medical system in the United States? Who are the main actors in that system and what are their motives? What institutions and procedures do these actors develop to perpetuate their control of the system? How do the main actors relate to each other? What are the implications of this system for the delivery of health care to rural people? Can the system be modified to meet the needs of rural people or must special rural health systems be constructed? What modifications must be made in the existing system to make it more compatible with the health-care needs of rural people? If a new system should be created, what are its characteristics and how should it relate to urban systems?

Because of its limitations for policy purposes, we have found it difficult to apply traditional economic analysis to health problems. These systems meet few of the traditional requirements for a competitive market. Entry is very restricted, and product demand and supply conditions are difficult to specify. The "product" supplied is hard to define and the costs of that product, as well as who must pay the costs, are difficult to specify. Consumers demand better health, but the system supplies medical care. Because of inadequate knowledge consumers are not likely to be able to specify the relationship between medical care and health. Utility analysis is of limited value because those who make direct payments for medical care often are not consumers but third parties whose motives are not necessarily identical with those of consumers.

Perhaps the main disadvantage of traditional economic analysis is its narrow focus. Orthodox analysis is likely to view decision making within the framework of *given* systems, while a systems approach is likely to suggest ways to change the system. Moreover, traditional analysis focuses on individual decision making, whereas we think that communities, organizations, governments, and groups also play a major role in structuring health systems.

Orthodox economics analyzes health markets in terms of "imperfections" in competitive market, but this analysis is frequently mechanistic and uninformative. For example, it is not "unnatural" for doctors or other actors in the system to attempt to establish organizations, rules, laws, and institutional arrangements to protect and advance their status, welfare, and control of the medical system. By the same token, it is natural that consumers and other actors in the health system should attempt to challenge the doctors' control of the system. Moreover, within the system, it is clear why there has been a trend toward specialization and the adoption of sophisticated technology, and these trends are not "unnatural" or "imperfections." Nor have competitive market forces directed by consumer demand been the main causes for these trends. Similarly, it is natural that doctors interested in family practice or primary care should challenge the trends and attempt to change the direction of the system. Indeed, attempting to use orthodox economics to analyze health problems is "unnatural" in the sense that analysis is forced into restrictive categories which do not fit the realities of the health system.

Besides its narrow focus, orthodox economic analysis is not very useful for health-policy purposes because perfectly competitive markets probably are neither possible nor desirable. Most people do not believe that health facilities and medical care should be distributed according to the ability to pay, or that the health of children should be determined by parents' ability to pay. Nor is it "unnatural" that the poor should attempt to substitute political power for their economic weaknesses by having health care distributed more equitably according to need rather than according to income or ability to pay. Indeed, it is very rational that all of the actors within the health system should attempt to accomplish through governments what they cannot do as individuals or collectively in the market. Some of these broader health questions can be treated as "externalities" by orthodox economics, which views the individual decisions as the main focus of analysis, but these are not "externalities" in a systems approach. Finally, a market-oriented health system under conditions of unequal distribution of income would not necessarily produce better health. Doctors would concentrate on those aspects of the system which were most "profitable," which probably would not be preventive medicine and environmental health care, nor care of disadvantaged members of society.

The remainder of this paper presents the results of a study of health problems in the rural South. It analyzes the implications of those problems, and evaluates various approaches or "models" for rural health-care delivery. Information for the project was collected through an extensive review of the literature, statistical data from a variety of sources, and detailed field interviews in approximately 70 rural health facilities in the South and with many people knowledgeable about rural health conditions. We are guided in our work by a board of advisers made up of doctors with various medical specialties. While our data and examples come mainly from the South, some of the generalizations probably are applicable to rural conditions outside the South.

III. RURAL HEALTH—HOW IS IT DIFFERENT?

Several characteristics distinguish the rural South from other areas, contributing to the severity of health problems and influencing the most prevalent types of health conditions. A major factor underlying many health problems is the high rate of poverty among rural Southerners with consequences both for the greater incidence of health problems and, through poor nutrition, greater vulnerability to disease and illness.

Even for more well-to-do rural people, however, limited availability of health professionals, poor telephone and communication services, bad roads and mountainous terrain impede easy access to medical services. Thus primary preventive services, particularly for children, are frequently neglected. Women are less likely to receive adequate prenatal care, cancer screening, and contraceptive information. Older rural people are less likely to follow proper maintenance and regular monitoring of chronic conditions such as hypertension, diabetes, and heart disease.

Poor dental health is a major problem for many rural Southerners. Individualized, unfluoridated water sources increase the incidence of dental caries. Lack of running water in some homes and limited education regarding good dental habits lead to poor dental hygiene. The limited availability of dental professionals compounds this problem, but even where dentists are within traveling distance, limited incomes frequently prevent ready use of these services. Loss of permanent teeth even among young adults is a shocking fact in many rural areas. Poor dental health has implications beyond its cosmetic effects, however. Increasingly it is recognized that infections in the mouth affect the whole body; pain from toothaches affects school and work performance; and missing teeth and false teeth compound nutritional and digestive problems.

Rural areas differ from urban ones in other significant ways. Water quality and sanitation are frequently more important sources of rural health hazards. Lack of acceptable municipal water and sewage disposal services leads to a greater incidence of diseases such as impetigo, diarrheal and gastrointestinal diseases, bacterial infections, parasitic diseases, and insect-borne diseases. Mobile homes with inadequate sewage disposal facilities abound in some rural areas not covered by urban plumbing codes. Lack of running water in some homes makes bathing and personal hygiene difficult. Lack of indoor plumbing or improperly constructed pit privies contributes to sanitation-related diseases.

Solid-waste disposal is another important health problem in some rural communities. While urban residents may come to expect regular, frequent garbage pickups, many rural communities are without such essential public services. Accumulations of tin and broken glass contribute to the rate of injuries. Abandoned cars and appliances are both a visual blight and a health hazard. Dumping refuse in streams is a common practice in some rural communities—contaminating water supplies for many others.

While rural areas are frequently viewed as blessed by clean air, occupational hazards of black lung disease and allergies to dust and fertilizer, all contribute to high rates of respiratory problems among rural adults. High accident rates in mining and farming have caused those occupations to be among the most hazardous of jobs.

Rural roads are an other source of accidents. Mountainous terrain makes travel extremely risky in some areas. Higher driving speeds and frequency of blind intersections contribute to serious accidents in flatter terrains.

Limited employment opportunities and the lack of cultural or recreational diversions contribute to the high prevalence of mental illness, depression, teenage pregnancy, child neglect, and alcoholism among rural Southerners. Shift work and irregular hours impose psychological hardships on those who can find work. Strenuous physical labor required in many rural industries wears out workers' health and ages many rural people well before their time.

These health problems, while alluded to time and time again in visits to Southern rural health centers in discussions with a variety of health professionals and community leaders, are inadequately documented in published statistical reports. Following, however, are some highlights of health problems of rural Southerners which are captured by existing records (see Tables 1-25 at end of paper for additional details).

(1) Infant and general mortality rates in the nonmetropolitan South are much higher than in other areas. In 1971, infant mortality rates in the nonmetropolitan 13-state South were 23.3 deaths per 1,000 live births compared with 19.0 nationally, or 23 percent higher than the national average infant mortality rate. General mortality rates were also higher in the nonmetropolitan South, averaging 10.4 deaths per 1,000 population in the nonmetropolitan South in 1971 compared with 8.5 per 1,000 in the metropolitan South and 9.3 deaths per 1,000 population nationally. Thus, general death rates were 22 percent higher in the nonmetropolitan South than the metropolitan South (age-adjusted death rates were not available for comparison between metropolitan and nonmetropolitan areas; some portion of the differences shown is undoubtedly attributable to the higher proportion of elderly people in rural areas of the South.)

(2) Infant mortality rates are 65 percent higher among nonmetropolitan black Southerners than among whites (33.1 deaths per 1,000 live births compared with 20.1 for whites). Infant mortality rates for each race were

higher in smaller nonmetropolitan counties than their counterparts in metropolitan counties.

(3) Infant mortality rates for both races are higher in counties with a greater incidence of poverty. Infant mortality rates in Southern nonmetropolitan counties with a poverty rate of 35 percent or more average 27.2 deaths per 1,000 live births, compared with 19.8 in nonmetropolitan counties with poverty rates below 15 percent. While infant mortality rates are generally higher in nonmetropolitan counties than in metropolitan counties, differences are most marked in high poverty areas.

(4) General mortality rates are also higher in high poverty areas. In nonmetropolitan Southern counties with poverty rates of 15 percent or less, the general mortality rate is 8.7; this increases to 11.2 for counties with poverty rates of 35 percent or more.

(5) The nonmetropolitan South has higher rates of morbidity and disability than other regions. Age-adjusted restricted activity days in the nonmetropolitan South are higher than other nonmetropolitan areas and higher than the metropolitan South. Age-adjusted work-loss days and bed disability days, however, are higher in the metropolitan South than the nonmetropolitan South—although both areas are above the national average. Age-specific figures indicate more bed disability among the elderly in the nonmetropolitan South than other areas. In 1969–70, the elderly in the nonmetropolitan South averaged 17.6 days of bed disability per person per year compared with 13.4 days nationally.

(6) Children in the nonmetropolitan South have a lower incidence of respiratory and infectious diseases. Adults, however, have a much higher rate of acute conditions in the nonmetropolitan South than in other areas. Injury rates are also higher for the nonmetropolitan South.

(7) The incidence of most chronic conditions is greater in nonmetropolitan areas than in the rest of the nation. Hypertensive heart disease, cerebrovascular heart disease, ulcers, emphysema, arthritis, and rheumatism are all more prevalent among nonmetropolitan residents.

(8) Nutritional levels of low-income rural Southerners lag behind those of other residents. Forty-three percent of low-income Southern farm housewives have poor diets compared with 36 percent of all low-income housewives in the nation.

(9) Sixty percent of substandard housing is located in rural areas. While only 5 percent of houses in the metropolitan South lack plumbing, 24 percent of housing in smaller nonmetropolitan Southern counties does not have plumbing. In Southern nonmetropolitan counties with high poverty rates, a third of houses lack plumbing.

(10) The nonmetropolitan South has fewer patient care physicians per capita than other areas, but slightly more general practice physicians. The

number of physicians choosing general practice, however, has declined in the last few decades so that many rural general practice physicians are now approaching retirement. Physician-population ratios are particularly low in smaller nonmetropolitan areas and in counties with high poverty rates.

(11) The nonmetropolitan South, like nonmetropolitan areas outside the South, receives fewer physician services and incurs more hospital stays (in 1973–1974 age-adjusted physician visit rates were 4.4 percent in nonmetropolitan areas and 5.2 percent in metropolitan areas of the United States). Thus, even though physicians in nonmetropolitan areas see more patients per week, this heavier workload does not entirely compensate for lower physician per capita ratios and rural residents lag behind urban residents in use of physician services. Since residents of the nonmetropolitan South have a higher incidence of health problems, they would appear to be underutilizers of ambulatory health services relative to their urban counterparts with similar health status. Hospital stays, however, are higher in nonmetropolitan areas, probably related to the fact that hospitals, while frequently substandard in the rural South, are in relatively greater supply due to the Hill-Burton program which financed hospital construction.

(12) Physician visits in nonmetropolitan areas, however, would be even lower if physicians did not adjust to their relative scarcity by spending more hours each week in patient care and seeing more patients per week than do urban physicians. To meet the patient loads they face, rural physicians employ more full-time personnel and, as a result, average higher practice expenses. Fees are lower, but the greater volume of patients results in both higher gross and higher net earnings of physicians in the East South Central region (Kentucky, Tennessee, Alabama, Mississippi) than in other areas.

(13) Dental visits nationally are 45 percent higher than in the nonmetropolitan South.

IV. OBSTACLES TO IMPROVED RURAL HEALTH CARE

While the health problems of the rural South are different from other areas, and generally more severe, there are considerable obstacles which confront any attempts to improve health of rural people. To start with, as shown in the last section, the health problems of rural people are more closely interrelated to the particular economic and environmental factors at play in rural areas. Thus, any single, narrow attack on medical care alone is unlikely to be effective.

Aside from the nature of rural health problems, however, several forces act to impede progress. These include: (1) inadequate financing of health services in rural areas; (2) characteristics of the nature of medical practice in rural areas; (3) incentives in the medical system and training of health professionals which mitigate against rural areas; (4) legal restrictions and opposition of the medical, nursing, and other health professions; and (5) racial barriers and discrimination that are particularly serious in rural areas where few alternative sources of care are available.

A. Financing of Health Services in Rural Areas

Purchasing power for health-care services in rural areas is a major barrier, impeding financial access to the health-care system:

(1) While about 11 percent of the nation's population falls below the poverty level, 23 percent of rural Southern families have below-poverty incomes. Over half of Southern rural black families are poor.

(2) Rural residents are less likely to be covered by private health insurance plans, and the plans they do have are less comprehensive than those of urban residents. Residents of the South are less likely to have hospital insurance coverage than others, and nonmetropolitan South residents have the lowest hospital insurance coverage of any group—about one-third of nonmetropolitan nonfarm residents have no hospital insurance and about one-half of farm residents in the South have no hospital insurance.

(3) Public programs have not responded by filling the gap in this private health insurance coverage. Instead, public programs also have less extensive coverage in the nonmetropolitan South than other areas. Half of all poor children in the nation are receiving Medicaid services. In the Southern states of Alabama, Arkansas, Louisiana, Mississippi, South Carolina, and Texas only one poor child in ten receives Medicaid services. Few rural families receive Medicaid benefits because, in the South, this program provides benefits largely to one-parent families while most rural families are two-parent families with low incomes from agriculture, small manufacturing, or public service jobs. Average Medicaid expenditure per poor child in nonmetropolitan areas is $5 compared with $76 in central city areas.

(4) Medicare also discriminates against rural areas. While a greater proportion of rural residents is elderly and Medicare has been of considerable assistance to them, the program systematically penalizes physicians practicing in rural areas by setting lower reimbursement levels for them. Average Medicare expenditure on physician services per person enrolled is $73 in the nonmetropolitan South compared with $100 nationally. Other data suggest that this reflects both the lower compensation for physician services in the nonmetropolitan South and the more limited

access of the elderly to physician services in the nonmetropolitan South. Hospital and post-hospital services expenditures are also lower in the nonmetropolitan South averaging $192 per person enrolled compared with $262 nationally—most of this difference, however, reflects the lower cost (and probably quality) of hospital care in the nonmetropolitan South.

B. Nature of Rural Medical Practice

A major problem in establishing an adequate health care system in the rural South is related to attracting health professionals, particularly physicians, to those areas. There are many reasons for this, including:

(1) Medical professionals are concerned about being isolated professionally if they establish rural medical practices. Few opportunities are available for the continued professional development of rural physicians. While some states are moving toward greater decentralization of medical education, few internships and residency positions are available in rural areas. Thus, rural physicians are not exposed to the latest in medical science.

(2) Because there are few health professionals in rural areas, those who do locate there tend to have very limited time for their families or for recreation. Rural physicians are normally obligated to be available 24 hours a day while their urban counterparts can tell patients to go to a hospital emergency room or find another doctor. Overwork is therefore a major cause of discontent among rural physicians.

(3) The limited availability of physicians in rural areas means that those who are there must see a lot of patients. To handle this load, physicians cannot spend as much time with each patient as he or she would in a less hectic practice. Patients recognizing this pace of practice are likely to come only with urgent medical problems. Preventive care is neglected. Fewer support services such as laboratories, physician specialists, mental health professionals, and social agencies are available in rural areas. Thus, rural physicians have fewer resources, and many essential aspects of complete health care may be inadequately addressed. Rural physicians often leave rural areas because they do not feel that they do as much for their patients as they could in other areas.

(4) Population densities also make it difficult to establish rural medical practices, because a minimum population is required to support a physician. It would be difficult to establish traditional medical practices in relatively small places. However, it might be possible to establish rural health systems using nonphysician health professionals (e.g., nurse practitioners and physician assistants) to extend medical care into relatively small communities. The population of a small town might not justify a

physician, but it might support a nurse practitioner supervised by a physician located in a larger town.

(5) Although rural doctors have net earnings equal to or higher than their urban counterparts, the costs of establishing rural medical practices apparently are much greater than the costs of establishing urban practices. All of the relative cost components are not clear, but a major reason for higher rural start-up costs is the necessity of building facilities and establishing components in rural places that are not necessary in urban places because support services are provided by other groups, laboratories are available, and medical office space can be rented. In rural areas, on the other hand, buildings are not likely to be available, utilities must often be brought in at considerable expense, and roads or parking lots might even have to be paved. In other words, a rural practice must internalize certain costs that are external to an urban practice.

(6) Rural areas often have trouble attracting health professionals because those communities lack the cultural, entertainment, educational, and housing facilities many professionals are likely to require. Moreover, the dominant value systems of many small towns and rural areas are likely to be incompatible with those held by many medical professionals. Special efforts, therefore, are required to match health professionals with rural communities.

Some new trends may affect some of the historic disadvantages of rural communities. The growing preference for rural life reflected in opinion polls appears to be spreading to health professionals. An increase in women pursuing professional careers may lead to more husband-wife teams interested in rural practice.

Most objections to rural practices can be overcome through specific policies, such as the development of group physician practices, team approaches to health care, promotion of nonphysician health professionals, and improved professional support services. It is possible, however, that the nature of the medical system will counteract any positive changes which are made to improve rural practice.

C. The Medical System and Legal Restrictions

The medical system is a system in the sense that it has certain interrelated values and institutions which condition the nature of its processes and outcomes. In the United States, this system has certain actors whose powers and interests cause the system to be what it is. The central actors in the system have been physicians who make most major medical decisions. Physicians, through local, state, and national medical societies, control medical practice through a variety of procedures, especially licensing and legal restrictions on the practice of medicine by others and control of medical education, hospitals, and the use of medical technology.

Although it has never been monolithic, and there are some encouraging trends toward a higher percentage of family practitioners, the medical system has had several dominant values which cause it to be biased against rural practice. One such value has been specialization. An increasing proportion of medical care is delivered by specialists who require dense populations and close association with medical centers. Even training programs for nonphysician health professionals have frequently been specialized to segments of the patient population. Rural areas are not likely to be very attractive to specialists nor are such specialists suitable for meeting the health-care needs of the entire rural population.

Similarly, there has been a proliferation of medical technology, much of which also must be located in urban areas or medical centers in order to be used effectively. Since medical role models are likely to be specialists and "good" medical practice requires considerable technology, even those medical students strongly inclined to rural practice tend to get socialized by the natural desire to conform with the values communicated in medical schools.

Other features of the present medical system that tend to be incompatible with the requirements of effective health-care delivery include:

(1) The emphasis on curative rather than preventive medicine, which will cause physicians to emphasize exotic medical problems rather than practicing preventive medicine and dealing with those environmental problems so important in rural areas.

(2) The restrictions on the use of nonphysician health professionals, who could perform many medical tasks.

(3) Emphasis on single practitioners who are likely to be overworked and professionally isolated in rural areas.

(4) The medical system has given little attention to the efficient use of resources for medical care, and the shortage of health professionals relative to the demand has made it possible for the system to ignore efficiency. Because of the greater incidence of poverty in rural areas and the rising costs of health care, there is a special need to emphasize efficiency in health-care delivery.

We do not wish to imply by the foregoing that the medical system in the United States has been oblivious to the needs of rural areas or even that it is consciously hostile to the health needs of rural people; rather, we merely wish to emphasize that what appear to us to be the dominant trends in American medical practice cause that system in the main not to address itself to the needs of rural people as effectively as it might.

D. Minorities and Rural Health Care

A surprising incidence of insensitive and/or discriminatory practices toward black, Mexican American, and other minorities still persists widely throughout the South. Some physicians still maintain segregated waiting rooms, and black patients are frequently restricted to certain hours of the day in seeing private physicians. Hospitals are built with private rooms to prevent racial mixing of patients, and in some instances hospital dining rooms are segregated. In one hospital visited, white nurses are prohibited from performing some types of nursing care for black male patients. Language barriers, ignorance of cultural traditions, and insensitivity are also problems encountered among health providers serving Mexican Americans.

Other practices are more subtle but may have serious consequences for the health of rural minorities. Cursory, inadequate physical examinations are frequently given to minority patients. In some places, rural blacks are unaware that it is customary to undress for medical examinations whereas this procedure is common among whites in the same area. Blood-pressure readings are taken through the clothing of black patients, thus increasing the risk of inaccurate measurements, a particularly serious problem for blacks with a high incidence of hypertension. Minority women are less likely to receive professional preventive services such as Pap smears and breast examinations. High rates of hysterectomies on minority women are also seen in some areas.

Instances of discriminatory or insensitive treatment are particularly burdensome for rural minorities, for whom few alternative sources of health care are available.

V. NEW APPROACHES TO RURAL HEALTH CARE: THE SOUTHERN EXPERIENCE

While the obstacles to improved health care for rural Americans are substantial, they are not overwhelming. Too frequently, pessimism pervades discussions of rural health care. Attitudes such as "No one wants to live there" and "Everything that's been tried has failed" preclude serious consideration of what will work to bring better health care to rural people.

These attitudes give rise to fatalism or to proposals to force all health professionals to take a tour of duty in rural areas, regardless of their interest in or suitability for such positions. Before endorsing either of these extreme positions, it seems fruitful to consider what is currently being tried in rural areas, learn which approaches have succeeded, and gain a better appreciation for the genuine obstacles to systematic improvements in rural health care.

The absence of strong rural media and communications networks makes such a summarization of rural experience particularly important. Success in one area often goes unnoticed or unheralded outside a narrow confine. Strategies which are successfully employed to overcome obstacles could be fruitfully applied by other groups in similar positions—if knowledge about these experiences were more broadly available.

Among new approaches to health care in the rural South which seem particularly promising are: (1) the development of new organizational structures designed to impart greater stability and continuity to the provision of primary health care; (2) comprehensive health centers providing a wide range of health and health-related services; (3) nurse practitioner or physician assistant primary care centers; (4) new types of group medical practices and team approaches; (5) changes in health professional education including area health education center programs, communication systems linking rural physicians with medical centers, emphasis upon preparation of students for rural practice, new roles for nonphysician health personnel, and family practice residency programs.

A. Sponsorship of Rural Primary Care Centers

One major difficulty with traditional medical practice in rural areas is the instability introduced by the loss of a physician. While turnover of health professionals may have no noticeable impact in a large, urban area, rural communities are much more vulnerable to movements of physicians, nurses, or other health professionals. Several approaches in providing continuity and stability to rural practice are being tried in the South. These approaches include the creation of a community-organized and controlled nonprofit corporation which takes the responsibility for attracting health professionals and maintaining a stable health-care center. Other approaches use the resources of health providers in nearby larger communities to sponsor extension of primary-care centers in rural communities.

A surprising diversity of organizational structures is being demonstrated. These may be broadly characterized as falling into one or two types: community or consumer sponsorship and provider sponsorship. But within each of these broad types is a wide range of possible alternatives:

Community or Consumer Sponsorship:
- Projects with an elected consumer board which takes a strong active role in policy setting.
- Projects with a community board composed of leading members of the community (local power structure—banker, head of school board, county commissioner, etc.)

- Projects which are sponsored by consumer organizations formed for other purposes (e.g., Federation of Southern Cooperatives, Welfare Rights Organizations, community development corporations).
- Projects sponsored by church groups.

Provider Sponsorship:
- Projects sponsored by medical schools.
- State or county health department sponsorship.
- Projects sponsored by area community hospitals.
- Projects sponsored by physicians or area medical practices.

Community or consumer sponsorship of rural health projects appears to have many advantages. Unlike urban areas which can recruit health professionals to expand existing practices, most rural communities have no health base on which to build. Formation of a nonprofit community corporation which takes responsibility for recruitment of health professionals and obtaining essential developmental financial support is one means of providing a stable, ongoing organization in rural areas. Thus, even if some turnover of health professionals occurs, patients have a permanent place equipped with their medical records to turn to for medical care.

Community people take a keen interest and deep pride in upgrading the quality of life in their community; their different efforts on behalf of a health project are important resources which can be tapped through this approach. This dedication often has financial payoff for evolving health centers—either through local fund-raising or through donations of labor and materials. All health centers funded by the State of North Carolina are required to raise $1 locally for every $5 contributed by the state for renovation or construction of a health facility. Methods used by community health projects there and in other states include: cookbook sales, barbecues, bluegrass jamborees, walk-a-thons, used-clothing sales, etc. One industrious restort community solicited contributions from summer tourists, and far exceeded its original fund-raising drive.

Community sponsorship has other important spinoff benefits. In some communities where feelings of helplessness and hopelessness have led to serious mental health problems, a successful community effort to sponsor a health project, raise developmental funds, and recruit health professionals has important impacts on the mental health of the community. Leaders of the project become recognized as "doers" and the community begins to feel that it can affect the quality of community life. Citizens who have learned to obtain local revenue-sharing funds from county commissioners for a health project begin to feel that other essential public improvements are also possible—from paving a road to improving local water supplies and sewage disposal. Citizens who have learned to unravel the secrets of Federal grantsmanship to obtain funding for a health project become sophisticated in seeking support for improved housing. The Lee County Cooperative Clinic was the major force behind the receipt of a $2 million water and sewage demonstration project for eastern Arkansas. Since health is an uncontroversial issue in most rural communities, it is an issue around which community citizens can unite and then act as a lever for change and community economic development generally.

Different types of community sponsorship appear to work well in different situations. In communities where needs of minorities or poor people have been neglected and improvement in their position opposed by local forces, an indigenous, patient-elected board has been extremely successful in acting as a lever for the improved economic and social position of these groups. These health projects in some cases contributed to the development of political leaders championing the cause of the poor and minorities. In other communities where poverty and racial discrimination are not factors, a community board made up of the local power structure—bankers, lawyers, and politically powerful figures—has been of assistance in obtaining requisite legal advice, financial assistance, and local and state governmental support. Whether such a constituted board membership is desirable or not depends largely on whether it identifies with and shares the goals of the health proejct.

A very different approach to sponsorship of a health project is sponsorship by area medical schools or by existing health facilities or personnel such as community hospitals, state or county health departments, or physicians in larger communities. Sponsorship by these provider groups usually brings more sophisticated management and professional expertise to the project. Hospitals and physicians are already adept at dealing with third-party reimbursement organizations. They are familiar with state laws affecting health delivery. They have sources which can be tapped to recruit health professionals to work for the project, on either a part-time or full-time basis.

Medical school sponsorship is one way of obtaining physician staff in towns that couldn't attract their own physicians. Faculty involvement in a rural health delivery project can provide at least part-time medical input. Students are exposed to rural practice through medical school involvement, and may have a greater inclination to pursue rural practice as a result of this experience. Participating in a rural health project may also induce some changes in the medical school making it more responsive to rural health needs—either through changes in its admissions policies or in its curriculum.

Provider sponsorship, however, can have quite negative effects. In one project which was site-visited, the medical school had withdrawn its support of a rural health project when it experienced a change of deans— leaving the community which had contributed heavily to the construction of a health facility to its own resources. In other cases medical school support of rural health delivery projects seems rather closely related to political forces, such as membership on the state medical school appropriations committee. Changes in these forces may alter the medical school's interest in, and continued support of, a particular rural health project.

Combining teaching with delivery of health services can also have disadvantages. Many aspects of teaching interfere with delivery; patients may complain of the time it takes to be seen first by a student and then seen again by physician staff. Patients tend to be deeply dissatisfied with turnover of health professional staff—which frequently occurs as interns and residents are rotated through a medical school sponsored project. Part-time involvement of university faculty located in a more distant medical center is not as acceptable to rural communities as someone who can be more closely identified as "their doctor." In many communities, a nurse practitioner living in that community is a more readily accepted source of care than an outsider physician.

Provider-sponsored health projects are more likely to take a narrower medical approach than community-sponsored projects. To the extent that rural health problems are closely related to nonmedical factors—such as water quality, sewage disposal, diet, housing, or occupational hazards—a narrow, medical approach may be largely ineffective in combating the basic causes of poor health.

B. Alternative Models of Rural Health Delivery

Considerable diversity also exists among innovative approaches to primary health care in the range of services provided and the mix of health professionals used to provide services. Three major types, however, seem to encompass the project sites visited: (1) comprehensive health centers (those that do more than provide medical care); (2) health centers staffed primarily by nurse practitioners or physician assistants; and (3) group practices consisting of two or more primary-care physicians or a team of health professionals including physicians and nonphysician health professionals.

1. Comprehensive Health Centers

Most comprehensive health centers receive some public support through federal or state programs. The three major sources of funding are the OEO-HEW community health centers, several Appalachian Regional Commission projects, and comprehensive children and youth projects funded under Title V of the Social Security Act. The field workers visited a number of examples of this approach to health care including: the Lee County Cooperative Clinic in Marianna, Arkansas; the Mountain Comprehensive Health Center in Hazard, Kentucky; the Beaufort-Jasper Community Health Center in Ridgeland, South Carolina; the Prospect Hill Center in Prospect Hill, North Carolina; the Delta Community Hospital and Health Center in Mound Bayou, Mississippi; the Jackson-Hinds Comprehensive Health Center in Utica and Jackson, Mississippi; the Central Virginia Community Health Center in New Canton, Virginia; Appalachian Regional Commission health projects in Evarts, Kentucky; Clairfield, Tennessee; Hot Springs, North Carolina; Farmington, North Carolina, and Briceville, Tennessee; and children and youth projects in Vicksburg, Mississippi, and Charlottesville, Virginia.

Common to all of these projects is concern with the causes of poor health, and an approach to health care that extends well beyond medical care alone. The OEO-HEW community health centers take the broadest approach including medical care, dental care, prescription drugs, mental health, outreach services, transportation services, environmental health services, home health services, nutrition programs, and child development programs. The Appalachian Regional Commission (ARC) projects tend to provide only some of these nonmedical support services; furthermore. ARC funding is required by law to terminate after five years so that projects are required to become self-supporting within that period.

Few sophisticated studies have been done evaluating the impact on health of these wide-ranging approaches. However, it is apparent in talking with health professionals and summarizing the available evidence that in many projects the nonmedical support services have been extremely effective. These projects, in contrast with smaller, narrower medical projects, respond to the types of health problems which are particularly severe in rural areas—such as dental, mental health, problems of the homebound elderly, preventive services, nutrition, and environmental services.

Not surprisingly, however, this approach to health care is also more expensive. Costs per encounter in many projects average $35 to $40—compared with $15 to $20 in more traditional medical projects. However, even in the comprehensive health centers the medical cost alone is roughly $20 per visit—competitive with other types of providers.

Financing has been a major problem for most comprehensive health centers. Appalachian Regional Commission funding ceases after five years, leaving many projects which have tried to provide fairly comprehensive services with huge deficits to meet on their own once funding ends. Cutbacks on services and staff at the end of funding cause great trials for the projects; and many go under at that point. The OEO-HEW community health centers do not automatically experience such a termination of funding, but cutbacks in this program pushed by the Administration in recent years have caused severe financial problems for many centers. Funding under the program is on a one-year basis, making it difficult for the projects, without certainty of long-run financial position, to recruit physicians and other health professionals.

Most of the comprehensive projects have found it difficult to obtain adequate reimbursement for patients covered under public programs. In some projects, Medicaid reimbursement is about $4 to $6 per visit—even though the costs considerably exceed that level. The Jackson-Hinds health center conducted a study and found that its costs of caring for Medicaid patients was well below the average spent by the state for those services to Medicaid patients—but it was unsuccessful in negotiating with the state for reimbursement at the average level paid by the state.

2. Nurse Practitioner Health Centers

Another major approach to primary health care in the rural South that is being tried extensively is rural health centers staffed with nonphysician health professionals, such as nurse practitioners, physician assistants, and nurse midwives. These heath centers take a variety of forms. Some are fixed facilities, while others use mobile vans to rotate through small communities on a scheduled basis. Some are free-standing health centers, others are satellites of a group practice in a larger town. Some health centers have affiliated with other health centers to share physician and administrative services. Nearly all arrange for some part-time physician services at the center—from area physicians, medical school faculty, National Health Service Corps physicians, or their own staff.

Health projects of this type site visited by the field workers include: the North Carolina state-funded rural health centers, the Georgia Health Access Stations, the East Tennessee mountain clinics in Briceville, Norma, and Clairfield; the Frontier Nursing Servie in southeastern Kentucky; the Tennessee state health department primary care clinics; and some of the Appalachian Regional Commission projects.

These health centers have been remarkably successful in getting professional staff. Those associated with training programs such as the North Carolina rural health centers or the Frontier Nursing Service have been particularly successful in recruiting staff. Of nurse practitioners trained at the University of North Carolina only seven out of 90 have failed to return to the rural area which they agreed to serve at the beginning of their graduate training. Recruiting registered nurses from rural areas who have ties there—family, husbands employed in farming or other industries, etc.—and training them near their homes provides a reliable, qualified source of health professionals capable of providing a wide range of health services to rural communities.

Nurse practitioner health centers are fairly low-cost operations. In contrast to the comprehensive health centers whose budgets may run from $500,000 to $4 million annually, rural health centers staffed by one or two nurse practitioners and part-time physicians have average annual budgets on the order of $60,000 to $80,000. These centers, however, provide far more limited services—typically excluding dental health, mental health services, prescription drugs, and nonmedical support services. The low cost of the centers, however, means that many rural communities which are too small or too poor to support a more expensive approach to health care can have access to primary care health services through this type of health center. Enhanced access to preventive services, proper monitoring of chronic conditions, and basic acute illness care are all important benefits which can be achieved by promoting the development of health centers which tap the resources of this type of health professional. Since nurses bring to their training as nurse practitioners a background emphasizing patient education and counseling, they are particularly well qualified to overcome some traditional barriers to health improvement.

The field work uncovered a wide range of settings in which nurse practitioners provide services. In North Carolina, the state has carefully thought through the implications of this model of health-care delivery and has taken a number of steps to insure the quality of care provided. The Nurse Practice and Medical Practice Acts were amended to outline conditions under which nurse practitioners could provide treatment—including provisions for adequate training (at least one additional year for an experienced registered nurse), provisions for physician backup (a physician must agree to sponsor the nurse practitioner and be available by telephone at any time she/he is seeing patients), and provisions for monitoring of nurse practitioner performance (written protocols must be in place and followed; all decisions requiring medical judgment must be countersigned by the sponsoring physician within a specified time period). In other instances, registered nurses without additional training are providing primary medical care services to patients with only limited physician involvement and monitoring.

Physician involvement in a manner similar to that required in North Carolina would seem desirable to ensure quality care. This does not imply that the nurse practitioners "work for" physicians. In North Carolina, the nurse practitioners are employed by rural health centers (controlled by nonprofit corporations with community boards) and physician services are obtianed by the health officer on a contractual basis. Thus, nurse practitioners as well as physicians "work for" the health center as a health professional team.

This approach to health care, while possessing substantial advantages for many communities, does have several potential drawbacks. One major difficulty is that major third-party insurance programs are quite restrictive about paying for services rendered by nurse practitioners when a physician is absent when services are rendered. Medicare does not pay for services under these conditions. Some states will cover the services under the Medicaid program, but even in those states covering the services, payments are frequently made directly to the sponsoring physician rather than to the health center—necessitating a negotiated agreement between the health center and the physician which often favors the physician. The Medicare program is currently engaged in a study considering possible liberalization of reimbursement policies, but opposition from organized medicine or other pressures to contain costs may make it difficult to achieve adequate compensation for these services.

Other difficulties are more long-range, and it will take time to see whether they actually occur. Rural health centers staffed by a single nurse practitioner eventually may face many of the difficulties currently confronting solo physicians. In some health centers, nurse practitioners have left because the demands on their time after regular office hours have been too heavy. In other centers, nurse practitioners have refused to take after-hours calls, and refer all requests to the sponsoring physicians. Other nurse practitioners have found it desirable to live outside the community in which they practice and commute to work—which spares them part of the demands on their time arising after hours. Isolated nurse practitioenrs also complain that they are not receiving the opportunities for continued professional development that they would like to have. These problems of heavy work loads and professional isolation are reduced considerably in projects which have employed two or more nurse practitioners and have established relationships with physicians for adequate support services and with medical and nursing schools for continued education.

3. Group Medical Practices

Another approach to rural health care which appears to be successfully working in a number of rural communities in the South is development of group medical practices. Again, this approach encompasses a number of varieties. Some groups, such as the Morehead Clinic in Kentucky, are organized on a for-profit basis with a board composed of the principal physicians in the group. It departs from traditional group medical practices, however, in that it is headed by a very capable administrator, makes heavy use of nurse practitioners, physician assistants, and nurse midwives, and is sponsoring a network of satellite clinics in smaller communities 20 to 30 minutes from the major facility.

Another type of group practice is one currently being tried in Hindman, Kentucky—the East Kentucky Health Services Center. This group practice has five primary-care physicians assisted by mid-level health practitioners working in a team with the physicians. The center is a nonprofit corporation with a board composed of leading members of the local community. It also emphasizes good management, and has become self-supporting within a three-year period after considerable start-up support from private foundations. Organized on a nonprofit basis, it plans to use surpluses to provide nonpaying health services, such as health screening and environmental health services.

Another type of group practice is represented by a new U.S. Department of Health, Education, and Welfare initiative called "integrated rural health demonstration grants." This program supports health centers staffed primarily by National Health Service Corps physicians and other health professionals who are Federal employees. The program, however, tries to emphasize a systems approach to health care establishing necessary relationships with county health departments, area medical schools, and specialized support services.

Other group practices provide the variation of promoting pre-payment or capitation methods of compensation. Among those site-visited are the health maintenance organization developed in Harlan, Kentucky—the Mountain Trails Health Plan—and family health centers funded by the U.S. Department of Health, Education, and Welfare including the Madison-Yazoo-Leake Family Health Center in Mississippi and the Triangle Health Plan in Apex, North Carolina. Family health centers are characterized as "moving toward" the health maintenance organization form and are required to have some portion of patients enrolled on a capitation reimbursement basis.

While considerable variety among group medical practices exists, their central common characteristic is that they emphasize medical services provided by a group of primary-care physicians. Their main emphases are finding characteristics of rural practice which will appeal to physicians and inducing them to locate in rural communities.

From the experience in the rural South to date, it would appear that this approach to health care is extremely attractive to physicians. Group practices can overcome most of the professional objections to rural practices including the long hours, heavy demands, and professional isolation. This approach provides opportunities for time off to pursue continuing education activities. Physicians in the group and their families frequently form their own social unit—thus overcoming some of the social and cultural isolation as well.

Emphasis upon good management provided by nonphysician-trained administrators also appears to be a major strength of this approach. In some projects visited, physicians were at first reluctant to add administrators for fear that this would reduce physician incomes. After trying this approach, however, physicians have become convinced that administrators add more to the practice than they cost—and that physician incomes have risen rather than having been spread more thinly through acquisition of a skilled administrator. Removal of the paperwork burden and duties of collecting patient revenues have also made physicians generally more satisfied with rural practice. Furthermore, efficient management of the practices has made them financially viable, even in fairly low income areas.

There are several potential disadvantages, however, with some types of group medical practice. These include exclusive emphasis upon profit-making medical problems to the neglect of less profitable environmental or other factors causing poor health. Another danger is that emphasis upon economic self-sufficiency will make the practice less sensitive to the needs of poor people, so that only a portion of the community benefits from the practice. More evidence on the experience of this approach should be obtained, and alternative variations of the group medical practice approach watched to see how some of these potential disadvantages can be minimized.

C. Health Professional Education

As noted earlier, a long-run trend in the prevailing medical system in the United States has been toward specialization, which causes the training of physicians to be biased against rural practice. Moreover, the values of the prevailing system have been such that students who were inclined to rural practice when they entered medical school became socialized by the prevailing system, inclining them toward urban medical systems. As a consequence, many physicians trained in modern medical schools are unable to practice rural medicine. In order to deal with this problem, traditional medical training must be changed or special rural training programs must be adopted.

There have been in recent years, however, several encouraging trends in medical education and training of nonphysician professionals. These include: (1) development of area health education centers (AHEC) programs; (2) communication systems linking rural physicians with medical centers; (3) new roles for nonphysician health personnel; and (4) emphasis upon preparation of medical students for primary care and rural practice.

1. Area Health Education Centers

One interesting innovation is the decentralization of medical education through area health education centers. The North Carolina Area Health Education Center program has established nine regional training centers throughout the state. Medical, dental, and other health professional students rotate through these regional centers, as a part of their training. Internship and primary-care residency positions are also available at the regional centers. Faculty support at the training centers is composed of local qualified rural practitioners and university faculty, some of whom are flown to the regional centers on a daily basis by a fleet of five airplanes maintained by the program. Such programs contribute to the professional development of rural physicians, acquaint medical and other health professional students with rural practice, and better prepare health professionals for the skills needed in rural areas.

2. Communication Systems

The University of Alabama at Birmingham has developed a relatively inexpensive telephone system to connect family physicians to specialists at the Medical School. Rural physicians throughout Alabama have used this system extensively to obtain consultations from specialists in the diagnosis and treatment of conditions encountered in rural practice with which the practicing physician was uncertain as to how to proceed.. In some cases, physicians place calls to specialists and obtain advice during the patient hours; at other times physicians consult, following patient visits, to assure themselves of appropriate continuing monitoring and therapeutic treatment of conditions.

3. Nurse Practitioners and Physician Assistants

One type of health professional which has successfully recruited and retained in rural areas is the nonphysician health professional. The University of North Carolina family nurse practitioner training program, with one-year additional training for experienced registered nurses available in regional centers, has been a reliable source of qualified health professionals for rural practice in that state. The Frontier Nursing Service Graduate School of Family Nursing and Nurse Midwifery continues to be one of the pioneering efforts in preparing qualified health professionals for rural practice. The University of Mississippi Nurse Midwifery program is another example.

Physician assistants have also been a source of health personnel in rural areas. A recent survey by the American Academy of Physician's Assistants shows that many of these professionals are selecting rural practice (see Table 23).

4. Family Practice Residencies

An encouraging trend in medical education, at least for those interested in rural health, has been the growth in the number of family practitioners since the mid-1960s when a number of investigations concluded that the traditional medical education system was not meeting the need for primary health care. A number of family practice residency programs were started in the 1960s as a result of special Federal support for such programs. The number of family practice (FP) programs increased from 30 in 1969 to 260 in 1975 and has reached some 340 in 1976. The number of residents in these FP programs increased from 290 in 1970 to 3,720 in 1975. Family practitioners are more broadly trained than specialists and many are likely to receive a good bit of their medical education away from medical schools in clinical situations. Indeed, in 1975 about 60 percent of the family practitioner residency training programs were away from teaching hospitals.

Family practice training differs from specialty training in emphasizing the synthesis of knowledge and skills from all areas of medicine to deal with whatever problem the patient has. In other words, the patient's problem rather than the doctor's training determines the treatment. Family practice training also emphasizes using all available data about patients and their families in the treatment. Although some medical educators in teaching hospitals are concerned about the quality of family practice training programs, most of these programs seem to be of high quality and serve a real need.

That the training of family practitioners is helping meet the need for rural health professionals is indicated by Tables 24 and 25. Table 24 shows that family practice graduates are concentrating in smaller communities and a majority are going into family group practices. Indeed, in 1973, about 25 percent of the population was in nonmetropolitan counties but they received 35 percent of the family practice residency graduates surveyed.

While this trend in family-practice training has been relatively rapid and is helping meet the need for rural physicians, these trends must be viewed in perspective. The graduates of all family-practice residency programs during the years 1970 to 1975 was 1,332. If we assume that 35 percent of these went into nonmetropolitan areas, the physician input from this source was about 466. The family practice residency programs are therefore only a small-scale source of rural physicians. The programs are also drawing medical students away from other primary-care fields rather than from narrow specialities.

VI. RECOMMENDATIONS

While many new rural health initiatives are in a pilot, experimental stage, it is apparent that some activities afford considerable promise. Recommended future directions for health policy to improve rural health include:

A. Changing the Training of Health Professionals

(1) Greater emphasis on training physicians and other health professionals specifically for rural practice.

(2) Special programs should be established to acquaint medical students with the realities of rural health problems and medical practice. The Vanderbilt Student Health Coalition and the Appalachian Leaders for Community Outreach (ALCOR) have provided useful experiences which

should be replicated in other places. These programs not only familiarized medical students with rural problems, but probably also had some impact on the attitudes of their respective medical schools toward training professionals for rural practice. Many of the students associated with ALCOR went into rural practice in Appalachia, mainly as a result of this experience.

(3) States should support the establishment of Area Health Education Centers and family practice residencies in rural areas of the state.

(4) Greater support should be given to the development of broadly trained nonphysician health professionals. Specialized training of new health professionals, such as pediatric nurse practitioners, geriatric nurse practitioners, child health associates, and so forth should be deemphasized as these types of health professionals can only be optimally employed in larger group or institutional settings found primarily in urban areas. Family nurse practitioner training programs should be widely available in rural areas, so that registered nurses from rural areas can receive additional training without relocating. In rural areas with shortages of locally trained registered nurses, additional training programs at the undergraduate level should be encouraged.

(5) Admission and scholarship procedures of medical, dental, and nursing schools should be reviewed to ensure that students desiring rural practice are sought and that such students are familiar with sources of financial support for education.

B. Changing the Nature of Rural Practice

While more experience is required to know with certainty those changes in rural practice which will be most successful in attracting qualified health professionals and in improving rural health, the following components of a rural health system are recommended:

(6) Emphasis on group practice where needed to prevent professional isolation and overwork of professionals. Groups of health professionals also frequently form their social unit, thus removing some of the social and cultural isolation of families of health professionals.

(7) Emphasis on nurse practitioner clinics with backup part-time physician support for smaller communities which cannot support or attract groups of physicians. Such clinics should be sponsored by stable, ongoing groups. The best experiences to date are with sponsorship by community organized nonprofit corporations and by group physician practices in nearby larger towns. Other possible sponsors which may be effective in some situations include churches, community development corporations, medical schools, community hospitals in nearby larger towns, and county or state health departments. Developmental funds and technical assis-

tance for such clinics should be provided through newly created Federal and /or state programs. Some provision for ongoing operating expense subsidies in low-income rural areas should also be made.

(8) Legal support and technical assistance should be given to promote the effective use of nonphysician health professionals. State Nurse Practice Acts and Medical Practice Acts should be amended similar to those of North Carolina to permit nurse practitioners with appropriate training to treat patients and write prescriptions subject to requirements on physician backup and supervision, written protocols, continuous auditing of nurse practitioner performance, and continuing education. Such nurse practitioners should be permitted to see patients without the physical presence of a physician, if the backup physician is available by telephone for consultation and such physician participates in a continuous auditing of nurse practitioner performance.

(9) Programs should be adopted to help meet the start-up costs of establishing rural group practices, if these practices meet certain conditions required for effective rural health-care delivery.

(10) Ideally, rural health care should be part of a system which (a) extends care into remote areas either through outposts or the use of mobile facilities, and (b) relates the particular practice to hospitals, laboratories, and other specialists in rural or urban areas.

(11) Provisions should be made for the continuing education of the health professionals involved in rural practice. This could be done by planning for periodic attendance at conferences, short courses, seminars held within the area, or interaction with members of the faculty on medical school staffs.

(12) Because health training is very expensive, medical professionals receive very little training in management, and it would not, in any event, be economical for health professionals to spend much time on management and administrative matters. Special attention, therefore, should be given to management systems. As a number of such systems are available, they should be studied very carefully to develop a model of particular practices. Moreover, a skilled administrator should be made an integral part of every rural health practice.

3. Changing the Content of Rural Health Care

(13) Rural health practices should be concerned with environmental health and preventive medicine. Because of the conflict within practices between their primary concern for providing medical care and attention to environmental health problems and community affairs, it is not at all clear that private medical professionals can or will provide the leadership for environmental health and preventive medicine. The following considerations flow from our study of this issue:

(a) Establishing nonprofit corporations with community representation on boards of directors could cause medical practices to be concerned with environmental health problems.

(b) Community outreach programs and transportation facilities improve the access of rural people to medical care, but these services increase the cost of providing health care. Since it is desirable to provide environmental and preventive health services as well as services facilitating access to health care, these costs should be borne by the public. Expenditures for environmental and preventive health make the immediate costs of medical care seem higher than would be the case if only traditional medical care were provided, but these expenditures probably are very cost-effective in the long run.

(14) An essential component of a model rural health program is comprehensive primary ambulatory care. Special attention should be given to meeting the dental-care needs of rural people. In many ways, dental care is relatively worse in rural areas than medical care. Mental health also appears to be a significant problem in many rural areas. Services of qualified mental health professionals should be a key part of rural health delivery.

(15) Rural areas have a much higher proportion of elderly people, and the incidence of chronic conditions and confinement to bed is much greater in the rural South than in other areas. Emphasis upon home health services which provide qualified nursing care to housebound elderly is important in the rural South.

(16) Attention to nutritional needs of rural Southerners should also be a part of the health system. Participation in Federal nutrition programs and nutritional counseling should be encouraged.

(17) Because of low educational levels, many rural residents are unfamiliar with good health habits. Effective patient health education, supplemented with visual aids where appropriate, should be a part of rural health care.

(18) Since preventive care has been long neglected in rural areas, special emphasis should be given to well-baby care, immunizations, contraceptive information, cancer screening, and prenatal services.

D. Minorities and Rural Health Care

Affirmative action programs in health training programs and Federal health programs are weak. Few minority women have been trained in the nurse practitioner training programs. The National Health Service Corps has few minority health professionals in its program. Since attitudes toward accomplishment are an important element in mental health, it is particularly important that role models be provided to rural minorities to demonstrate what can be achieved.

While these findings are tentative and not systematic, the evidence available suggests that several additional steps should be taken to improve health care for rural minorities. These include:

(19) A systematic study of discriminatory or insensitive practices in the provision of health care in rural areas, the training of health professionals for rural areas, and the administration of Federal, state, and local health-care programs should be conducted to determine the extent, severity, and form of discriminatory practices.

(20) Local medical societies should not be permitted to veto Federal or state rural health projects. The Black Belt Community Health Center sponsored by the Federation of Southern Cooperatives in Epes, Alabama, has been unable to receive Federal funding because of local medical opposition.

(21) The National Health Service Corps should conduct a vigorous affirmative action program in the provision of scholarships for medical training and in the placement of health professionals in rural areas in order to increase the supply of qualified Spanish-speaking and black health professionals.

(22) The Medicare program should enforce nondiscriminatory practices in the provision of hospital care, nursing home care, private physician care, and other covered services. Currently, the Medicare program does not require physicians to be in compliance with Title VI of the Civil Rights Act to receive Medicare funds.

(23) Programs should be undertaken to increase the sensitivity of health professionals dealing with minority groups. Community aides and outreach workers may be particularly important complements of medical services in areas where language or cultural barriers exist between patients and health professionals. More information should be obtained on services and advice given by *curanderos* and other sources of folk medicine. Detrimental health practices should be discouraged, but legitimate counseling services building upon intimate knowledge of cultural traditions should be encouraged.

E. Changing the Financing of Rural Health Care

Current Federal and Federal/state health programs have proved to be of limited assistance to rural Southerners. Changes in existing programs and implementation of new ones designed with rural areas in mind are required to correct the imbalance in present policies:

(24) Implementation of national health insurance would greatly benefit

rural residents who are not now well covered by private health insurance and public programs. Specific features which would help insure that rural residents receive a fair share of benefits include:

(a) Establishment of fee schedules for physicians that reward rather than penalize physicians for practicing in underserved areas.

(b) Reimbursement for services of nonphysician health professionals at rural health centers whether a physician is physically present or not when service is rendered.

(c) Recognition of community-sponsored rural health centers meeting specified standards as providers of health services eligible for direct reimbursement.

(d) Coverage of all people regardless of family composition, eligibility for welfare, employment status, or other conditions. Minimal or nonexistent direct patient charges for low-income persons.

(e) Creation of health resources development board with sufficient funds targeted on personnel who desire to locate in rural communities and on the development of innovative approaches to health-care delivery in rural areas.

(f) Supplementary programs should be developed to overcome specific barriers to improved health in rural areas—such as transportation services, outreach services, environmental health services, home health services, patient education services, and nutritional services.

(25) If existing financing programs are not soon replaced by national health insurance, amendments to current programs would provide some much needed relief to rural residents. Changes include:

(a) Amend the Medicare and Medicaid programs to provide for reimbursement of nurse practitioner services whether or not a physician is physically present at the time service is provided.

(b) Designate rural health centers as participating providers under Medicare and Medicaid with a separate reimbursement policy based on average expenditures of Medicaid recipients and Medicare enrollees in the state.

(c) Amend the Medicare and Medicaid programs to provide for reimbursement of rural physicians on the same basis as urban physicians within the state. Explore moving toward a uniform physician reimbursement fee schedule under Medicare for the nation.

(d) Revise the Medicaid program to include low-income two-parent families regardless of welfare or employment status. Require all states to cover rural health center services and the medically needy.

(26) Comprehensive health centers currently funded by the U.S. Department of Health, Education, and Welfare should be maintained. The Medicare and Medicaid programs should be amended to permit comprehensive health centers to receive capitation payments from these programs based upon average expenditure levels for all persons covered by Medicare and Medicaid in the state. Attempts should be made to upgrade the environmental health, home health, patient education, dental health, mental health, and nutrition activities of existing centers. Administrators should have opportunities to visit other centers which make effective use of these support services. Better technical assistance from the federal and regional offices of the U.S. Department of Health, Education, and Welfare should be provided to existing centers. Evaluation studies regarding the payoff of different types of support services for different populations should be conducted. Consideration should be given to establishing additional comprehensive health centers in rural areas with particularly severe health problems.

(27) The National Health Service Corps should continue to experiment with a greater variety of approaches to rural health including more emphasis on nurse practitioner clinics, group practices, greater role for community residents in the management of practices, and better technical assistance to Corps practices. The Integrated Rural Health Demonstration grant program sponsoring the Corps, the comprehensive health center program, the migrant health project, and the Appalachian Regional Commission, is an approach promoting the development of county-wide or multicounty systems of health care in underserved areas. The experience of this program should be carefully monitored for possibly broader application to rural areas.

FOOTNOTES

1. This paper is based on the Rural Health Project of the Task Force on Southern Rural Development, of which the authors are codirectors. The project was funded by the Robert Wood Johnson Foundation. The views expressed in this paper are those of the authors and not necessarily those of the Robert Wood Johnson Foundation, the Task Force on Southern Rural Development, the Brookings Institution or the University of Texas.

*Karen Davis is currently Deputy Assistant Secretary for Planning (Health), Department of Health, Education, and Welfare.

**Ray Marshall is currently Secretary of Labor.

Table 1. Infant Mortality Rate and General Mortality Rate by Race, U.S.
and South, 1971. (Deaths per 1,000 Live Births and Deaths
per 1,000 population.)

	Infant Mortality Rate [a]			General Mortality Rate		
	Total	White	Black	Total	White	Black
United States	19.0	16.6	32.5	9.3	9.4	9.2
South (13 states)	21.4	18.2	31.1	9.4	9.1	10.6
Nonmetropolitan	23.3	20.1	33.1	10.4	10.3	11.2
Smaller areas[b]	24.2	21.3	34.0	11.3	11.4	11.3
Larger areas[b]	22.9	19.5	32.5	9.8	9.6	11.1
Metropolitan	19.8	16.7	29.3	8.5	8.2	10.1

Source: Calculated from data published in Southern Regional Council, *Health Care in the South: A Statistical Profile,* June 1974. United States totals from: U.S. Department of Health, Education, and Welfare, National Center for Health Statistics, "Final Mortality Statistics, 1973, Summary Report."

[a] Excludes counties with no infant deaths. State totals, therefore, differ slightly from published figures.

[b] Smaller areas include all nonmetropolitan counties with population under 25,000. Larger areas include all nonmetropolitan counties with population of 25,000 or more.

Table 2. Infant Mortality Rates in the South by Residence and Race,
by Percent of the Population Below the Poverty Level in County, 1971[a]
(Deaths per 1,000 Live Births)

	Total	:	Percent population below poverty level			
			Under : 15.0	15.0- : 24.9	25.0- : 34.9	35.0 : and over
Infant mortality rate —all races						
South (13 states)	21.4		19.0	21.1	23.2	26.4
Nonmetropolitan	23.3		19.8	22.1	23.3	27.2
Smaller areas[b]	24.2		18.9	22.7	22.7	27.5
Larger areas[b]	22.8		20.0	21.8	23.7	26.8
Metropolitan	19.8		18.8	20.4	22.9	20.9
White infant mortality rate						
South (13 states)	18.2		16.5	18.7	19.2	20.9
Nonmetropolitan	20.1		18.5	20.4	19.7	21.1
Smaller areas	21.3		18.8	21.3	20.7	22.6
Larger areas	19.4		18.4	20.1	18.9	19.0
Metropolitan	16.7		16.1	17.3	15.8	20.1
Black infant mortality rate						
South (13 states)	31.1		29.7	29.3	33.3	34.1
Nonmetropolitan	33.1		30.9	30.5	34.0	34.2
Smaller areas	34.0		51.1	29.0	34.2	35.2
Larger areas	32.5		30.2	31.0	33.9	33.0
Metropolitan	29.3		29.6	28.7	31.2	31.4

Source: Calculated from data published in Southern Regional Council, *Health Care in the South: A Statistical Profile,* June 1974.

[a] Excludes counties with no infant deaths.

[b] Smaller areas includes all nonmetropolitan counties with population under 25,000. Larger areas include all nonmetropolitan counties with population of 25,000 or more.

Table 3. General Mortality Rates in the South by Residence, by Race, by Percent Population Below the Poverty Level in County, 1971 (Deaths per 1,000 People, Not Adjusted for Age Composition)

All persons	:	Under 15.0 :	15.0-24.9 :	25.0-34.9 :	35.0 and over
		Percent population below poverty level			
		Total mortality rate – all persons			
South total – 13 states	9.4	8.4	9.3	10.8	10.9
Nonmetropolitan	10.4	8.7	10.0	10.9	11.2
Smaller areas*	11.3	9.4	11.0	11.6	11.6
Larger areas*	9.8	8.6	9.7	10.4	10.5
Metropolitan	8.5	8.3	8.7	10.3	7.8
		White general mortality rate			
South total	9.1	8.2	8.9	10.9	10.7
Nonmetropolitan	10.3	8.6	9.9	11.0	11.1
Smaller areas	11.4	9.4	11.1	11.7	11.7
Larger areas	9.6	8.5	9.4	10.3	10.0
Metropolitan	8.2	8.2	8.1	10.0	7.6
		Black general mortality rate			
South total	10.6	9.2	10.8	11.2	11.2
Nonmetropolitan	11.	9.8	11.0	11.3	11.3
Smaller areas	11.3	10.1	11.0	11.2	11.4
Larger areas	11.1	9.8	10.9	11.4	11.2
Metropolitan	10.1	9.1	10.7	10.9	9.1

*Smaller areas include all nonmetropolitan counties with population under 25,000. Larger areas include all nonmetropolitan counties with population of 25,000 or more.

Table 4. Characteristics of Women Admitted to Maternal and Infant Care Projects and Infant and Maternal Mortality and Low Birth Weight, by Regions, United States, First Half of 1970[a]

Characteristics	United States	North-east	North Central	South	West
Live births (Rates per 1,000 live births)	40,583	7,775	10,923	18,605	3,280
Neonatal death rate	15.4	13.5	10.0	18.2	22.3
Birth weight under 2,500 grams	133	91	132	143	104
Maternal deaths (number)	17	2	3	12	0
Women admitted	56,748	12,441	15,080	24,449	4,778
Percent unmarried	49	47	55	47	41
Percent under age 16	6	6	7	6	4
Percent age 35 and over	4	5	5	3	3
Percent black	68	56	77	76	25
Percent initiating care after:					
first trimester	84	79	84	87	76
second trimester	36	19	38	45	31

Source: U.S. Department of Health, Education, and Welfare, Maternal and Child Health Service, "Statistical Summary of Patients Served Under Maternity and Infant Care Projects," processed 1970.

[a] Based on 50 projects reporting data.

Table 5. Age-Adjusted Percent of Persons Limited in Activity, by Geographic Region: United States, 1973, 1974.

	All areas	SMSA Central City	SMSA Non-Central City	Non SMSA
All regions	13.8	14.2	12.7	14.7
Northeast	12.8	13.8	11.5	14.2
North Central	13.2	13.7	12.3	13.6
South	14.7	14.1	13.4	15.8
West	14.6	15.4	14.2	14.2

Source: U.S. Department of Health, Education, and Welfare, National Center for Health Statistics, unpublished tabulations.

Table 6. Age-Adjusted Days of Restricted Activity per Person per Year, by Geographic Region: United States, 1973, 1974.

	All areas	SMSA Central City	SMSA Non-Central City	Non SMSA
All regions	16.8	18.3	15.7	16.7
Northeast	14.3	16.6	12.9	13.6
North Central	15.9	17.2	15.4	15.2
South	18.8	19.1	17.1	19.4
West	18.6	21.1	18.4	15.0

Source: U.S. Department of Health, Education, and Welfare, National Center for Health Statistics, unpublished tabulations.

Table 7. Age-Adjusted Number of Days of Bed Disability per Person per Year, by Geographic Region: United States, 1973, 1974.

	All areas	SMSA Central City	SMSA Non-Central City	Non SMSA
All regions	6.6	7.6	6.0	6.1
Northeast	5.9	7.5	5.1	5.0
North Central	5.9	7.0	5.9	5.0
South	7.5	8.4	6.7	7.4
West	6.8	7.8	6.5	5.8

Source: U.S. Department of Health, Education, and Welfare, National Center for Health Statistics, unpublished tabulations.

Table 8. Age-Adjusted Number of Work-Loss Days per Currently Employed Persons per Year, by Geographic Region: United States, 1973, 1974.

	All areas	SMSA Central City	SMSA Non-Central City	Non SMSA
All regions	5.2	5.8	4.9	4.8
Northeast	4.9	5.9	4.3	4.9
North Central	4.9	5.9	4.6	4.5
South	5.5	5.7	5.5	5.4
West	5.2	5.6	5.4	3.8

Source: U.S. Department of Health, Education, and Welfare, National Center for Health Statistics, unpublished tabulations.

Table 9. Number of Acute Conditions per 100 Persons per Year, and Number of Persons Injured per 1,000 Persons per Year, 1969 - 1970.

	United States	South, SMSA	South, Non SMSA
All acute conditions	202.1	202.7	193.9
By age			
Under age 17	289.5	283.7	264.7
17-44 years	189.6	195.3	172.4
45 years and over	119.7	114.0	139.6
By type			
Infective and parasitic			
Respiratory	24.5	34.3	23.1
Upper respiratory	64.7	62.0	58.3
Influenza and other			
respiratory	45.3	37.8	43.5
Other acute conditions	67.5	68.5	68.9
Injury rates	26.3	25.0	27.1
Work	4.0	4.2	4.3
Home	10.4	9.1	11.5
Other	12.8	12.4	12.6

Source: U.S. Department of Health, Education, and Welfare, *Health Characteristics, by Geographic Region, Large Metropolitan Areas, and Other Places of Residence, United States 1969 - 1970* (HRA) 74-1513, January 1974.

Table 10. Incidence of Selected Chronic Conditions, Rates per 1000 Population, by place of residence, U.S., selected years between 1968 and 1972.

	U.S.	SMSA	Non-SMSA	Ratio, Non-SMSA to SMSA
Conditions relatively more prevalent in nonmetropolitan areas[a]				
Chronic Digestive Conditions				
Ulcer of stomach and duodenum	17.2	15.9	19.4	1.22
Upper GI disorders	13.1	11.7	15.6	1.33
Gallbladder	10.3	9.0	12.6	1.40
Constipation	23.8	20.9	28.9	1.21
Chronic Respiratory Conditions				
Emphysema	6.6	5.4	8.7	1.61
Sinusitis	103.0	96.3	115.3	1.20
Pleurisy	3.4	2.9	4.5	1.55
Chronic Circulatory Conditions				
Hypertensive heart disease	10.5	9.6	12.1	1.26
Cerebrovascular disease	7.5	6.8	8.8	1.29
Chronic Skin and Musculosketal Conditions				
Disease of nails	22.9	20.2	28.3	1.40
Arthritis	92.9	86.0	106.2	1.23
Rheumatism	6.1	5.2	7.8	1.50
Displaced disc	8.6	8.0	9.6	1.20
Conditions relatively more prevalent in metropolitan areas[b]				
Chronic Respiratory Conditions				
Deflected nasal septum	4.0	5.2	1.8	.35
Laryngitis	5.7	6.3	4.8	.76
Chronic Circulatory Conditions				
Congenital abnormalities	4.4	4.9	3.6	.73
Chronic Skin and Musculosketal Conditions				
Psoriasis	6.5	7.1	5.3	.75
Gout	4.8	5.2	4.1	.79

Sources: U.S. Department of Health, Education and Welfare, National Center for Health Statistics, *Prevalence of Selected Chronic Digestive Conditions, United States, July-December 1968,* Series 10, No. 83; *Prevalence of Chronic Skin and Musculoskeletal Conditions, United States 1969,* Series 10, No. 92; *Prevalence of Selected Chronic Respiratory Conditions, United States 1970,* Series 10, No. 84; *Prevalence of Chronic Circulatory Conditions, United States 1972,* Series 10, No. 94.

[a] Those reported chronic conditions for which rates in nonmetropolitan areas exceeded metropolitan areas by 20 or more percent.

[b] Those reported chronic conditions for whihc rates in metropolitan areas exceeded nonmetropolitan areas by 20 or more percent.

Table 11. Patient Care Physicians by Type of Practice per 100,000 Population, U.S. and Southern States, by Metropolitan-Nonmetropolitan Areas, 1973.

	Total patient care	General practice	Medical specialities	Surgical specialties	Other specialties	Hospital-based practice
United States	133	23	23	30	19	35
SMSA	151	21	28	35	23	45
Non SMSA	69	27	10	17	8	7
South	103	21	18	27	15	22
SMSA	130	18	24	35	20	30
Non SMSA	60	26	8	15	6	8
Alabama	45	21	6	12	5	1
Arkansas	54	31	5	11	6	2
Florida	74	23	12	22	10	7
Georgia	63	23	9	16	8	7
Kentucky	56	26	7	13	6	4
Louisiana	45	25	4	29	3	3
Mississippi	58	25	7	16	6	2
North Carolina	62	23	11	18	6	4
Oklahoma	58	26	9	14	7	3
South Carolina	60	26	8	17	8	2
Tennessee	50	24	6	13	5	3
Texas	56	33	6	11	4	2
Virginia	98	27	15	21	12	23

Source: American Medical Association, *Distribution of Physicians in the U.S., 1973.*

Table 12. Patient Care Physicians per 100,000 Population, by Residence, by Percent Population Below the Poverty Level in County, 1971.

		Percent population below poverty level			
	Total	Under 15.0	15.0-24.9	25.0-34.9	35.0 and over
South (13 states)	98	126	100	74	45
Nonmetropolitan	63	76	74	56	44
Smaller areas[a]	43	45	49	44	36
Larger areas[a]	75	81	84	66	57
Metropolitan	130	135	121	165	57

Source: Calculated from data published in Southern Regional Council, *Health Care in the South: A Statistical Profile,* June 1974.

[a] Smaller areas are nonmetropolitan counties with population under 25,000. Larger areas are nonmetropolitan counteis with population of 25,000 or more.

100

Table 13. Characteristics of Physician Practices, U.S., Non-SMSA, South, 1973.

	U.S.	U.S., Non SMSA	South Atlantic	South East South Central	West South Central
Hours of direct patient care per week	46.1	49.7	46.8	50.9	49.5
Average number of weeks per year	47.2	47.0	47.5	48.2	47.9
Patient visits per week	137.7	175.9	148.8	182.9	151.1
Office visits per week	97.9	127.5	n.a.	n.a.	n.a.
Hospital visits per week	39.0	49.6	n.a.	n.a.	n.a.
Average net annual income	$49,415	47,284	50,408	57,466	50,301
G.P.	42,336	43,613	n.a.	n.a.	n.a.
Non-SMSA	47,284	47,284	53,000	55,480	46,577
Average professional expenses	33,066	34,464	32,695	39,507	38,189
G.P.	36,228	35,968	n.a.	n.a.	n.a.
Non-SMSA	34,464	34,464	32,270	38,404	36,521
Average number of full-time personnel					
Registered nurses	0.58	0.62	n.a.	n.a.	n.a.
Licensed practical nurses	0.31	0.45	n.a.	n.a.	n.a.
Nurses' aides	0.37	0.43	n.a.	n.a.	n.a.
X-ray and other technicians	0.92	0.87	n.a.	n.a.	n.a.
Secretaries, receptionists, clerks	1.13	1.20	n.a.	n.a.	n.a.

Source: American Medical Association, *Profile of Medical Practice, 1974.*

Table 14. Age-Adjusted Number of Dental Visits per Person per
Year, by Geographic Region: United States, 1973, 1974.

	All areas	SMSA		Non SMSA
		Central City	Non-Central City	
All regions	1.6	1.6	1.9	1.3
Northeast	2.0	2.0	2.1	1.6
North Central	1.6	1.5	1.8	1.4
South	1.3	1.3	1.6	1.1
West	1.9	1.8	2.1	1.6

Source: U.S. Department of Health, Education, and Welfare, National Center for Health
Statistics, unpublished tabulations

Table 15. Age-Adjusted Number of Physician Visits per Person per
Year, by Geographic Region: United States, 1973, 1974.

	All areas	SMSA		Non-SMSA
		Central City	Non-Central City	
All regions	5.0	5.2	5.2	4.4
Northeast	5.0	5.4	4.9	4.3
North Central	4.9	5.1	5.3	4.3
South	4.8	4.8	5.1	4.5
West	5.4	5.8	5.7	4.5

Source: U.S. Department of Health, Education, and Welfare, National Center for Health
Statistics, unpublished tabulations.

Table 16. Age-Adjusted Number of Short-Stay Hospital Discharges per
1,000 Persons per Year, by Georgraphic Region: United States, 1973, 1974.

	All areas	SMSA		Non-SMSA
		Central City	Non-Central City	
All regions	140.5	134.5	129.1	160.4
Northeast	122.5	125.7	111.9	143.5
North Central	148.4	151.7	136.4	159.3
South	153.4	135.9	142.8	171.6
West	130.4	122.4	129.4	144.4

Source: U.S. Department of Health, Education, and Welfare, National Center for Health
Statistics, unpublished tabulations.

Table 17. Percent of Persons Under Age 65 Years, *without* Hospital
Insurance Coverage, by Region and Place of Residence, 1968.

	U.S.	North East	North Central	South	West
All areas	20.5%	14.8%	14.6%	28.3%	24.0%
SMSA	17.4	15.0	12.2	22.4	22.0
Nonmetropolitan					
Nonfarm	24.2	13.8	16.1	32.1	30.1
Farm	36.8	21.7	28.2	48.8	29.9

Source: U.S. Department of Health, Education, and Welfare, National Center for Health Satistics, *Hospital and Surgical Insurance Coverage, United States, 1968,* Series 10-No. 66, DHEW Pub. No. (HSM) 72-1033, Table 14, p. 34.

Table 18. Medicaid Payments per Recipient and per Poor Person, and Ratios of Recipients to Poor, by Age, Selected Southern States, 1970.

	Children under age 21			Adults, age 21-64			Adults, age 65 and over		
	Medicaid payments per child recipient	Ratio of recipients to poor children	Medicaid payments per poor child	Medicaid payments per adult recipient	Ratio of recipients to poor adults	Medicaid payments per poor adult	Medicaid payments per aged recipient	Ratio of recipients to poor aged	Medicaid payments per poor aged
United States	$126	0.55	$69	$408	0.61	$250	$527	0.69	$363
Alabama	97	0.10	10	446	0.11	48	511	0.49	253
Arkansas	56	0.06	4	179	0.10	17	68	0.19	13
Florida	68	0.20	13	192	0.25	48	351	0.43	150
Georgia	87	0.26	23	447	0.31	139	416	0.71	296
Kentucky	76	0.38	29	262	0.37	96	231	0.68	158
Louisiana	112	0.08	9	260	0.18	46	245	0.94	230
Maryland	118	0.73	86	376	0.83	313	464	0.68	316
Mississippi	43	0.11	5	264	0.07	20	181	0.49	89
North Carolina	a	a	a	a	a	a	a	a	a
Oklahoma	201	0.37	75	402	0.43	174	583	0.64	372
South Carolina	65	0.09	6	325	0.19	60	475	0.38	180
Tennessee	66	0.16	10	222	0.17	37	166	0.32	53
Texas	215	0.08	17	738	0.09	69	326	0.66	213
Virginia	98	0.20	19	374	0.18	69	250	0.28	69
West Virginia	87	0.38	33	183	0.39	71	135	0.19	25

Sources: Karen Davis, "National Health Insurance," in Barry Blechman, et al., Setting National Priorities: the 1975 Budget (Washington, D.C.: The Brookings Institution, 1974), Chapter 8.

Table 19. Mean Expenditure for All Personal Health Services per Low Income Person by Source of Payment by Age, by Residence, 1970.

| | Total Mean Expenditures | | | Medicaid and other free care | | | Percent of expenditures paid by Medicaid or free care | | |
Age	SMSA Central city	Other urban	Rural	SMSA Central city	Other urban	Rural	SMSA, Central city	Other urban	Rural
Low income [a]									
Birth to 17	$101	$124	$ 46	$ 76	$ 58	$ 5	75.2%	46.8%	10.9%
18 - 64	360	352	281	158	83	52	43.9	23.6	32.9
65 and over	446	329	407	54	38	27	12.1	11.6	6.6

Source: Ronald Andersen et al., Expenditures for Personal Health Services: National Trends and Variations, 1953-1970, U.S. Department of Health, Education, and Welfare, Health Resources Administration, October 1973.

[a] Low income defined as family income below $6,000.

Table 20. Medicare Reimbursement per Enrollee, U.S. and Southern States, by Metropolitan and Nonmetropolitan Residence, 1971.

	All Medicare benefits	Hospital and post-hospital services	Physician and other medical services
United States	357	262	100
SMSA	395	287	114
Non SMSA	280	212	73
South	296	212	92
SMSA	329	230	109
Non SMSA	260	192	73
Alabama	247	181	72
Arkansas	236	173	68
Florida	282	199	88
Georgia	251	174	82
Kentucky	249	196	57
Louisiana	245	184	70
Mississippi	260	195	71
North Carolina	255	200	60
Oklahoma	303	220	89
South Carolina	204	145	62
Tennessee	237	178	64
Texas	310	221	95
Virginia	224	177	51

Source: U.S. Department of Health, Education, and Welfare, Social Security Administration, Office of Research and Statistics, *Medicare 1971, Reimbursement by State and County,* DHEW Pub. No. (SSA) 73-11704.

Table 21. Percentage of Low-Income Women with Poor Diets, by Region and Residence, 1965[a]

	U.S.	North East	North Central	South	West
All areas	36%	32%	36%	40%	26%
Urban	35	32	41	38	26
Rural nonfarm	38	35	31	42	26
Rural farm	36	17	28	43	23

Source: U.S. Department of Agriculture Agricultural Service, 1968; cited in National Academy of Science, *The Quality of Rural Living,* 1971, p. 38.

[a] Low-income is defined as family income below $3,000. Poor diet is defined as a diet meeting less than two-thirds of the recommended daily allowance for 1 to 7 nutrients.

Table 22. Percent Housing Without Plumbing, by Residence, by Percent Population Below the Poverty Level in County, 1971

	Total population	Percent population below poverty level			
		Under 15.0	15.0- 24.9	25.0- 34.9	35.0 and over
South (13 states)	11.7	3.8	9.5	19.3	32.3
Nonmetropolitan	19.3	8.5	13.5	21.3	33.1
Smaller areas[a]	24.2	9.3	16.3	22.6	35.1
Larger areas[a]	16.2	8.3	12.4	20.1	30.1
Metropolitan	5.0	3.0	6.3	9.4	23.8

Source: Calculated from data published in Southern Regional Council, *Health Care in the South: A Statistical Profile,* June 1974.

[a] Smaller areas are nonmetropolitan counties with population under 25,000. Larger areas are nonmetropolitan counties with population of 25,000 or more.

Table 23. Graduates of Physician Assistant Programs by Type of Practice as a Function of Size of Community in Which Practicing.

Type of Practice	Size of Community										Totals
	Under 10,000		10-19,999		20-49,999		50-99,999		Over 100,000		
Family Practice	177	83%	72	75%	44	49%	28	37%	64	31%	385
Gen. Int. Med.	9	5%	8	8%	20	22%	6	8%	31	15%	74
Emer. Med.	7	3%	4	4%	3	3%	4	5%	25	12%	43
Gen. Surg.	6	3%	3	3%	9	10%	7	9%	9	4%	34
Gen. Ped.	3	1%			2	2%	3	4%	12	6%	20
Adm.	5	2%			1	1%	4	5%	25	12%	35
Other	6	3%	10	10%	12	13%	24	32%	42	20%	94
Totals	213		97		91		76		208		685

Source: Donald W. Fisher, "Physician Assistant: A Profile of the Profession," American Academy of Physicians' Assistants, April 16-18, 1975.

Total Graduates — 562
Surveyed
Total Responses — 507 (90%)

Population of Community	Number of graduated residents	Percentage of Grads entering practice	Percentage of total grads
Smaller than 5,000	72	17.4%	14.2%
5,000 to 15,000	106	25.5	20.9
15,000 to 30,000	61	14.7	12.0
30,000 to 100,000	59	14.2	11.6
100,000 to 500,000	72	17.4	14.2
Over 500,000	45	10.8	8.9
Other			
Another Residency	2		
Undecided	7		
Foreign	12		
Military (with orders)	67		
Military (no orders)	4 92		18.2%
Totals	507		100.0%

Summary of Distribution of Graduating Residents (1975)
Practice Profile.

Practice Type	Number of graduated residents	Percentage of grads entering practice	Percentage of total grads
Solo	73	15.6%	14.4%
Family Practice Group	247	52.8	48.7
Multi-Specialty Group	47	10.0	9.2
Teaching	30	6.4	5.9
Military	71	15.2	14.0
Other			
Entering another residency	2		
Indian health	2		
Emergency Medicine	7		
NRSC	3		
Not applicable	25 39		7.8%
Totals	507		100.0%

Source: American Academy of Family Physicians.

Table 25. Summary of Distribution of Graduating Family Practice
Residents (1975) by County Classification.

Total questionnaires distributed   562
Total responses   507 (90%)
    Total into practice or teaching   415 = 81.9%
    Total into military   71 = 14.0%
    Other (undecided, outside USA or
      unknown)   21 = 4.1%

Demographic County Classification	Number of FP Graduates locating within such areas	Percentage of FP Graduates locating within such areas	Percentage of U.S. Population within such areas
1	16	3.9%	2.2%
2	29	7.0%	7.2%
3	51	12.3%	7.7%
4	45	10.8%	7.7%
5	3	.7%	2.0%
6	102	24.6%	18.6%
7	41	9.9%	13.2%
8	106	2.55%	30.0%
9	22	5.3%	11.4%
Total	415	100.0%	100.0%

Demographic County Classification

1 — Nonmetropolitan Counties with 0 to 9,999 Inhabitants
2 — Nonmetropolitan Counties with 10,000 to 24,999 Inhabitants
3 — Nonmetropolitan Counties with 25,000 to 49,999 Inhabitants
4 — Nonmetropolitan Counties with 50,000 or more Inhabitants
5 — Counties Considered Potential SMSA's
6 — Counties in SMSA's with 50,000 to 499,999 Inhabitants
7 — Counties in SMSA's with 500,000 to 999,999 Inhabitants
8 — Counties in SMSA's with 1,000,000 to 4,999,999 Inhabitants
9 — Counties in SMSA's with 5,000,000 or more Inhabitants

Note: The county classification schema used in this compilation was that from 1973, while
the resident location information is 1975 data. Since some counties may have changed their
classification code between 1973 and 1975, the final analysis of data will need to use 1975
county classification codes matched with 1975 resident location. This will be available in
the final data analysis form.
Source: American Academy of Family Physicians.

A DISAGGREGATED MODEL OF MEDICAL SPECIALTY CHOICE*

Jack Hadley, THE URBAN INSTITUTE

I. INTRODUCTION AND BACKGROUND

One of the foremost issues of current health manpower policy is the apparent specialty maldistribution of physicians. As can be seen from Table 1, the proportion of physicians in general and family practice declined from 73.7 to 27.9 percent between 1949 and 1973. Although partially offset by an increase in the proportion of general internists from 7.7 to 19.3 percent, substantial differences in physician productivity imply fewer patient encounters with primary contact physicians.[1] Over the same time period, the proportion of general surgeons and surgical specialists increased from 14.7 to 27.8 percent of all physicians. The view that there is

Research in Health Economics, Vol. 1, pp 111–152.

Table 1. Distribution of Physicians by Specialty, 1931 - 1973 (percent)

Specialty	1931 [a]	1940 [a]	1949 [a]	1958 [b]	1967 [c]	1973 [d]
Total physicians	150,358	156,970	173,129	179,485	247,256	270,412
Physicians per 100,000 pop.	119.8	118.4	115.6	102.7	124.5	130.0
Population in 100,000	1240.4	1325.9	1497.7	1748.8	1986.3	2090.9
Gen. & fam. prac.	82.4	90.6	73.7	39.2	36.2	27.9
General internal med.	4.1	4.9	7.7	9.9	16.6	19.3
General pediatrics	3.1	1.8	2.9	5.3	7.2	8.0
Internal med. subspec.	NA	.5d	1.3e	2.1e	2.0e	4.3
Pediatric subspec.	NA	NA	NA	NA	.1	.3
Dermatology	.8	.7	1.1	1.4	1.6	1.8
Neurology & psychiatry	1.7	1.8	3.2	4.6	8.5	9.5
General surgery	10.7f	5.0f	8.1f	13.0g	13.9g	14.3
Neurosurgery	NA	NA	NA	.5	1.0	1.2
Obstetrics & gynecology	5.2	1.9	3.4	7.3	8.0	8.8
Orthopedic surgery	.7	.8	1.4	2.1	3.7	4.5
Plastic surgery	NA	NA	NA	.3	.6	.9
Ophthalmology	NA	NA	NA	NA	4.1	4.8
Otolaryngology	6.8	5.7	6.2	6.0	2.5	2.3
Urology	1.9	1.3	1.5	1.9	2.4	2.7
Anesthesiology	.4	.2	.8	2.4	4.3	5.2
Pathology	.6	.7	1.2	1.6	3.5	4.0
Radiology	1.4	1.2	1.9	2.7	4.7	6.2
Physical med. & rehab.	NA	NA	.2	.2	.4	.5
Others	NA	1.2	1.2	2.2	2.2	2.5

Source: "Medicare-Medicaid Reimbursement Policies," Report prepared by the Institute of Medicine under DHEW Contract No. SSA-PMB-74-250, March 1976: p. 231.

Note: M.D.'s only

[a] All physicians; specialists are full-time in their specialty.

[b] Non-Federal general practitioners and full-time specialits in the United States.

[c] Non-Federal physicians in the United States listing patient care as their primary professional activity; specialists not necessarily full-time.

[d] Pulmonary disease only.

[e] Pulmonary disease, allergy, cardiology, and gastroenterology.

[f] Occupational medicine and general surgery.

[g] General surgery, thoracic surgery, and colon and rectal surgery.

excess surgical capacity is further buttressed by several studies of surgical workloads, which found surgeons to be performing fewer operations (adjusted for complexity) than normatively determined full case loads [Hughes et al. (1975) p. 379; Nickerson et al. (1975), p. 10]. In general the perceived dimensions of the maldistribution problem can be summarized by the findings of a recent and comprehensive study which was commissioned by the U.S. Congress. "Primary care appears generally to be undersupplied, and would benefit from an increase in the total number and proportion of 'contact' physicians. Surgery appears to be oversupplied and should have no further increase in ratio of surgical specialists to population . . ." [Institute of Medicine (1976), p. 8]. Among the recommendations of this study were (1) changing Medicare-Medicaid reimbursement policies so as to provide more funds for training in ambulatory care, (2) making direct grants to training institutions (medical schools and teaching hospitals) in support of training for primary contact specialties (general and family practice, general internal medicine, and general pediatrics), and (3) freezing the number of residency training positions in nonprimary contact specialties at the levels of filled positions as of July 1, 1975, while expanding the number of training positions in the primary contact specialties [Institute of Medicine (1976), pp. 9–10].

Federal legislation in this area has traditionally focused on the adequacy of the aggregate supply of physicians [Reinhardt (1975), ch. 1]. However, with the passage of the Health Professions Educational Assistance Act of 1976 (Public Law 94-484), the U.S. Congress declared that there is no longer an insufficient number of physicians and surgeons in the United States and enacted measures which specifically address the specialty maldistribution problem. In particular, medical school's receipt of Federal capitation grants is made contingent upon meeting target

. . . percentages of filled first-year residency positions in direct or affiliated residency programs in primary care. . . . The required percentages of primary care positions are: 35% for FY 1978 grants, 40% for FY 1979 grants, and 50% for FY 1980 grants. Unless this requirement is met by a national average of all schools on July 15 before a fiscal year begins, . . . schools individually must meet requirements on July 15 of the following year ("The Blue Sheet," October 27, 1976, p. S-13).

Implicit in this legislation is the assumption that medical colleges can in fact influence specialty choices. However, there are no guidelines or requirements as to how such decisions should be affected, nor does the legislation employ extra-educational financial incentives as a policy tool.

This study poses two questions germane to choosing policy instruments for altering medical specialty choices. First, what impact do various specialty, personal, and institutional characteristics have on the probabilities of choosing alternative specialties? Second, which are most important in terms of their influence on a policy maker's ability to predict specialty choices? The purposes of the latter are to offer a criterion for evaluating the study's results in addition to the traditional tests of statistical significance and to provide guidance for identifying the type of information which should be collected.[2]

These questions are addressed by specifying and estimating a set of linear probability functions which have their conceptual roots in the various economic theories of occupational choice. The dependent variables consist of nine alternative specialty choices. Independent variables are measures of relative specialty characteristics, individual physician data, and information on the physician's medical college and internship hospital. The model is estimated using longitudinal data on a cohort of physicians who graduated from medical school in 1960. Specialty choices are measured by the physicians' self-designated specialties in 1972. The predictive power of the model is tested with data for a subsample of the cohort which was held in reserve, and assessment of the importance of groups of variables is based upon the change in the model's predictive ability when those variables are deleted.

The study of physician specialty choice is, of course, not a recent phenomenon. Most of the prior research on specialty choice has been by noneconomists who primarily focused on the personal characteristics of physicians choosing various specialties and on the influence of medical education. Analytic techniques predominantly involved bivariate statistics and tabular presentations, and sample sizes were frequently small, e.g., a sample of students from a single medical school. Although this limits the utility for drawing policy inferences, results from these studies nevertheless suggest a number of hypotheses. One common finding is that different medical schools produce consistently different specialty distributions of graduates, which raises the question of whether this is due to variations in the characteristics of the medical schools or of their students [Fein and Weber (1971), pp. 15, 21, 23; *Journal of Medical Education* (1970), p. 716; Lyden et al. (1968), p. 93]. Along these lines, it has been argued that the increasing proportion of careers in specialty, research, and/or academic medicine is associated with a number of factors: shifts in medical school faculty composition toward full-time medical specialists and Ph.D. holders [Kendall and Selvin (1957), p. 159; Powers et al. (1962), p. 1084], high Medical College Admissions Test (MCAT) scores [Lyden et al. (1968), pp. 178–185; Glaser (1959), pp. 351–352; Fein and Weber (1971), pp. 22–23], high research budgets and expenditures per student [Fein and Weber (1971), pp. 20–21], and internships in privately controlled, university-affiliated teaching hospitals [Mumford (1970), pp. 63–68; Perlstadt (November 1972), p. 86].

Other findings related sociodemographic, cognitive, and noncognitive personal characteristics to specialty choices. For example, students choosing general practice tend to be older, marry before completion of medical school, come from small towns, score lower on the MCAT, and have lower class rank than students choosing specialty practices [Lyden et al. (1968), pp. 62, 65, 78, 91–92, 97; Paiva and Haley (1971), p. 285; Coker et al. (1960), pp. 97–98; Monk and Terris (December 13, 1956), pp. 1136–1138]. Studies which focused on sex differences found women more likley to enter pediatrics, psychiatry, public health, and certain hospital-based specialties (anesthesiology, radiology, pathology), presumably because of preferences for shorter and more stable work weeks, societal sex role pressures, and/or discrimination in obtaining residencies in certain specialties [Kosa and Coker (1965), p. 295; Westling-Wikstrand et al. (1970), pp. 275–276; Lopate (1968), pp. 127–129]. Financial constraints have also been examined and were found to affect primarily the decision to seek additional residency training, thereby making the choice of general practice more likely [Lyden et al. (1968), pp. 145–163; Glaser (1959), p. 350; Coker et al. (1969), p. 97]. Finally, a number of studies have examined the relationships between personalities, values, specialty stereotypes, and specialty choices [Otis and Weiss (1972), pp. 19–20]. While there has been less consistency and comparability across studies of this type than in those looking at sociodemographic variables, there do appear to be significant personality and value differences between choosers of various specialties. Based on this work, one can construct specialty stereotypes which medical students may try to match with their own personalities and values.[3]

Prior economic research on physician specialty choice has emphasized the importance of the internal rate of return to residency training as an allocation device [Sloan (1970); Lindsay (1973); American Medical Association (1973), pp. 88–98]. However, even after adjusting for differences in hours worked, considerable variations were found in the rate of return to specialization relative to general practice. These findings are at odds with the conditions of a competitive equilibrium under the assumption that the rate of return is the central allocation mechanism. Monopoly power, suggested by some writers [Friedman and Kunznets (1946); Kessel (1970); Rayack (1964)], is not a likely explanation of the variations in rates of return because of the general excess supply of residency training positions. Sloan has suggested that nonmonetary market signaling mechanisms may be more significant, although this proposition has not been explicitly tested [Sloan (1970), pp. 53–54].

The next section of this paper describes the specification of the model: its theoretical basis, dependent and independent variables. Section III describes the data and the estimation method. Results are presented in section IV, and in the last section the study is summarized and conclusions are drawn.

II. MODEL SPECIFICATION

A. Conceptual Underpinnings

The study proceeds on the assumption that choice of a medical specialty may be treated as a special case of the general occupational choice process. As such, one may start with any one of three basic theoretical formulations of the underlying process: the maximization of a utility function with income and leisure as arguments over some relevant time horizon, treating different occupations as alternative streams of earnings/leisure combinations [Gallaway (1967), pp. 14–24; Boskin (1974), p. 390]; the human capital approach, which views the choice of an occupation as an investment decision that requires foregoing current consumption in favor of future returns [Becker (1964), Weis (1971), pp. 833–387]; and Lancasterian utility maximization over a discrete characteristics space, with occupations treated as bundles of characteristics, such as income, leisure, prestige, intellectual challenge, etc. [Lancaster (1966); Freeman (1971), pp. 4–5]. Although these theories start with somewhat different assumptions and employ different analytic manipulations, their empirical implications are really quite similar. Namely, holding constant preferences and abilities, the choice of an occupation should be positively related to its expected monetary and nonmonetary returns and inversely related to the expected monetary and nonmonetary costs [Rottenberg (1956)].

One may extend this notion by positing that the physician engages in an implicit (or "as if") calculation process which requires accumulating information or data about alternative specialties. Assuming that only some subset of all specialties is seriously considered, each physician then forms expectations of the relevant psychic and monetary returns and costs, compares alternatives, and presumably makes a choice which leads him/her to be better off. The notion of comparison is used here in an imprecise fashion, in that it is not assumed that calculations are made for all possible alternatives and the highest net total return chosen, nor that net monetary returns dominate the decision-making process. It is assumed, however, that, *other things equal,* physicians would prefer more income to less, lower costs to higher, shorter training periods to longer, etc.

In translating this conceptualization of the general process into an empirical model, it is important to point out several of the factors which make this a special case. First is the fact that medicine is a professional occupation, which implies that the nonpecuniary component of the alternatives is likely to be more important than if nonprofessional occupations were under consideration. Second, it is a profession which requires an extremely long training period, generally a minimum of five years following college, with seven to eight years not at all uncommon. This suggests that the training institutions themselves may play an important role in the choice process. Third, the choice objects, medical specialties, are neighboring activities within a particular occupation, so that the types of factors which usually influence choices among distinct occupations may be less discriminating in this type of analysis. Finally, as a corollary of the last observation, just about all physicians regardless of specialty tend to wind up in the upper tails of both the income and prestige distributions.

The implications of these observations are twofold. On the one hand, the model should attempt to account explicitly for the effects of variations in preferences and institutions. On the other hand, it may be the case that some of the theoretical predictions based on the general occupational choice model will be less likely to hold, if at all. In the next two subsections the definition and construction of the dependent and independent variables will be discussed. The latter draws heavily on both the prior literature and considerations raised in this subsection.

B. Dependent Variables

Given the objective of explaining how an individual physician chooses his/her medical specialty, a convenient procedure for representing possible choices is to create specialty groupings which are mutually exclusive and which exhaust all possible choice outcomes. Each group may then be represented by a dichotomous variable which takes the value one if the physician selects a specialty in the corresponding choice group, and zero if he/she selects a specialty from some other group. Dichotomous variables have the useful properties that their means are equivalent to the sample proportions of physicians choosing alternative specialties and, for large samples, that they can be interpreted as relative frequencies, or the probabilities of choosing particular specialty groups. In this study, the number of possible specialty outcomes is limited by the fact that income data were available for only nine specialties.[4] Therefore, there are nine dichotomous dependent variables, one corresponding to each possible specialty choice. The variable corresponding to the physician's actual specialty in 1972 takes the value one, while the other eight dependent variables take the value zero. Table 2 presents data on the specialty choices of the Association of American Medical College's Longitudinal Study cohort, which is used as the study's principal data set. The third column of Table 2 corresponds to the mean values of the nine dependent variables for the subsample of physicians used to estimate the model's parameters.

C. Independent Variables

Central to the conceptual model outlined above is the notion that specialty choice is the result of comparing the pecuniary and nonpecuniary

Table 2. Specialty Choices of the Longitudinal Study Cohort
(percent)

Specialty	All Physicians (2,524)	Study Physicians (1,269)[h]	Variable Name
General practice	.118	.228	GP
Medical specialities			
Allergy·	.008		
Cardivoscular	.025		
Dermatology	.024		
Family practice	.016		
Gastroenterology	.010		
Internal medicine	.135	.201	IM
Pediatrics[a]	.057	.076	PED
Pulmonary disease	.006		
Surgical specialities			
General surgery	.061	.109	SRG
Neurological surgery	.008		
Obstetrics gynecology	.057	.090	OBG
Ophthalmology	.042		
Orthopedic surgery[b]	.044		
Otorhinolaryngology	.023		
Plastic surgery	.007		
Colon & rectal surgery	.001		
Thoracic surgery[c]	.010		
Urology	.025		
Additional specialities			
Anesthesiology	.038	.060	ANES
Neurology[d]	.025		
Pathology[e]	.044	.043	PATH
Psychiatry[f]	.106	.123	PSY
Radiology[g]	.055	.068	RAD
Other	.055		

Source: Association of American Medical Colleges, "The Longitudinal Study of Medical Students of the Class of 1960," p. 14.

Notes:

[a] Pediatrics, allergy; pediatrics, cardiology

[b] Hand surgery

[c] Cardiovascular surgery

[d] Child neurology

[e] Clinical pathology; forensic pathology; hematology

[f] Child psychiatry; psychoanalysis

[g] Diagnostic roentgenology; nuclear medicine; pediatrics, radiology; therapeutic radiology

[h] Physicians in direct patient care who are not subspecialists

costs and returns associated with some set of possible choice outcomes. Ideally, one would like to have direct observations of physicians' expectations of incomes, costs, prestige, work hours, etc., for each of the specialties under consideration. In the absence of such data, however, it is necessary to make some simplifying assumptions. The most critical of these is that physicians' expectations are based on current population values of the relevant proxy variable. In effect, this is equivalent to assuming an expectation formation function of the form $EX_{it} = f(X_t)$, where EX_{it} is the expected value of X for the *ith* individual in period t, and X_t is the value for some reference population. Thus, for example, it is assumed that expected specialty incomes can be represented by the mean net incomes of all physicians in each specialty.

A second major assumption is that the choice process consists of a series of pairwise comparisons, each of which is independent of any other comparison [Boskin (1974), p. 390]. This permits one to specify a separate estimation equation for each dependent variable, with each equation involving only two specialties. One consequence of this assumption is that the independent variables are permitted to have different impacts on the probabilities of choosing each specialty. Thus, for example, a 10 percent increase in general practitioners' income may have a different effect on the probability of choosing general practice than a similar increase in, say, pediatricians' incomes might have on the probability of choosing pediatrics. If one believes that the choosers of different specialties either have different preference functions and/or make their final selections from different subsets of specialties, then this consequence seems acceptable.

Thirdly, it is assumed that the choices depend on relative rather than absolute differences between specialties.[5] The last assumption raises the question of how the pairs of specialties are selected for each equation. First, the specialty corresponding to the numerator value of an independent variable is the same as the specialty represented by the equation's dependent variable. Taking relative mean net incomes, for example, the numerator value in the general practice equation is general practitioners' mean net income, pediatricians' mean net income in the pediatrics equation, surgeons' income in the surgery equation, etc.

The selection of a specialty for the denominator value depends on whether the dependent variable takes the value zero or one. Consider, for example, the general practice equation for a physician who in fact chose internal medicine. (In terms of the dependent variables, IM = 1, GP = 0, SRG = 0, PED = 0, etc.) Since this physician is not a general practitioner, the implicit question being asked by the equation is why some other specialty was chosen instead. Clearly, the alternative specialty in this case is the physician's actual specialty in 1972, internal medicine. Therefore, for each specialty not chosen (dependent variable equals zero), the denominator value corresponds to the physician's actual specialty.

If the dependent variable equals one, then which of the other eight specialties was most likely to have been the alternative against which it was compared? One feature of this data file is that it contains information on specialty preferences in 1960, 1961, and 1965. The assumption made, therefore, is that the alternative to the physician's actual speciality is the last different specialty in the longitudinal record. For example, if internal medicine is both the current and 1965 specialty, but general practice was indicated in 1961, then general practice is the denominator or alternative specialty.[6]

Given these assumptions, what are the model's independent variables? For convenience, these variables may be grouped into three sets: measures of expected returns, expected costs, and preferences and abilities. The first two contain relative specialty characteristics, constructed as described above. The last set includes both personal characteristics and medical school and internship hospital characteristics. (In the Results section below, these variables will be grouped into financial incentive, admissions criteria, and institutional-structural categories in order to facilitate drawing policy inferences.)

The choice of a specialty is hypothesized to be a positive function of both the expected monetary and nonmonetary returns. The principal measure of the former is the ratio of mean net incomes in 1965 of the two specialties in each equation (RELY).[7] In addition certain personal characteristics may affect earnings expectations. Older physicians may anticipate shorter practice careers and, therefore, a lower return to any given investment in specialty training. Thus, age at graduation (AGE) should be positively related to choosing general practice and generally negative in the specialty equations. There is some evidence that, in the past, female physicians were subject to discrimination in obtaining first quality residency training in certain specialties, particularly surgery [Lopate (1968), pp. 127–129]. It has also been argued that the demands of child-rearing make it relatively more difficult to successfully establish private, office-based practices, so that women may anticipate greater returns, other things equal, in specialties which are either hospital-based or permit greater scheduling of hours [Kosa and Coker (1965), p. 295; Lowenstein (1971), p. 735]. Therefore, the dichotomous variable FEMALE (1 if female) should be negative in the surgery equation and positive in the radiology, pathology, anesthesiology, and psychiatry equations. The expected signs for the other specialties are ambiguous. Third, to the extent that a physician has a particular ability or skill in a specialty, one might expect the physician to have higher expected earnings in that specialty. An indirect measure of this type of ability is given by scores from the National Board of Medical Examiners (NBME) test, Part II, which attempts to measure clinical skills. In particular, scores from the medicine (MEDCN), surgery (SURG), pediatrics (PDTRC), and obstetrics/ gynecology (OBGYN) portions of the test should be positively related to choosing their respective specialties. The effects on choosing other specialties are ambiguous. (The score from a fifth test section, public health and physical medicine (PHPM), is also included in the NBME variables, though without any prior expectations.)

The nonmonetary returns of a specialty are assumed to depend on its perceived prestige, intellectual rewards, and other subjective factors, and on how closely the characteristics of the specialty match the physician's individual preferences for various aspects of medical practice. Since there are no generally accepted measures of prestige for a sufficiently large number of specialties, a proxy variable will be constructed: the proportion of filled residency positions in affiliated hospitals for the specialties for which these data are available (RELPCT). The implicit assumptions made are that there are no effective supply-side constraints on physicians' residency training choices and that the proportion of filled residencies measures aggregate preferences for various specialties.[8] In general, it is expected that a relatively high proportion of filled residencies will be positively related to choosing a specialty.

The second aspect of nonmonetary returns is the extent to which the subjective dimensions of practicing each specialty are consistent with the individual physician's preferences for those dimensions or characteristics. Thus, for example, a physician who enjoys interacting with patients should have a higher psychic return from a patient-contact specialty such as pediatrics or general practice than from specialties such as pathology or radiology, which involve little direct patient contact. One of the unique aspects of the AAMC Longitudinal Study data file is that it includes direct measures of physicians' preferences for various aspects of medical practice. The Career Attitudes Inventory Test [Association of American Medical Colleges (1974), pp. 3162–3169] is a questionnnaire which asks respondents to rate a number of medical practice situations on a five-unit scale, from highly desirable to highly undesirable. Using factor analysis, these rankings were converted into five indices measuring the desires for prestige, recognition, and reward (PRESTIGE), intellectual challenge (INTELECT), patient contact (PATCNTCT), pressure (PRESSURE), and teamwork (TEAMWORK). Hypotheses regarding the signs of the variables can be regarded as tentative at best because of the lack of any objective measures of how integral these characteristics are in each of the specialties. However, so-called specialty stereotypes [Otis et al. (1972), pp. 19–20] do provide the basis for forming general expectations.

Since these variables are measured on a continuous scale, low values may be interpreted as either an aversion or indifference to a particular

characteristic. Therefore, these same variables will also be used to measure the nonmonetary or psychic costs associated with alternative specialties. This means, for example, that a physician who has a low value for
patient contact (PATCNTCT) should be more likely to select a specialty
such as radiology or pathology. In other words, the variable will take a
negative sign when it represents a psychic cost.

The monetary costs associated with entering a particular specialty are
the opportunity costs (foregone earnings) and direct expenses incurred
while in training, plus the specialty's practice expenses. However, the
latter are subsumed in the expected income variable, which measures net
rather than gross earnings. For convenience, direct training expenses (and
stipends) are assumed to be reasonably constant across specialties.
Therefore, the major cost of choosing a specialty is the earnings foregone
while in training. If it is further assumed that the opportunity cost can be
approximated by what would have been earned as a general practitioner
and that this varies relatively little across individuals, then the total opportunity cost is primarily a function of the length of the residency training period. Therefore, relative opportunity costs are approximated by the
modal lengths of training, adjusted for military service and board certification, of the two specialties in each equation (RELTRN).[9] This variable is
hypothesized to be negatively related to the choice of any particular specialty.

A second type of cost is implicit in the budget constraint for financing
additional years of graduate training. Even if annual training expenses are
similar, as assumed above, inability to finance those expenses will limit
the amount of training undertaken, and thereby influence specialty
choice. Three indirect proxies for access to education funds are
employed. The first is the dichotomous variable which takes the value one
if the physician reported a debt of $5,000 or more in 1960 (HIDEBT). The
second proxy measures the proportion of medical college expenses financed by zero cost funds, such as parental gifts, scholarships, or trust
funds (SCHGIFT). These variables should have opposite signs, with the
former having a negative sign for specialties which generally require
longer training periods. Finally, parental resources are approximated by
three dichotomous variables measuring the father's occupation: physician
or dentist (DADMED), other professional or managerial (DADMANAG),
and blue collar or not in the labor force (DADBLCOL). To the extent that
these three variables represent access to training funds, DADBLCOL
should have a negative effect on the choice of specialties with relatively
longer training periods, and should be opposite in sign to DADMED and
DADMANAG.

The model's remaining variables are personal and institutional characteristics which are assumed to affect either physicians' preferences or

ability. One factor which may affect specialty choice is the so-called rate of time preference, which is a measure of the willingness to forego current earnings in order to undertake additional training. Although this cannot be observed directly, physicians who are married, particularly if they have children, are hypothesized to have a higher rate of time preference (i.e., are less willing to give up current consumption). Two dichotomous variables, MAR56 (1 if married in 1956) and MARKIDS (1 if married and children present in 1960), are used to represent marital and family status. Due to their hypothesized influence on the length of training, married physicians with children should be more likely to choose general practice. Being married without children, however, may have the opposite effect, if a spouse's earnings make it easier to finance additional residency training. Therefore, MARKIDS is constructed as an interaction term with MAR56, and the expected signs in the specialty equations are ambiguous.[10]

A final personal characteristic employed as a preference measure is the size of the physician's home town, represented by the dichotomous variable NONMETRO (1 if he/she comes from a town of fewer than 10,000 people, excluding suburbs of large cities). This variable frequently has been used in earlier studies, which found it to be positively related to choosing general practice [Lyden et al. (1968), p. 62; Monk and Terris (1956), p. 1136]. This may reflect either a greater exposure to general practice as a model of medical practice and/or a higher probability of practicing in a similar-size community.

It was hypothesized above that a physician's clinical skills could be partly measured by scores on Part II of the NBME. A measure of more general academic ability is the average score on the Medical College Admissions Test (MCATAVG). Since this is a general rather than specific ability measure, one cannot readily form hypotheses as to how it might influence the probabilities of choosing particular specialties. However, it will be of some interest to test whether this group of ability variables jointly has a significant effect in any of the specialty choice equations.

Finally, medical school and internship hospital variables are included to test whether they have any impact on specialty choices. Although there have been a number of papers suggesting the nature of the relationship between choices and institutional characteristics, most of these hypotheses would be extremely difficult to test, primarily because of difficulties with measuring the appropriate conceptual variable. Therefore, rather than speculating about specific mechanisms, the approach taken here simply treats the institutions as black boxes whose internal workings are not well understood. The specific hypothesis to be tested is simply whether the variables describing the institutions have any effect on specialty choice.

The medical school variables are divided into two groups. The first measures two characteristics of the school's student body, since this is certainly an integral part of the medical school environment. One variable is the average Medical College Admission Test score for the school (SCHMCAT). The other is the proportion of first-year acceptances who are out-of-state residents (PCTOUT). The latter may be thought of as an indirect measure of student quality, since schools with relatively high proportions of out-of-state students may be more likely to have larger applicant pools from which to select. Separate variables are included for public and private schools by means of interaction variables with the form of control variable described below.

The second group of medical school variables are referred to as structural characteristics. These include form of control (PRIV = 1 if a private school), budget per student (BGTSTUD), faculty per student (FACSTUD), the ratios of Ph.D. to M.D. faculty (PHDMD) and basic science to clinical science faculty (BASCLIN), and research expenditures per faculty member (RSCHFAC). As stated above, no hypotheses regarding the signs of individual variables are developed.

Similarly, there are no strong priors regarding the signs of the internship hospital characteristics. Three variables are used: a dichotomous variable measuring medical school affiliation (MAJAFIL = 1 if hospital has a major medical school affiliation), the proportion of deaths which undergo autopsy (PCTAUTOP), and a dichotomous variable measuring whether half or more of the internships offered are straight, as opposed to rotating (HALFSTRT). These variables may be thought of as crude proxies for the quality of the hospital's teaching program.

To sum up, the model's variables represent measures of expected returns and costs associated with alternative specialties;, personal information about physicians as proxies for the rate of time preference, academic ability, and practice preferences; and institutional characteristics which may have an effect on the specialty choice process. In terms of policy variables, expected earnings and the costs of medical training may be subject to direct intervention; personal characteristics of medical students may be affected via the admissions process; and institutional structure could be manipulated by medical education administrators, possibly in response to financial or other incentives.

Table 3 presents the definitions, mean values, and standard deviations of the independent variables. Note that the relative specialty characteristics variables, RELY, RELTRN, and RELPCT take on different values in each equation, since the pairwise comparisons vary across both physicians and equations. However, the values of the personal and institutional variables are identical across equations.

Table 3. Definitions, Mean Values, and Standard Deviations
of the Independent Variables

A. Relative Specialty Characteristics[a]

    1. RELY — the ratio of mean met specialty incomes specific to the state in which the physician was located when the 1972 specialty first appeared in the longitudinal record.

    2. RELTRN — the ratio of modal lengths of post medical school training, adjusted for military service and board certification.

    3. RELPCT — the ratio of the proportions of filled residencies in hospitals with major medical school affiliations.

	GP	IM	PED	SRG	OBG	PSY	RAD	ANES	PATH
RELY[b]	1.014	1.046	1.010	.997	.978	1.024	1.007	1.020	1.028
	(1.185)	(1.63)	(.126)	(.135)	(1.54)	(.165)	(.155)	(.149)	(.221)
RELTRN[b]	.461	1.660	1.123	1.669	1.619	1.454	1.369	1.165	1.582
	(.234)	(1.254)	(.847)	(1.281)	(1.331)	(1.190)	(1.053)	(.872)	(1.264)
RELPCT[b]	.554	1.351	1.249	1.273	1.321	1.147	1.162	1.052	1.265
	(.038)	(.395)	(.368)	(.369)	(.377)	(.339)	(.334)	(.311)	(.375)

B. Personal Characteristics

	Variable	Definition	Mean[c]	S.D.[e]
4.	AGE	Age at graduation	26.95	2.66
5.	FEMALE[d]	1 if female	.04	
6.	MAR56[d]	1 if married in 1956	.28	
7.	MARKIDS[d]	1 if married with children in 1960	.14	
8.	NONMETRO[d]	1 if from place of less than 10,000 pop	.30	
9.	DADMED[d]	1 if physician or dentist father	.14	
10.	DADMANAG[d]	1 if professional or manager father	.47	
11.	DADBLCOL[d]	1 if blue collar father	.12	
12.	HIDEBT[d]	1 if debt greater than $5,000 in 1960	.12	
13.	SCHGIFT	percent of medical school expenses financed by gifts	42.75	34.36
14.	MCATAVG	average score on Medical College Admissions Test	52.23	8.09
15.	MEDCN	medicine score on NBME[f]	80.34	4.84
16.	SURG	surgery score on NBME	80.46	5.17
17.	PHPM	public health and physical medicine score on NBME	80.77	5.16
18.	OBGYN	obstetrics-gynecology score on NBME	80.07	5.48
19.	PDTRC	pediatrics score on NBME	80.30	4.99
20	PRESTIGE	prestige, recognition, and reward, from CAIT[g]	29.77	3.20
21.	INTELECT	intellectual challenge, from CAIT	36.84	5.61
22.	PATCNTCT	patient contact, from CAIT	23.90	3.58
23.	PRESSURE	pressure desirable, from CAIT	27.32	4.62
24.	TEAMWORK	teamwork, from CAIT	13.92	2.15

Table 3. (Continued)

C.   Institutional Variables — Medical School

	Variable	Definition	Mean[c]	S.D.[e]
25.	PRIV[d]	1 if private medical school	.48	
26.	SCHMCAT	average MCAT score for medical		
		school (Pub.)	51.73	2.60
		(Pri.)	55.16	3.82
27.	PCTOUT	percent of entering class which is from		
		out-of-state (Pub.)	9.70	8.43
		(Pri.)	44.20	21.37
28.	BGTSTUD	budget per student (thousands)	.97	.49
29.	FACSTUD	total faculty (in full time equiv.)		
		per student	.50	.21
30.	PHDMD	ratio of Ph.D to M.D. faculty	.48	.17
31.	BASCLIN	ratio of basic to clinical science		
		faculty	.42	.13
32.	RSCHFAC	research budget per full-time faculty		
		(thous.)	8.13	4.32

D.   Institutional Variables — Internship Hospital

33.	MAJAFIL[d]	1 if major affiliation with a medical		
		school	.47	
34.	PCTAUTOP	percent of deaths undergoing		
		autopsy	.60	.16
35.	HALFSTRT[d]	1 if half or more of internships are		
		in straight services	.18	

Notes:

[a]   The following three variables are defined as the ratios of values for two specialties in each equation. For every equation, the numerator value corresponds to the specialty represented by the dependent variable. The denominator value depends on whether the dependent variable equals zero or 1. If it equals 0, then the denominator refers to the physician's actual specialty in 1972. If it equals 1, then the denominator is assumed to refer to the last different specialty in the physician's longitudinal record. Means and standard deviations vary across equations. Data are available for 1,269 direct patient-care physicians who are not subspecialists.

[b]   Standard deviations appear in parentheses.

[c]   Samples for means vary from 955 to 1,269 physicians, depending on the number of missing values. Physicians who are subspecialists or not in direct patient care are excluded.

[d]   Dichotomous variable.

[e]   Standard deviations are shown only for continuous variables.

[f]   National Board of Medical Examiners, Part II, administered in 1960.

[g]   Career Attitudes Inventory Test, administered in 1960.

III. DATA AND ESTIMATION METHOD

A. *Data Sources*

The data required for this study refer to three units of observation: individual physicians, medical schools and internship hospitals, and medical specialties. Information on individuals is provided by the Longitudinal Study of Medical Students of the Class of 1960 [Association of American Medical Colleges, (1972, 1974)]. In 1956, twenty-eight medical schools agreed to participate in a longitudinal study of physicians' career choices. Accordingly, the entire entering classes, approximately 2,800 individuals, were surveyed in 1956 about their background characteristics, during their undergraduate medical educations, at graduation in 1960, again in 1961, which was the internship year for most, and in 1965. In 1972, information from the American Medical Association's Physician Masterfile was added to the records of those physicians who could be located. The 1972 data includes self-designated specialty, practice location, type of practice, certification status, military training, and residency training history.

The two outstanding characteristics of this data file are its richness of information about each physician and its longitudinal nature. There is extensive information about each physician's family background, premedical school education, and direct measures of ability and preferences derived from a variety of tests administered to the cohort. (These tests included the Medical College Admissions Test (MCAT), the National Board of Medical Examiners test (NBME), the Allport-Vernon-Lindsay Study of Values (AVL), the Edwards Personal Preference Scale (EPPS), and the Career Attitudes Inventory Test (CAIT).)

The benefit of the longitudinal feature is that in the 1960, 1961, and 1965 rounds, physicians were asked to express their specialty preferences (or current specialty if already decided). Thus, for physicians for whom all data are available, there are four observations of specialty over a twelve-year period.

Institutional data describing the 28 medical schools are included in the Longitudinal Study data bank. Among the variables available are measures of faculty composition, budget size and structure, and numerous student body characteristics, particularly scores from the various tests (MCAT, NBME, CAIT, etc.) administered to the individual medical students.

Also included as part of the Longitudinal Study are codes identifying physicians' internship hospitals. Data on affiliation, autopsy rates, and the proportion of rotating and mixed internships offered were obtained from the *Directory of Approved Internships and Residencies,* 1961, and merged to the individual observations.

Finally, data describing the specialties themselves were from three sources. Mean net incomes in 1965 by state for nine specialties were taken from a study of physicians' incomes [Dyckman (1976), Table 15]. Modal lengths of training, defined as the first practice year less the year of graduation, controlling for military service and certification status, were computed for the 50-plus specialties recognized by the AMA from information on physicians graduated from medical school between 1955 and 1965. Third, the proportion of filled residencies in hospitals affiliated with medical schools was found in the annual survey of graduate medical education [*Journal of the American Medical Association* (1962)].

B. Estimation Method

It is now well known that the preferred method of estimation for models with dichotomous dependent variables is some type of multinomial logit or probit procedure. These methods constrain predicted values to fall within the zero-one interval, eliminate the inefficient (nonminimum variance) estimates which result from the heteroskedasticity of the error term, and generate unbiased estimates of the variance of the error term (and thus unbiased t-statistics). However, the available computer programs tend to be expensive to run, and their robustness and validity across different data sets, computing facilities, and internal algorithms have not been fully established.

Goldberger (1964) has suggested that the use of generalized least squares is an appropriate method of dealing with the problems of heteroscedasticity and biased t-statistics.[11] Although one cannot in general determine the direction or the extent of the resultant bias in the t-statistic, empirical experience with dichotomous dependent variables suggests that, for large samples, the bias in the standard errors tends to be small and positive, thereby making the computed hypotheses tests more conservative [Bowen and Finegan (1969), pp. 644–648; Comay (1971), p. 336]. Using the Monte Carlo method, another study of this problem confirmed the proximity of the ordinary and generalized least squares estimates of the standard errors for large (i.e., greater than 100) samples under a variety of assumed values for R^2 and the mean value of the dichotomous dependent variable [Smith and Cicchetti (1972)].

Use of generalized least squares does not address the problem of predicted values of the dependent variable falling outside the zero-one interval. However, the objective of this analysis is not to make point predictions of the values of the probabilities. Rather, the main purpose is to draw qualititive inferences regarding the marginal effects of small changes in the values of the independent variables. Since these effects will be evaluated around the observed mean values of the independent variables, behavior of the functions at extreme values does not seem critical.

Therefore, it will be assumed that over the relevant range of observation, a linear function is an acceptable approximation to the true functional form. Second, given the relatively large sample available (over 700 observations), the prior evidence regarding the similarity between ordinary and generalized least squares results, and the computational cumbersomeness of the latter, the former will be the principal estimation method.

The final matter to be described in this section is the drawing of the sample for the estimation of the model's parameters. Although there were approximately 2,800 physicians in the cohort initially, attrition from the cohort and nonresponse on individual variables have the effect of substantially reducing the number of usable observations. For example, only 2,524 physicians were located by the American Medical Association. The usable sample is further restricted by limiting it to physicians who practice direct patient care (as defined by the American Medical Association) since this is the professional activity with which policy is primarily concerned but who do not designate themselves as being subspecialists within a major specialty area. The latter restriction is imposed in order to increase the conformity between the specialties of the physicians in the sample and the specialties defined by the available physician income data.

The result of these various limits is to produce a final sample of 767 physicians. Although considerably smaller than the initial cohort, this sample is of sufficient size to invoke large sample properties for the estimated parameters. Further, it leaves an ample residual sample which will be used to test the validity of the model's predictions. Other than testing the model's predictions on the residual sample, however, no attempts are made either to identify the presence of systematic differences between the two subsamples or to analyze the consequences of such differences if they exist.

IV. RESULTS

A. Parameter Estimates and Hypothesis Tests

The hypothesis testing strategy chosen is based upon the study's objective of identifying factors which significantly influence physicians' specialty choices. Since the lack of an ideal data set requires the use of groups of operational variables to represent a single conceptual variable, each null hypothesis takes the form of a set of exclusion restrictions imposed on the coefficients of the relevant operational variables. For example, the hypothesis that academic ability has no effect on specialty choices is tested by assuming that the coefficients of each of the ability variable proxies [average MCAT score (MCATAVG), and the scores from the National Board of Medical Examiners test, Part II, i.e., medicine (MEDCN), surgery (SURG), public health and physical medicine (PHPM), pediatrics (PDTRC), and obstetrics/gynecology (OBGYN)] are *jointly* equal to zero. Multiparameter hypotheses of this sort are tested in two steps. First, the model is estimated under the alternative hypothesis, which is that all coefficients are free to take on any value. Then the null hypothesis is imposed by deleting the variables of interest and the model is reestimated. The null hypothesis is rejected if an F-statistic computed from the sums of squared residuals of the constrained and unconstrained equations exceeds some critical value.[12] This approach also has the advantage of lessening the impact of multicollinearity on the inferences which can be drawn. In particular, the use of groups of related operational variables to represent each of the model's conceptual variables could result in the presence of multicollinearity among the related variables. Using a well known test for assessing the degree of multicollinearity [Kmenta (1971), pp. 389–391], this in fact turned out to be the case, particularly for the so-called medical college structural variables. As such, the variances of the individual parameter estimates may be unduly large and, consequently, the associated t-statistics may be biased downward. Although the parameter estimates themselves remain unbiased, the general quality of the data and the uncertainty of the model's specification preclude placing undue emphasis on the point estimates themselves. However, the F-statistics used to test the multiparameter hypotheses are computed from the sums of squared residuals of the constrained and unconstrained regressions and, therefore, should be unaffected by the degree of multicollinearity.

Since the model consists of nine separate equations, each hypothesis must be tested for each equation. In order to conclude that a particular factor does not have a statistically significant effect on specialty choice, it is necessary to accept the null hypothesis in each of the nine specialty choice equations. Eight general null hypotheses were tested. These were:

(1) Access to funds for graduate training has no effect on specialty choice.

(2) Sociodemographic characteristics have no effect on specialty choice.

(3) Academic ability is unrelated to specialty choice.

(4) Preferences for various types of practice situations do not influence specialty choice.

(5) Medical college form of control and student body characteristics have no effect on specialty choice.[13]

(6) Medical college structural variables have no impact on specialty choice.

(7) The quality of the internship hospital teaching program has no effect on specialty choice.

(8) The characteristics of the alternative specialties are unrelated to specialty choice.

Following the procedure just outlined, the model was first estimated including the full set of variables listed in Table 3. The parameter estimates and individual tests of significance are presented in Table 4. Each of the above hypotheses was tested by deleting the appropriate subset of variables, reestimating the equations, and computing the relevant F-statistic. Table 5 presents the values of F computed for each hypothesis and equation. Only hypotheses (1) and (6), which relate access to training funds and medical school structure, respectively, to specialty choice, were not significant at the 5 percent level of confidence in all nine equations. The subsequent hypothesis that both sets of variables are jointly insignificant was formulated and tested, and, as can be seen from row 9 of Table 5, was not rejected in any of individual equations. Accordingly, the proxy variables measuring access to training funds (DADMED—physician or dentist father; DADMANAG—managerial or other professional father; DADBLCOL—blue collar or unskilled father; HIDEBT—debt greater than $5,000 in 1960; and SCHGIFT—proportion of medical college expenses financed by gifts, scholarships, grants, etc.) and medical school structure (BGTSTUD—budget per student; FACSTUD—full-time equivalent faculty per student; PHDMD—ratio of Ph.D. to M.D. faculty; RSCHFAC—research budget per full-time equivalent faculty; and BASCLIN—ration of basic to clinical science faculty) were deleted from the model and the equations reestimated with the remaining variables. These final parameter estimates, presented in Table 6, form the basis of the remaining discussion.

The first thing to consider is the model's overall validity. This is done by examining the percentage of variation explained by the independent variables, i.e., the R^2 statistic, adjusted for degrees of freedom. With the exceptions of obstetrics/gynecology and radiology, the R^2s range from .127 for pathology to .309 for internal medicine (Table 6). Given that the individual is the unit of observation, these values are quite reasonable. For the other two equations, even though the R^2s are low, .041 and .049, respectively, the hypothesis that all parameters are jointly equal to zero is rejected at the one percent confidence level.

Although performance of the model based on the R^2 criterion seems acceptable, it has been shown that when the dependent variable is

Table 4. Initial Parameter Estimates[a]

Variable	CP	IM	PED	SRG	OBG	PSY	RAD	ANES	PATH
AGE	.0209*	-.0075	-.0117*	-.0035	-.0077	-.0027	-.0074	-.0027	-.0012
FEMALE[b]	.0298	-.0804	.1217**	-.0443	-.0406	-.0768	-.0772	.2137**	.0284
MAR56[b]	.0451	-.0393	-.0255	-.0528	.0672**	-.0072	-.0097	.0337	-.0293
MARKIDS[b]	.1188**	-.0835	-.0238	.0096	-.0513	.0551	.0038	.0291	.0490
NONMETRO[b]	.0848*	-.0388	-.0306	.0372	-.0428	-.0077	-.0216	-.0360	.0216
DADMED[b]	.0284	-.0368	-.0374	.0482	.0116	.0202	-.0010	-.0160	-.0066
DADMANAG[b]	.0175	.0224	-.0295	.0034	.0276	.0138	.0076	.0020	-.0054
DADBLCOL[b]	.0169	-.0343	.0095	-.0029	.0248	.0140	-.0000	.0028	-.0088
HIDEBT[b]	.0472	-.0423	-.0247	-.0053	-.0040	.0528	-.0515	-.0066	-.0144
SCHGIFT	-.0005	.0005	.0004	-.0002	.0001	.0003	-.0007*	.0001	-.0004
MCATAVG	.0011	-.0038	-.0014	.0018	-.0016	.0040**	-.0004	.0010	-.0001
MEDCN	-.0011	.0101**	-.0006	-.0058	-.0015	-.0061	-.0021	.0021	.0014
SURG	.0104**	-.0065	-.0065**	.0049	-.0038	-.0014	.0017	-.0035	.0005
PHPM	-.0073	.0033	.0002	-.0003	.0059**	-.0056	-.0005	.0033	.0046**
OBGYN	-.0037	.0050	.0027	-.0055	-.0040	.0091*	.0019	.0012	.0011
PDTRC	.0003	-.0012	.0028	.0028	-.0000	-.0014	-.0014	-.0047	-.0055**
PRESTIGE	-.0038	.0065	-.0024	-.0009	-.0016	.0001	.0022	.0043	-.0020
INTELECT	-.0074*	.0087*	.0020	-.0017	-.0068*	.0097*	.0001	-.0006	.0034**
PATCNTCT	.0047	-.0012	.0047	-.0010	-.0003	.0150*	-.0124*	-.0134*	-.0125*
PRESSURE	.0053	-.0013*	-.0013	.0197*	.0089*	-.0241*	-.0037	.0039**	-.0009
TEAMWORK	.0008	.0078	-.0022	-.0010	-.0001	-.0135*	-.0016	.0058	.0001
PRIV[b]	.6933	-.0019	-.1006	-.1767	-.0522	-.0320	-.0852	.2605	.1720

132

SCHMCAT[c] (Pub.)	-.0094	.0138	.0028	.0078	.0061	-.0030	-.0037	.0005	-.0035
SCHMCAT[c] (Priv.)	-.0232	.0129	.0042	.0125	-.0070	-.0006	-.0018	-.0043	-.0071
PCTOUT[c] (Pub.)	-.2341	.1540	-.1213	.4222	.0903	.0918	.0756	-.0448	-.0252
PCTOUT[c] (Priv.)	-.0331	.1972	-.0439	-.0448	-.0448	-.1226	-.0158	.0710	.0209
BGTSTUD	.0057	-.0214	.0639	-.0247	-.0630	-.0212	.0173	-.0004	.0099
FACSTUD	-.1491	-.0164	-.0797	.2997**	.0412	.1639	.0053	.0403	-.0180
PHDMD	-.0137	-.0137	-.0963	.2471**	-.0669	.0313	.0161	.0312	-.1226
BASCLIN	-.1418	-.1428	.1000	.2503	-.0946	.0141	-.0170	.0480	.0684
RSCHFAC	.0141**	-.0038	-.0034	-.0123*	.0009	-.0033	.0013	.0014	.0025
MAJAFIL	-.1026*	.0473	.0542*	.0224	.0250	-.0173	.0406	-.0392**	.0086
PCTAUTOP	-.0273	.0451	.0274	.0020	.0850	-.0033	-.0536	-.0334	.0079
HALFSTRT[b]	-.0325	-.0017	.0340	.0773**	-.0183	-.0241	-.0440	-.0505**	-.0320
RELY	-.1351	.2156**	.0251	-.1208	.0080	-.0924	-.0491	.0277	-.0316
RELTRN	.1842*	.0413*	.0334**	.0195	.0054	.0823*	.0545*	.0655*	.0395*
RELPCT	-2.7145*	.4025*	.2172*	-.1240*	-.0603	-.1544*	-.1668*	-.0143	-.1831*
(CONSTANT)	1.9930	-2.0255	.0484	-.4792	.4421	.7947	1.0760	.0985	.5732
Adj. R²	.242	.311	.154	.119	.035	.233	.047	.118	.123
F	7.625	10.347	4.774	3.809	1.741	7.279	2.033	3.772	3.912

Notes:

a   767 observations
b   dichotomous variable
c   individual test of significance not computed
*   significiant at 1% level of confidence
** significant at 5% level of confidence

133

Table 5. Values of F for Null Hypotheses

Variables in Null Hypothesis	Equation								
	GP	IM	PED	SRG	OBG	PSY	RAD	ANES	PATH
1. Access to funds for graduate training (DADMD, DADMANAG, DADBLCOL, HIDEBT60, SCHGIFT)	.738	.983	1.313	.477	.326	.627	1.367	.145	.726
2. Sociodemographic preference proxies (AGE, FEMALE, MAR56, MARKIDS, NONMETRO)	8.995^a	3.838^*	5.349^*	1.603	2.101	1.323	1.752	6.297^*	1.179
3. Ability (MCATAVG, MEDCN, SURG, PHPM, OBGYN, PDTRC)	1.361	2.602^b	1.317	1.227	1.763	5.022^a	.254	1.231	1.750
4. Direct preference measures (PRESTIGE, INTELECT, PATCNTCT, PRESSURE, TEAMWORK)	16.433^a	21.519^a	18.647^a	28.541	19.373^a	44.983^a	20.281^a	22.764^a	23.608^a
5. Medical school student body variables (PRIV, SCHMCAT, PCTOUT)	2.634^b	2.344^b	.598	1.477	.326	.615	.127	.992	.835
6. Medical school structure (BGTSTUD, FACSTUD, PHDMD, BASCLIN, RSCHFAC)	2.018	1.418	.857	2.077	.646	.498	.000	.119	.712
7. Internship hospital quality (MAJAFIL, PCTAUTOP, HALFSTRT)	20.065^a	16.345^a	19.008^*	17.949^a	16.081^a	15.712^a	3.212^a	19.174^a	16.318^a
8. Specialty characteristics (RELY, RELTRN, RELPCT)	19.233^a	82.987^a	36.650^*	3.615^b	.894	13.925^a	7.111^a	12.153^*	15.214^a
9. Hypotheses 1 and 6	1.416	1.232	1.170	1.582	1.179	.946	1.459	.136	.711

[a] Significant at 1% level of confidence.
[b] Significant at 5% level of confidence.

Table 6. Final Parameter Estimates[a]

Equations

Variable	GP	IM	PED	SRG	OBG	PSY	RAD	ANES	PATH
AGE	.0221*	-.0087	-.0121*	-.0038	-.0080	-.0030	-.0063	-.0026	-.0004
FEMALE[b]	.0174	-.0641	.1265*	-.0583	-.0368	-.0736	-.0807	.2149*	.0307
MAR56[b]	.0568	-.0520	-.0347	-.0471	.0609	-.0115	.0065	.0302	-.0184
MARKIDS[b]	.1175**	-.0849	-.0220	.0128	-.0525	-.0417	-.0140	-.0285	.0420
NONMETRO[b]	.0938*	-.0502	-.0381	.0411	-.0418	-.0049	-.0187	-.0364	.0212
MCATAVG	.0008	-.0036	-.0013	.0018	-.0017	.0040**	-.0004	.0011	-.0000
MEDCN	-.0028	.0115*	-.0001	-.0056	-.0017	-.0054	-.0025	-.0021	.0017
SURG	.0119*	-.0073	-.0068**	.0043	-.0037	-.0022	.0018	-.0034	.0005
PHPM	.0064	.0029	-.0001	-.0009	.0058**	-.0054	-.0002	.0030	.0047**
OBGYN	-.0038	.0047	.0026	-.0054	-.0040	.0094*	.0020	.0014	.0009
PDTRC	.0002	-.0008	.0026	.0031	.0007	-.0022	-.0013	-.0046	-.0057**
PRESTIGE	-.0041	.0069	-.0023	-.0010	-.0076	.0000	.0016	.0042	-.0020
INTELECT	-.0079*	.0085*	.0019	-.0007	-.0070*	.0099*	.0003	-.0006	.0035**
PATCNTCT	.0057	-.0015	.0045	-.0018	-.0003	.0149*	-.0119*	-.0134*	-.0123*
PRESSURE	.0054	-.0110*	-.0014	.0196*	.0091*	-.0242*	-.0038	.0037**	.0010
TEAMWORK	-.0000	.0087	-.0023	-.0013	-.0000	-.0132*	-.0018	.0055	.0004
PRIV[b]	.7831	-.0855	-.2661	-.1762	.0413	-.0464	-.0490	.2597	.1951
SCHMCAT[c](Pub.)	-.0000	.0082	-.0013	.0018	.0058	-.0012	-.0003	-.0004	-.0026
SCHMCAT[c](Priv.)	-.0154	.0098	.0038	.0049	.0048	.0009	.0007	-.0054	-.0060
PCTOUT[c](Pub.)	-.1309	.2586	-.0257	.0827	-.0093	.0664	.1053	-.0854	.1097
PCTOUT[c](Priv.)	-.0702	.1503	-.0528	.0762	-.0275	-.0905	-.0069	.0862	-.0042
MAJAFIL[b]	-.1005*	.0542**	.0520*	.0146	.0299	-.0152	.0348	-.0407**	.0048
PCTAUTOP	-.0064	.0132	.0188	-.0003	.0725	.0028	-.0433	-.0337	.0195
HALFSTRT[b]	-.0544	.0128	.0503	.0788**	-.0282	-.0151	-.0451	-.0479**	.0369
RELY	-.1178**	.2185**	.0223	-.1673**	.0206	-.0943	-.0621	.0242	-.0276
RELTRN	.1784*	.0386*	.0314	.0187	.0063	.0823*	.0530*	-.0653*	.0382*
RELPCT	-2.5678*	.4078*	.2191*	-.1241*	-.0614	-.1584*	-.1597*	-.0161	.1790*
(CONSTANT)	1.3044	-1.8779	.3102	.2228	.4091	.8223	.8537	.2082	.4130
Adj. R[2]	.238	.309	.152	.113	.041	.237	.049	.128	.127
F	9.870	13.680	6.095	4.597	2.214	9.817	2.474	5.180	5.118

Notes:

[a] 767 observations
[b] dichotomous variable
[c] individual test of significance not computed
*   significant at 1% level of confidence
** significant at 5% level of confidence

dichotomous, the R^2 is subject to bias [Goodman (1976), pp. 5–6]. There-fore, an alternative and perhaps more appropriate method for assessing the model's validity is to test how well it predicts physicians' specialty choices. Using the estimated parameters from Table 6 and values of the independent variables specific to each physician, estimates of the prob-abilities of selecting each specialty were calcualted for each physician. The decision rule adopted was that the physician selects the specialty which has the largest predicted value. The distribution of predicted specialties can then be compared to the distribution of actual specialty choices, and the proportion of correct predictions used to assess validity.

Tables 7 and 8 compare the predicted and actual specialty choices based on the parameter estimates of Table 6. In testing the predictive ability of a model, it is generally desirable to use a sample which was not involved in the parameter estimation. There are two sources of additional observations: physicians who had missing information for one or more variables and physicians who were subspecialists within a broader spe-cialty. These groups were sequentially added to the initial sample, result-ing in sample sizes of 1,266 and 1,770 physicians for the purpose of mak-ing predictions.[14] Mean values from the base sample were substituted for variables with missing values.

For both samples of physicians the model seems to perform quite well, with over 50 percent of the specialty choices correctly predicted. This compares quite favorably to prediction based on random allocation to each specialty with equal probabilities, which on average would correctly predict about 11 percent of the specialty choices.[15] Within individual specialties, the proportion of correct predictions varied from 34.7 percent for obstetrics/gynecology to 74.7 percent for internal medicine (Table 7). It is also of some interest to examine the pattern of incorrect predictions. This gives some indication of how actual choices deviated from predicted choices. In particular, 33.4 percent of predicted general practitioners selected either general surgery or obstetrics/gynecology. On the other hand, 22.9 percent of predicted internists, 51.1 percent of predicted pediatricians, and 26.7 percent of predicted anesthesiologists chose gen-eral practice. Third, general surgery and obstetrics/gynecology appeared to be closely related. The other specialties had less distinctive patterns of incorrect predictions.

Before turning to the substantive findings of the model, a number of caveats should be raised. First, this study's results are based on the behavior of only a single cohort of physicians who graduated from medi-cal school in 1960. Since that time there have been a number of dramatic changes in both the medical care and medical education systems, e.g., Medicare and Medicaid, the abolition of free-standing internships, and large increases in the total numbers of physicians, medical students,

Table 7. Comparison of Actual and Predicted Specialties: Primary Specialists Only[a]

Actual Choice	Predicted Choice[b]									N	%
	GP	IM	PED	SRG	OBG	PSY	RAD	ANES	PATH		
GP	*52.9*	22.9	51.1	0.0	2.7	5.3	0.0	26.7	1.0	289	22.8
IM	6.3	*74.7*	0.0	7.6	2.7	11.7	14.5	1.1	13.3	255	20.1
PED	2.9	0.0	*46.7*	2.3	4.2	6.4	3.9	3.3	3.1	97	7.7
SRG	16.3	0.4	0.0	*45.8*	19.4	2.3	7.9	4.4	8.2	138	10.9
OBG	17.1	0.0	0.0	15.3	*34.7*	2.9	14.5	3.3	8.2	114	9.0
PSY	1.7	0.4	1.5	13.0	6.9	*60.2*	11.8	5.6	9.2	156	12.3
RAD	2.1	0.8	0.7	7.6	12.5	7.6	*44.7*	1.1	10.2	86	6.8
ANES	0.8	0.0	0.0	4.6	12.5	2.9	2.6	*51.1*	5.1	76	6.0
PATH	0.0	0.8	0.0	3.8	4.2	0.6	0.0	3.3	*41.8*	55	4.3
N	240	245	137	131	72	171	76	90	98	1,266[c,d]	100%
%	19.0	19.4	10.8	10.3	5.7	13.5	6.0	7.1	7.7	100%	

Notes:

a Each column shows the percentage distribution of physicians predicted to choose a particular specialty by their actual specialty. Thus, the second element of the first column indicates that 6.3 percent of the physicians predicted to choose general practice in fact chose a medical specialty. The diagonal elements of the table are the proportion correctly predicted by specialty.

b Column percentages may not sum to 100% due to rounding.

c 53.95 percent of all physicians are correctly classified.

d This sample excludes subspecialists but includes physicians with missing data.

137

Table 8. Comparison of Actual and Predicted Specialties: All Physicians in Direct Patient Care[a]

Actual Choice	Predicted Choice[b]									N	%
	GP	IM	PED	SRG	OBG	PSY	RAD	ANES	PATH		
GP	34.2	17.5	52.6	0.3	1.7	2.8	0.0	25.0	0.0	289	16.3
IM	9.2	80.7	1.2	5.7	5.1	9.8	16.9	3.0	12.8	387	21.9
PED	2.3	0.0	43.9	2.2	0.0	4.5	1.1	2.0	1.4	106	6.0
SRG	30.9	0.3	0.6	68.4	42.4	17.9	27.0	9.0	35.5	464	26.2
OBG	12.2	0.0	0.0	12.0	25.4	2.8	6.7	3.0	5.0	113	6.4
PSY	4.9	0.0	1.2	2.8	6.8	52.0	9.0	6.0	3.5	177	10.0
RAD	3.6	0.6	0.6	4.4	8.5	7.3	37.1	2.0	9.2	99	5.6
ANES	2.0	0.0	0.0	2.2	6.8	2.4	2.4	47.0	2.1	75	4.2
PATH	0.7	0.9	0.0	1.9	3.4	0.4	0.0	3.0	30.5	60	3.4
N	304	342	173	316	59	246	89	100	141	1,770[c,d]	100%
%	17.2	19.3	9.8	17.9	3.3	13.9	5.0	5.6	8.0	100%	

Notes:

a   Each column shows the percentage distribution of physicians predicted to choose a particular specialty by their mutual specialty. Thus, the second element of the first column indicates that 9.2 percent of the physicians predicted to choose general practice in fact chose a medical specialty. The diagonal elements of the table are the proportion correctly predicted by specialty.

b   Column percentages may not sum to 100% due to rounding.

c   53.00 percent of all physicians are correctly classified.

d   Includes both subspecialists and physicians with missing data.

foreign medical graduates, and the proportions of female and minority medical students. These types of changes limit the extent to which findings can be applied directly to current problems. Second, some variables, especially proxies for expectations of specialty characteristics, may be measured with error. Again, caution is in order. Third, all conclusions and inferences will be implicitly prefaced by the condition that other factors are held constant. This is particularly important when findings are to be compared with other studies which may have used simple bivariate correlations or tabular relationships which do not hold constant the influence of other variables. Therefore, this research should be considered primarily an exploration of a method (the specification and estimation of a micro choice model) for studying physicians' specialty choice. Its results must be considered tentative in the absence of corroborative findings based on other, hopefully better suited data and more appropriate estimation techniques.

The first general question posed at the beginning of this paper was "What factors affect specialty choices?" Given an interest in designing policies to influence these choices, it is useful to group the model's variables into financial factors, institutional factors, and personal factors (which could be related to admissions criteria at both the undergraduate and graduate medical education levels). The following three subsections will discuss inferences pertinent to formulating policies directed at manipulating these types of variables.

A.1. Financial Variables

Variables measuring financial factors included proxies for access to training funds (father's occupation, represented by the three dichotomous variables DADMED, DADMANAG, DADBLCOL, whether more than $5,000 debt in 1960, HIDEBT, and the proportion of medical school expenses financed by gifts from parents, scholarships, trust funds, etc., SCHGIFT), the ratio of mean net incomes for pairs of specialties, RELY, and the ratio of modal lengths of postmedical school training for pairs of specialties, RELTRN, as a proxy for opportunity costs. From Table 5, it can be seen that the access to training funds variables were statistically insignificant in each of the nine equations. On its face, this suggests that loan-forgiveness programs tied to debt-financed medical education would have little influence on specialty choices. However, it must be pointed out that this particular sample was highly homogeneous and fairly well off financially to begin with. Table 2, for example, indicates that 44 percent of these physicians had fathers in medical, other professional, or managerial occupations; only 12 percent reported debts (of all types) greater than $5,000 in 1960; and the average proportion of medical school expenses financed by gifts was over 40 percent. Therefore, the composition of this sample makes it difficult to predict the effects of large increases in indebtedness, say on the order of $10,000 per year of medical education, for students with more heterogeneous financial backgrounds.

Perhaps more surprising are the results regarding relative income, RELY, and relative length of training, RELTRN. Only one of the nine relative income variables (in the equation for internal medicine, IM) was both positive and statistically significant as hypothesized. This finding must be tempered, however, by the potential bias arising from the measurement error due to the inability to directly observe expected relative incomes. In particular, it is plausible that a physician might have higher than average income expectations for his/her chosen specialty and lower than average expectations for rejected specialties. Therefore, a variable measuring the ratio of average specialty incomes would systematically understate the value of the true variable which is based on expectations.

An alternative explanation of this result, however, is that physicians make their specialty choices subject to an income constraint or minimum acceptable income level. If on average physicians expected to attain this income *regardless* of which specialty was chosen, then relative income would not affect specialty choices. It would follow, then, that policies such as paying subsidies to physicians choosing shortage specialties or altering relative reimbursement rates would amount to little more than pure income transfers to physicians who would have made those choices anyway.

The hypothesis that financial factors are not significant is also supported by the parameters of RELTRN, the ratio of modal lengths of postmedical school training. It was hypothesized that with the influence of income, prestige, and ease of access to residency training positions (RELY and RELPCT) held constant, choices should be inversely related to the relative length of training. However, RELTRN is positive in eight of the nine equations and is statistically significant at the one percent confidence level in five of the eight. This suggests that, other things being equal, a physician is more likely to select a specialty with a longer training period. To the extent that longer training is correlated with increased specialization and higher skill attainment (across specialties, since subspecialists were excluded from the sample), then this finding is quite consistent with the frequently cited trend of the 1950s and 1960s toward greater specialization. It is also consistent with the results of three other economic analyses of specialty choice which found the monetary rate of return to specialty training to be negative in some cases [Sloan (1970), pp. 53–54; Lindsay (1973), pp. 333–334; American Medical Association (1973), p. 97]. One might speculate, therefore, that psychic returns and preferences may be more important than financial factors.

A.2. Institutional Variables

Interest in institutional variables stems primarily from the potential policy of altering institutional structure in order to influence specialty choices. This could be done either directly by private decision makers within the medical education system, or indirectly by public decision makers through the use of either financial incentives and disincentives or direct regulation. [Both approaches are included in the Health Professions Educational Assistance Act of 1976 (PL 94-484).] Perhaps one of the more surprising results of the hypothesis tests reported in Table 5 is that the set of medical school structure variables (budget per student, faculty per student, research budget per faculty, and the ratios of Ph.D. to M.D. and clinical to basic science faculty) is statistically insignificant. However, one should not necessarily interpret this to mean that undergraduate medical education has no effect on specialty choice. What is suggested, rather, is that this particular set of variables does not seem to be systematically related to specialty choice. The true relationship may be more complex and difficult to represent than can be done by these easily observable structural variables. Another possible factor, explored below, is that variations in medical student characteristics are more important than variations in medical school characteristics in explaining specialty choices. If true, then it may be the case that medical schools can make decisions about these types of structural variables without having to consider possible consequences for specialty distribution.

The three proxy measures of internship hospital quality, major affiliation with a medical school (MAJAFIL), the autopsy rate (PCTAUTOP), and whether half or more of the internships are in straight services (HALFSTRT) were generally significant. Since the free-standing internship no longer exists, the implications of these variables have little direct relevance to current policy formulation. (One probable consequence of eliminating internships is that more specialty decisions are made before medical school graduation.) It may be interesting to note, however, that to the extent that these variables are related to teaching program quality, all three were negatively related to the choice of anesthesiology and positively related to choosing pediatrics, internal medicine, and pathology. Signs were mixed for the other five specialties.

A.3. Personal Characteristics

Physicians' personal characteristics may be loosely associated with admissions policies in the sense that they are pertinent to the process of allocating medical school applicants to various medical schools and graduates to residency programs. These criteria are presumably subject to manipulation by either private and/or public policy makers. The issue of whether factors other than ability ought to be considered in medical school admissions decisions is both controversial and beyond the scope of this paper. The purpose here is merely to investigate whether personal characteristics are systematically associated with certain specialty choices on a *ceteris paribus* basis.

The most statistically significant set of variables were those measuring preferences for various aspects of medical practice (PRESTIGE, IN-TELECT, PATCNTCT, PRESSURE, TEAMWORK). As described earlier, these variables are based on a factor analysis of individuals' ratings of a number of practice-related characteristics. Table 9 reproduces the scoring key which allocates the individual items to their respective factors and indicates the direction of their effects. By and large, the relationships implied by the parameter signs appear quite consistent with at least a layman's view of specialty stereotypes. Desire for intellectual challenge (INTELECT) is positively related to choosing internal medicine, psychiatry, and pathology, and negatively related to general practice and obstetrics/gynecology. Patient contact (PATCNTCT) is negative in the radiology, anesthesiology, and pathology equations and positive in the psychiatry equation. Finally, desire for pressure (PRESSURE) has a positive effect on choosing surgery, obstetrics/gynecology or anesthesiology, but a negative effect on internal medicine and psychiatry. Although preferences cannot be directly observed, this finding tends to reinforce the hypothesis raised above that nonmonetary factors are more important determinants of specialty choices than financial considerations.

Academic ability was measured by the average score on the Medical College Admissions Test (MCATAVG) and scores from the National Board of Medical Examiners, Part II (MEDCN, SURG, PHPM, OBGYN, PDTRC). Although this set of variables was statistically significant, no clear pattern emerges from the pattern of parameter signs. For some of the coefficients, the implied elasticities are quite large. For example, a 1.0 percent increase in the medicine score of the NBME (MEDCN) would increase the probability of choosing internal medicine by 4.04 percent, and a 1.0 percent increase in the surgery score (SURG) would increase the probabilities of choosing general practice or surgery by about 3.65 percent. However, these figures probably overstate the true effect of an exogenous change in these scores, since a physician who *plans* to enter either internal medicine or surgery would be expected to concentrate on the medicine and surgery portions of the NBME, respectively.

The coefficients of the demographic variables tend to be quite consistent with both hypothesized effects and prior research. Age at graduation (AGE) is positively related to choosing general practice, and has a negative effect on each of the other eight specialties. (The elasticity associated with the coefficient of AGE in the GP equation implies that an increase of one year in the average age at graduation to 27.95 would increase the

Table 9. Scoring Key for the Career Attitudes Inventory Questionnaire

Factor I – Prestige, Recognition, and Reward

Item No.	Item	Direction of Effect
14.	ample recognition for what you do	
13.	high prestige in medical profession	Positive
7.	standard of living above average for M.D.	
11.	patients really appreciate effort	
39.	not received recognition for efforts	
40.	only average prestige in medical profession	Negative
34.	only moderate financial rewards	
38.	seldom know if efforts appreciated	

Factor II – Intellectual Challenge

19.	uncertainties in diagnosis and therapy	
35.	many opportunities to contribute to knowledge	
41.	extensive reading and study	Positive
5.	difficult diagnostic problems	
45.	develop new treatment procedures	
32.	straightforward diagnostic problems	
46.	few uncertainties in diagnosis or therapy	
20.	treatment procedures well established	Negative
10.	few opportunities to contribute to knowledge	
16.	minimum amount of reading and study	
33.	effects of treatments assessed immediately	

Factor III – Patient Contact

29.	work closely with patient and family	
51.	see patients many times	Positive
1.	know patients well	
28.	close relations with patients not required	
26.	rarely see patient more than once or twice	Negative
4.	little contact with patient's family	

Factor IV – Pressure Desirable

42.	frequently required to meet emergencies	
49.	important decisions made rapidly	Positive
21.	frequently have patient's life in hands	
17.	considerable degree of manual skill required	
30.	"on call" at all hours	
48.	rarely have patient's life in hands	
15.	rarely meet emergency situations	Negative
44.	little manual skill required	
24.	ample time before important decisions	

Source: Association of American Medical Colleges, "Instruments Used in Collecting the Data and Tape Documentation Manual," Vol. II: "An Archive of Research Publications, Notes, and Data Reports." Report prepared under U.S. Department of Health, Education, and Welfare, Contract No. HSM 110-72096 (Washington, D.C.: Association of American Medical Colleges, 1972).

probability of choosing general practice by about 9.7 percent.) Female physicians are more likely than male physicians to select pediatrics or anesthesiology, by about 13 and 21 percent, respectively. Physicians who came from small towns (NONMETRO), were married at entry to medical school (MAR56), and had children by 1960 (MARKIDS) are about 27 percent more likely to choose general practice than a physician who did not fit any of the above conditions. Although none of these variables have large quantitative impacts individually, the fact that there is an oversupply of medical school applicants, many of whom are considered to be academically qualified, suggests that systematic preferences for one type of applicant over another may be a highly *cost-effective* policy tool for affecting specialty distribution. As stated earlier, however, implementation of such a policy depends on the resolution of the legal definition of discrimination.

Two final variables pertinent to admissions policies are a medical school's student body average score on the Medical College Admissions Test (SCHMCAT) and the proportion of accepted applicants who are out-of-state residents (PCTOUT). Since public schools may differ systematically from private schools with regard to accepting nonresident applicants, separate variables for SCHMCAT and PCTOUT were entered for public and private schools. From Table 5, one might conclude that the influence of these variables is small, based on their statistical significance. However, the quantitative effects implied by the elasticities of SCHMCAT suggest otherwise. For private schools, a 1.0 percent increase in the average MCAT score, from 55.16 to 55.71, would reduce the probability of choosing general practice by 3.72 percent and increase the probabilities of choosing internal medicine, surgery, pediatrics, or obstetrics/gynecology by between about 2.5 and 3.0 percent. For public schools the effects are less significant.

B. Inferences Based on Predictive Ability

Most of the above discussion concerning the impacts and inferences of various types of variables has been based on the traditional criteria of statistical significance and quantitative impact. A second approach is to ask how important certain variables are to making accurate predictions of specialty choices. This is one way of estimating the cost of not knowing certain information.

In order to address this question, groups of variables were deleted from the model and the parameters of the remaining variables were reestimated. The new set of parameters were then used to predict specialty choices following the method described above for generating Table 7. The difference in the proportion of correct predictions was then computed for all specialties combined and for each separate specialty, using Table 7 as a baseline. Table 10 displays the changes in predictive power for several such prediction simulations.

Based on this exercise, it appears that the most important type of information for predicting specialty choices is the characteristics of the specialties themselves. Deletion of the three specialty variables RELY, RELTRN, and RELPCT resulted in an overall reduction in predictive accuracy of 16.0 percent. The next most important set of variables by this criterion is the direct preference measures, which results in a 4.4 percent reduction in predictive accuracy. Deletion of the academic ability variables and the medical school admissions variables results in negligible reductions in the overall rate of correct predictions.

Since data collection and research on specialty choice are not costless activities, it is hoped that this last exercise might provide some evidence for evaluating the relative importance of alternative data collection strategies. In particular, it seems that the highest payoffs might come from information about expectations regarding the characteristics of specialties. These should include both the objective (income, hours worked, opportunity costs) and subjective (prestige, patient contact, pressure, etc.) aspects of specialties. Such information should be collected from both medical students and practicing specialists. Comparisons of the two would tell us how changes in practice conditions affect medical students' expectations, and that in turn should enable better predictions of how changes in specialty characteristics might influence specialty choices.

V. SUMMARY AND CONCLUSIONS

The objectives of this study were twofold: to identify factors which may affect specialty choices and to evaluate their importance in terms of the ability to predict specialty outcomes. The methodology employed was based upon a micro-behavioral model of intra-occupational choice. Possible choice outcomes were represented by a set of nine dichotomous dependent variables, whose corresponding equations embodied pairwise comparisons between alternative specialties. The independent variables measured specialty, individual, and institutional characteristics.

The model's parameters were estimated using a sample of 767 physicians who graduated from medical school in 1960. (Physicians who were subspecialists, not in direct patient care, or had missing values for at least one variable were not included in the sample.) The model was specified to be linear in the parameters and was estimated by ordinary least squares. After deleting a number of variables found to be statistically insignificant in each of the nine equations, the estimated parameters were used to predict specialty choices for two expanded samples. In both cases, over

Table 10. Absolute Changes in Percent Correctly Predicted[a]

Variables Deleted	ALL SPECS	GP	IM	PED	SRG	OBG	PSY	RAD	ANES	PATH
1. PRESTIGE, INTELECT, PATCNTCT, PRESSURE TEAMWORK	- 4.4	- 6.0	- 1.5	- 0.8	-10.5	-10.4	- 8.0	- 4.4	4.7	- 1.6
2. MCATAYG, MEDCN, SURG, PHPM, OBGYN, PDTRC	0.2	- 2.1	- 1.1	2.1	1.0	- 9.2	2.5	- 5.4	1.5	3.9
3. PRESTIGE, INTELECT, PATCNTCT, PRESSURE, TEAM-WORK, MCATAVG, MEDCN, SURG, PHPM, OBGYN, PDTRC	- 4.9	- 8.9	- 4.0	4.8	- 3.5	-20.4	- 5.1	-10.0	2.2	- 2.1
4. PRIV, SCHMCAT, PCTOUT, MAJAFIL, PCTAUTOP, HALFSTRT	- 1.8	- 2.9	- 5.3	- 1.1	- 5.5	- 1.8	0.0	8.7	4.6	- 2.4
5. RELY, RELTRN, RELPCT	-16.0	- 0.2	-24.4	-21.7	-13.1	- 91.7	-22.5	-16.1	-24.5	-15.0

a Based on 1,266 physicians and the distribution of correct predictions from Table 7.

146

50 percent of the choices were correctly predicted. This suggests that the model successfully identified a substantial portion of the specialty choice process.

From the point of view of policy, the major findings were that financial factors did not appear to have a significant effect on choices. Rather, preferences for various nonfinancial aspects of medical practice and for increased specialization in general seemed to be more dominant factors. However, these conclusions must be conditioned upon likely measurement errors in the data and substantial changes in students' backgrounds and medical education costs over the last 16 years.

Second, a set of variables approximating medical school structure was also found not to be significant. This does not necessarily imply that medical schools don't matter, but that manipulation of these particular variables would probably not have much impact on specialty outcomes. If there is an effect of medical education institutions independent of student characteristics, then it is apparently too complex to be captured via easily observable proxy variables.

Third, physicians' personal chraacteristics, especially preferences for various aspects of medical practice, appeared to have a statistically significant effect on specialty choices. Since there is a considerable oversupply of medical school applicants, changes in admissions criteria could be a highly cost-effective method of affecting future specialty distribution. This of course begs the question of how preferences can be measured and how they are affected by external, background, and institutional factors.

Finally, a simple policy simulation revealed that exclusion of the relative specialty characteristics variables had the largest impact on the model's predictive ability. Next most important were the direct preference measures. Failure to include the academic ability or institutional variables resulted in only negligible decreases in the rate of correct predictions.

What has been learned from this effort? Hopefully, it has been demonstrated that micro data and micro choice models can be usefully applied to the study of specialty choices and, by extension, to other aspects of medical career choice, such as location and practice mode. Since this approach has expensive data demands, the question of what types of information are most important is certainly relevant. Based on the findings, data on expectations of specialty characteristics, both monetary and nonmonetary, and their relative importance to each physician would seem to be the key ingredients for successful use of this method as a predictive tool. A critical part of this process would be collection of corresponding data from practicing specialists in order to determine the link between current practice conditions and expectations formation.

While much remains to be learned about the specialty choice process, two areas seem particularly important. One is the relation between financial factors, primarily education financing and expected earnings, and specialty choice. For several reasons enumerated above, the findings of this study can be considered only tentative. The potential costs of such policies and the relative ease with which they can be implemented require that more extensive research be carried out with multiple data sets.

The second is the area of preference formation and measurement. Failure to include such factors in economic models of physicians' career choices may be a serious omission which results in biased implications for other policies. Since ecomomists are not likely to have a comparative advantage in this line of inquiry, this would seem a fruitful realm for collaboration between economists, sociologists, and psychologists.

FOOTNOTES

*Computer work for this study was performed while the author was employed by the Division of Intramural Research, National Center for Health Services Research, U.S. Department of Health, Education, and Welfare (HEW). All conclusions and statements, however, are solely the responsibility of the author and do not necessarily represent either the policy or position of any office of HEW.

1. In 1971, general practitioners averaged 171.5 patient visits per week compared to 127.2 for internists [Vahovich (1973), p. 59].

2. The other side of the coin, of course, is the normative question of what should the physician specialty distribution look like. This study, however, limits itself only to the positive research issues posed in the text.

3. Examples of stereotypes are the following [Geertsma and Grinols (1972), p. 510]:

Medicine:	Sensitive to a wide rane of factors when evaluating a medical problem and deeply interested in intellectual problems.
Psychiatry:	Deeply interested in intellectual problems, emotionally unstable, confused thinker.
Surgery:	Domineering and arrogant, aggressive and full of energy, and mainly concerned with own prestige.
General Practice:	Deeply interested in people, aggressive and full of energy, extremely patient, friendly, pleasing personality, and sensitive to a wide range of problems when evaluating a medical problem.

4. However, this is a larger choice set than in any previous study of specialty choice. The nine specialties are general practice, internal medicine, pediatrics, general surgery, obstetrics/gynecology, psychiatry, radiology, anesthesiology, and pathology.

5. Becker discusses the issue of whether variables should be constructed as ratios or differences [Becker (1964), pp. 52–53]. Neither argument appears to be clearly preferred in this particular case. However, in an earlier study of specialty choice, a similar model was estimated in both ratios and first difference form [Hadley (1975), pp. 168, 324]. There was little difference in either statistical significance or quantitative implications.

6. In a number of cases, reported specialties were identical in all four observation periods. The assumption made, therefore, was that this type of physician was most likely to have considered the alternative specialty most frequently reported by other physicians who had the same current specialty and were from the same medical school.

7. In order to increase the amount of variation in this variable, it was assumed that the appropriate reference population was limited to physicians in the state in which the individual physician was located when he/she first indicated a preference for the specialty actually chosen. This would be either a medical school, internship, or residency training state. Further, state means were normalized by dividing through by the appropriate national specialty mean value.

8. Aggregate preference, of course, will be a function of both prestige and all other factors which make a specialty choice desirable, including expected income. Unfortunately, these influences cannot be separated in this variable.

9. Each physician's actual length of training is issued for the current specialty. Modal lengths of training were derived from distributions of the lengths of training by specialty, controlling for board certification and military status, of all 1955–1965 U.S. medical school graduates.

10. Age at graduation (AGE) may also affect the rate of time preference, i.e., older physicians may be less willing to postpone current consumption. This effect, however, works in the same direction as the hypothesized effect of age on the expected monetary return, and, therefore, cannot be separately identified.

11. This involves a two-stage procedure. In the first stage one estimates a linear probability function using ordinary least squares regression analysis in order to generate estimates of the predicted values of the dependent variables, $\hat{y}_1$. Each observation is then multiplied by $\dfrac{1}{\sqrt{y_i(1-y_i)}}$ and the model is reestimated with ordinary least squares. It can be shown that this transformation produces both efficient parameter estimates and unbiased t-statistics [Goldberger (1964), pp. 245–250].

12. The particular formula for F is

$$F(r,n\text{-}k) = \frac{(Q_0 - Q_a)/r}{Q_a/(n\text{-}k)}$$

where Q_0 is the sum of squared residuals under the null hypothesis (that certain coefficients are equal to zero), Q_a is the sum of squared residuals under the alternative hypothesis (that all variables belong in the equation), r is the number of variables deleted, and n-k is the number of degrees of freedom.

13. The form of control variable, PRIV, is included with this hypothesis because interaction variables are constructed between PRIV and average school MCAT score, SCHMCAT, and the proportion of out of state acceptances, PCTOUT, in order to determine whether the effects of these variables are different in public and private medical colleges.

14. The particular computer program used made sequential addition of extra blocks of observations considerably more convenient than separate predictions for each group.

15. In Hadley (1975), a simple prediction routine was devised for allocating physicians into five specialty groups using the proportion of physicians known to be in each group as the allocation probabilities. For 50 iterations of this model, the average proportion of correct predictions was .21, only slightly better than random allocation with equal probabilities.

REFERENCES

American Medical Association, Center for Health Services Research and Development (1973), "Contributions to a Comprehensive Health Manpower Strategy," report prepared for the Office of the Secretary, U.S. Department of Health, Education, and Welfare, Chicago: American Medical Association.

Association of American Medical Colleges (January 1974), "The Longitudinal Study of Medical Students of the Class of 1960," Washington, D.C.: Association of American Medical Colleges.

—— (1972), "Instruments Used in Collecting the Data and Tape Documentation Manual, Vol. II: An Archive of Research Publications, Notes, and Data Reports," report prepared under U.S. Department of Health, Education, and Welfare contract No. HSM 110-72-96, Washington, D.C.: Association of American Medical Colleges.

Becker, G. S. (1964), *Human Capital*, New York: National Bureau of Economic Research.

Boskin, M. J. (March-April 1974), "A Conditional Logit Model of Occupational Choice," *Journal of Political Economy* 82: 389–398.

Bowen, W. G. and Finegan, T. A (1969), *The Economics of Labor Force Participation*, Princeton, N.J.: Princeton University Press.

Coker, R. E., Miller, N., and Back, K. W. (March 1960), "The Medical Student, Specialization and General Practice," *North Carolina Medical Journal* 21: 96–101.

Comay, Y. (Summer 1971), "Influences on the Migration of Canadian Professionals," *The Journal of Human Resources* 6: 333–344.

Dyckman, Z. (1976), *study of Physicians' Incomes in the Pre-Medicare Period*, Washington, D.C.: U.S. Department of Health, Education, and Welfare, Social Security Administration.

Fein, R. and Weber, G. I. (1971), *Financing Medical Education*, New York: McGraw-Hill Book Co.

Freeman, R. B. (1971), *The Market for College-Trained Manpower: A Study in the Economics of Career Choice*, Cambridge, Mass.: Harvard University Press.

Friedman, M. and Kuznets, S. (1946), *Income from Independent Professional Practice*, New York: National Bureau of Economic Research.

Gallaway, L. E. (1967), *Interindustry Labor Mobility in the United States 1956 to 1960*, U.S. Department of Health, Education, and Welfare, Social Security Administration, Office of Research and Statistics, Research Report No. 18, Washington, D.C.: Government Printing Office.

Geertsma, R. H. and Grinols, D. R. (July 1972), "Specialty Choice in Medicine," *Journal Medical Education* 47: 509–517.

Glaser, W. A. (December 1959), "Internship Appointments of Medical Students," *Administrative Science Quarterly*, 4:337–356.

Goldberger, A. S. (1964), *Econometric Theory*, New York: John Wiley & Sons.

Goodman, J. L. (March 1976), "Is Ordinary Least Squares Estimation with a Dichotomous Dependent Variable Really That Bad?" Working paper 216-23, Washington, D.C.: The Urban Institute.

Hadley, J. L. (October 1975), "Models of Physicians' Specialty and Location Decisions," Technical Paper Series Number 6, National Center for Health Services Research, Health Resource Administration, U.S.D.H.E.W.

Hughes, E. F. X., Lewit, E. M., and Lorenzo, F. V. (March 1975), "Time Utilization of a Population of General Surgeons in Community Practice," *Surgery* 77:371–383.

Institute of Medicine (March 1976), "Medicare-Medicaid Reimbursement Policies," contract no. SSA-PMB-74-250, Office of Research and Statistics, Social Security Administration, U.S. D.H.E.W.

Journal of the American Medical Association (November 17, 1962; November 12, 1960).

Journal of Medical Education (September 1970), "Datagram" 45: 716.

Kendall, P. L. and Selvin, H. C. (1957), "Tendencies Toward Specialization in Medical Training," in *The Student Physician,* pp. 153–174, edited by R. K. Merton, G. G. Reader, and P. L. Kendall, Cambridge, Mass.: Harvard University Press.

Kessel, R. A. (Spring 1970), "The A.M.A. and the Supply of Physicians," *Law and Contemporary Problems* 35: 267–283.

Kmenta, J. (1971), *Elements of Econometrics,* New York: The Macmillan Company.

Kosa, J. and Coker, R. E. (March 1965), "The Female Physician in Public Health: Conflict and Reconciliation of the Sex and Professional Roles," *Sociology and Social Research* 49: 294–305.

Lancaster, K. J. (April 1966), "A New Approach to Consumption Theory," *Journal of Political Economy* 74: 132–157.

Lindsay, C. (Summer 1973), "Real Returns to Medical Education," *Journal of Human Resources* 8: 331–348.

Lopate, C. (1968), *Women in Medicine,* Baltimore: The Johns Hopkins University Press.

Lowenstein, L. M. (April 1971), "Who Wants Lady Interns?" *New England Journal of Medicine* 284: 735.

Lyden, F. J., Geiger, H. J., and Peterson, O. L. (1968), *The Training of Good Physicians.* Cambridge, Mass.: Harvard University Press.

Monk, M. A. and Terris, M. (December 13, 1956), "Factors in Student Choice of General or Specialty Practice," *New England Journal of Medicine* 255: 1135–1140.

Mumford, E. (1970), *Interns: From Students to Physicians,* Cambridge, Mass.: Harvard University Press.

Nickerson, R. J. Colton, T., Peterson, O. L., Bloom, B. S., and Hauck, W. W. (April 1975), "Physicians Who Do Operations," Contract no. NOI-MI-24078, Bureau of Health Resources Development, Health Resources Administration. U.S. D.H.E.W.

Otis, G. D. and Weiss, J. (May 1972), "Explorations in Medical Career Choice," Contract no. 71-4066, National Institute of Health, U.S. D.H.E.W.

Paiva, R. E. A., and Haley, H. G. (April 1971), "Intellectual, Personality, and Environmental Factors in Career Specialty Preferences," *Journal of Medical Education* 46: 281–289.

Perlstadt, H. (November 1972), "Internship Placements and Faculty Influence," *Journal of Medical Education* 47: 862–868.

Powers, L., Whiting, J. F., and Opperman, K. C. (October 1962), "Trends in Medical School Faculties," *Journal of Medical Education* 38:1065–1091.

Rayack, E. (October-December 1964), "The A.M.A and the Supply of Physicians: A Study of the Internal Contradictions in the Concept of Professionalism," *Medical Care* 2: 244–252.

——— (January-March 1965), "The A.M.A. and the Supply of Physicians: A Study of the Internal Contradictions in the Concept of Professionalism," *Medical Care* 3: 17–25.

Reinhardt, U. E. (1975), *Physician Productivity and the Demand for Health Manpower,* Cambridge, Mass.: Ballinger Publishing Co.

Rottenberg, S. (January 1956), "On Choice in Labor Markets," *Industrial and Labor Relations Review* 9: 83–199.

Sloan, F. (October 1970), "Lifetime Earnings and Physicians' Choice of Specialty," *Industrial and Labor Relations Review* 24: 47–56.

Smith, V. K. and Cicchetti, C. J. (1972), "Regression Analysis with Dichotomous Dependent Variables," paper presented at the Annual Meeting of the Allied Social Science Association, Toronto, Canada.

"The Blue Sheet" (October 27, 1976), Washington, D.C.: Drug Research Reports.

Vahovich, S. G., ed. (1973), *Profile of Medical Practice,* Chicago: American Medical Association.

Weiss, Y. (December 1971), "Investment in Graduate Education," *American Economic Review* 61: 833–852.

Westling-Wikstrand, H., Monk, M. A., and Thomas, C. B. (November 1970), "Some Characteristics Related to Career Status of Women Physicians," *Johns Hopkins Medical Journal* 127: 273–286.

RETENTION OF MEDICAL SCHOOL GRADUATES: A CASE STUDY OF MICHIGAN

Gail Roggin Wilensky,[1] NATIONAL CENTER FOR HEALTH

SERVICES RESEARCH, DEPARTMENT OF HEALTH,

EDUCATION, AND WELFARE

The geographic distribution of physicians and the "determinants" of the location decisions of physicians have been a focus of concern for policy makers inside the outside the health profession. More recently, one group of these policy makers—Michigan legislators—have given some practical urgency to an understanding of these issues. They have begun to question the wisdom of subsidizing medical schools if a large number of their graduates are likely to migrate to other states. Legislators in Michigan as well as other states have also begun considering the subsidization of graduate training as a way of attracting and retaining a higher proportion of physicians. Any attempt to answer these concerns of the legislators immediately leads us to an analysis of the factors which influence physi-

Research in Health Economics, Vol. 1, pp 153–183.
Copyright © 1979 by JAI Press, Inc.
All rights of reproduction in any form reserved.
ISBN 0-89232-042-7.

cians' location decisions. The purpose of this study is to understand and explain the location decisions of one set of recently trained physicians.

There is another reason for focusing on the location decisions of new physicians. Any serious attempts to alter the existing distribution of physicians rest with the location decisions of new physicians. This is because established physicians have too many location specific intangible assets to be regarded as a potentially mobile group. Understanding the factors which influence new physicians' location decisions is the first step to providing legislators with the leverage they need to influence these location decisions. This assumes that at least some of the variables influencing location decisions are subject to policy intervention—an assumption which needs to be empirically verified.

EARLIER STUDIES

There have been several studies which have described or explained location decisions of recently trained physicians including those done by Weiskotten et al. (1960), Fein and Weber (1971), Yett and Sloan (1974), Held (1972), and Hadley (1976). Two trends of thought can be distilled from these studies and are implemented in this study. The first is that there is a relationship between the location of events in the physician's past such as birth, medical school, residency, etc., and the place that the physician decides to locate his practice. Weiskotten et al. were the first to comment on the relationship between "contact events" and location choice. Looking at 1945 and 1950 graduates of medical schools, they noted that almost 60 percent of the medical school graduates with residency training were practicing in the same states as their residency and that more than 42 percent were practicing in the same state as their medical school.[2] Because the study relied on a simple cross-tabular presentation of the data, causation is difficult to infer and few attempts were made to infer causation.

Two different causal hypotheses have arisen out of the observed Weiskotten relationships. Fein and Weber argue that physicians choose their residency in states where they plan to practice since this allows them to establish professional contacts and minimize any barriers to entry which otherwise might exist. As part of their empirical analysis, they regress the fill rate for residency programs in a state against the number of residencies offered relative to the number of medical graduates from 1950-1959 classes who were practicing in the state in 1967, weighted average residency stipend and the percent of residencies in nonaffiliated hospitals. They interpret the negative sign on the first variable as support for their hypothesis.[3] If their interpretation is accepted, the policy significance of this finding is that subsidization of graduate medical education is not an effective way of increasing the number of physicians locating in a particular state. The reason is that physicians would continue to choose residencies in areas they regarded as desirable for practice, with the practice location guiding the residency location rather than the reverse.

Yett and Sloan propose alternative hypotheses to explain the Weiskotten observation. They hypothesize that the more contacts a physician has with a state before his first practice location, the more likely he is to locate in that state and that more recent events will have a stronger effect than less recent events. Using *Medical Economics* data on physicians who first established a practice in 1966, they tested their hypotheses by calculating the probabilities that a physician will locate in a state of prior contact given various contact frequencies and sequencing, and by estimating various state retention probability equations given various contact and socioeconomic variables. Their findings supported the first part of their hypothesis that increasing the number of contacts increases the probability of locating in a given place. Their findings for the second part of the hypothesis were mixed but in general supportive.[4] They also retested the Fein and Weber hypothesis. Their interpretation of the estimated equation is that most physicians do not choose the state they intend to practice in and then seek out a residency in the same area. They do, however, recognize that the reason a physician may experience a large number of medical training events in a state is that he already has a strong personal attachment to the area. The latter possibility is not the same as the Fein and Weber hypothesis but some of the policy implications are similar, i.e., subsidizing graduate training as a way of increasing the marginal retention probability may not be as effective as it appears it would be from the correlation between residency location and practice location.

The second trend to emerge from these previous studies involves the use of a more explicit economic model to explain physician location choices. In addition to their contact variables, Yett and Sloan include several socioeconomic variables in an estimation of state retention probabilities which clearly reflect an implicit economic model. These include variables measuring income, barriers to entry, opportunity for professional development, effort, and general environmental factors. Held and Hadley postulate more explicit economic models which are based on economic models of migration and are derived from models of individual labor market equilibrium. Held estimated migration probability equations incorporating both the Weiskotten, Sloan and Yett contact hypotheses with economic variables reflecting expected supply and demand. Held found that for physicians who graduated from medical school between 1955 and 1965, migration was generally toward the coasts and to areas characterized by high growth rates, high physician-population ratios, and high nonmonetary benefits. He also found that physicians were as likely to locate in states with no previous contact as they were to locate in states with which they had multiple contacts.[5] The Hadley model focuses on a more explicit choice process which incorporates both the Weiskotten, Yett-Sloan contact variables and an economic theory of migration. Hadley uses four binary dependent variables which collectively describe the set of possible choices: a state of no contact, medical-school-only contact, graduate-training-only contact, and medical school and graduate contact. Each choice is viewed as being made with respect to a specific alternative—in his case, the most recent contact state which is different from the practice state. The primary reason for restricting the choice to a binary variable was a practical one rather than a theoretical one. He didn't have direct observations on the other choices considered and he also lacked an estimation procedure which allowed for the simultaneous comparison of more than two choices. His results imply that physicians who choose states with which they have had substantial contact do so primarily because of close personal ties, that physicians who choose states they have had only graduate contact with seem more attracted by nonpecuniary rewards than pecuniary rewards, and that physicians who choose states with which they have had no previous contact behave more like a traditional economic person, being attracted by high monetary and nonmonetary returns.[6]

The study reported here contines the effort to explain location choices of recently trained physicians. It is restricted to a limited group—a subset of those who received part of their medical training in Michigan. The purpose of the study is to estimate and explain the probability of this group's staying in Michigan as a function of the number and mix of contact events and of the net monetary and nonmonetary returns from alternative locations. An analysis is also made of the probability of staying in an SMSA that the physician had contact with as a resident and the probability of staying in an SMSA the physician had contact with as a medical student. Viewing the SMSA as th focus of the location choice should be of considerable policy interest, since it seems intuitively reasonable that physicians are more likely to choose to locate in a particular localized area than in a particular state. Finally, several specific policy issues will be examined in the context of this new data set.

DATA

A short questionnaire was sent to a sample of Michigan-trained physicians in the summer of 1975. The sample of physicians included all physicians who graduated from Michigan medical schools during the years 1960,

1965, and 1968, plus all residents who were in training in Michigan hospitals during 1968. One thousand eighty-nine questionnaires were returned. Excluding the nondeliverables, this implied a response rate of 72 percent of the former medical students, a response rate of just under 50 percent of the former residents and a response rate of just under 60 percent of the group as a whole. No attempt has been made to analyze the nonresponses.

The first section of the questionnaire asks the respondent to specify the place (city and state) where various events occurred from birth and childhood to college, medical school, internship, residency, armed services, and practice location. This is followed by several questions about the physician and his practice at the time his practice was initially established including certification, type of practice, specialty, marital status, expected income, etc. An attempt was then made to establish minimum and crucial characteristics regarding their location choices, the degree of importance associated with various factors thought to influence location, second choice of location, and other alternatives considered, at what point in his career the physician chose his specialty and the location of his practice, and whether the prospect of full cost tuition coupled with an appropriate loan forgiveness program might have influenced his location decision. A copy of the questionnaire is shown in Appendix 1. Data reflecting the supply conditions as well as some summary data on economic and demographic characteristics of the alternatives considered were merged into the basic data files.

DESCRIPTIVE ANALYSIS

Because of the unique nature of the data set, we begin with a brief descriptive analysis of the physicians in the sample in terms of their geographical background. We then reexamine the Yett and Sloan hypotheses regarding retention probabilities as a function of the number and mix of contact events.

The percent of the sample which experienced various contact events, from birth through practice, in each of six specified states is shown in Table 1. From Table 1 we can see that 44.6 percent of the sample were born in Michigan, 5 percent in Ohio, and so forth. These six states were chosen because they represented the states with the highest shares of Michigan-trained physicians from sample and/or they border Michigan and were regarded as somewhat more likely places of migration because of proximity. Two foreign countries, not shown in the table, served as significant sources of physicians for our sample. Six percent of the sample were born in the Philippines and remained there through medical school; 4

Table 1. Percent of Physicians Experiencing Specified Events in 6 States

(Percent)

Event	California	Ohio	New York	Wisconsin	Illinois	Michigan
Birth	1.3	5.0	3.4	.8	2.8	44.6
Childhood	1.3	5.1	3.3	.5	2.2	49.8
College	1.4	3.0	2.0	.5	1.6	52.3
Medical School	1.0	1.1	1.9	.5	1.7	61.6
Internship	10.0	5.0	4.9	1.1	3.8	52.3
Residency	6.0	1.7	2.2	.4	1.6	69.8
Practice	11.2	2.5	1.6	1.6	2.3	44.3

percent of the sample were born in India and remained there through medical school. Physicians who responded from our sample are now practicing in every state except Alaska and Delaware and in at least 20 countries. It is interesting to note that the share of the sample practicing now in Michigan is almost identical to the share born in Michigan and is 10 to 25 percentage points smaller than the percent who received some training in Michigan. This does not imply that people who are born in Michigan are more likely to practice in Michigan, since there is no way of knowing from such a table how many of the people who experienced one event in Michigan also experienced various other events in Michigan. This is considered next. Two things Table 1 does show, however, is that a substantial share of those who went to medical school or did their residency in Michigan during the years under consideration do not practice in Michigan (55 percent) and that 11 percent of our sample practice in California, although prior to internship only 1 percent had any contact with California. It should not be inferred from these two statements that Michigan is a net exporter of physicians trained in Michigan. In order to answer that question, we would also have to know the number of physicians who practice in Michigan who were not trained in Michigan. This is beyond the scope of the present study.

The present sample provides us with an opportunity to reexamine the Yett and Sloan hypotheses. According to Yett and Sloan (1974), the more recent the contact and the more frequent the contact, the more likely is the physician to locate in a particular state. Tables 2 and 3 are conditional probability tables which show the probability of American medical school graduates and foreign medical school graduates (FMG's) locating in Michigan given a particular mix of contact events experienced in Michigan. We can see from Table 2, for example, that the probability of an American medical school graduate who has done only a residency in Michigan and has otherwise not had contact with Michigan is .17. The 66 shown below indicates that 66 American graduates in our sample did only their residency in Michigan. We have separated FMG's from the non-FMG population since it is clear from casual observation that their responses to contact with Michigan are of a different order of magnitude.

In general, it appears that the Yett and Sloan (1974) hypotheses are confirmed, although there clearly are some exceptions. The probability of staying in Michigan for physicians who have experienced all five events in Michigan is substantially higher than most other probabilities. There are three combinations with higher probabilities, RICB, RIMB, RIC; but in each of these cases there are very few observations with that combination of events, which leads us to suspect the reliability of those figures. One probability that seems surprisingly high is the .62 associated with RIM. Residency, internship, and medical school are the last three events which

Table 2. Probability of Staying in Michigan Given Various Contacts
American Medical School Graduates

	RIMCB	IMCB	RMCB	RICB	RIMB	RIMC	MCB	IMC	RMC	RIC	RIM	MC	IM	RM	RI	M	R
Probability	.67	.35	.37	.88	.75	.5	.12	.2	.2	.75	.62	.11	.28	.28	.33	.12	.17
Number of People Having Only That Event	226	72	63	8	43	30	177	5	2	4	45	18	18	25	73	51	66

Where

R — Residency
I — Internship
M — Medical School
C — Childhood
B — Birth

Table 3. Probability of Staying in Michigan Given Various Contacts
FMG's

	RI	R	I
Probability	.74	.63	.33
Number of People Having Only That Event	87	133	6

Where

R — Residency
I — Internship
M — Medical School
C — Childhood
B — Birth

occur there. We should expect a high probability, but it is not obvious why the probability should be so much higher than what we observe for RMCB and RIMC. It also appears that having residency as one of the component events increases the probability of staying relative to combinations with the same number of events which do not have residency as one of the components. This is precisely what Yett and Sloan would lead us to expect. In contrast, it appears that having medical school as one of the components does not increase the probability of staying relative to other combinations with the same number of events. The policy which suggests itself is that there is more payoff in terms of retention in attracting residents rather than in attracting medical students. This is a very strong policy statement and the analysis on which it is based is not strong enough to warrant such a conclusion. The probabilities which are presented in Table 2 cannot be interpreted as marginal probabilities since we have not held constant other factors which we think may be important in determining a physician's location decision. We will consider marginal probabilities when we discuss the results of the regression analysis.

From Table 3 it is clear that FMG's who obtain postgraduate training in Michigan have a relatively high probability of staying. The policy which suggests itself here is that attracting FMG's into a state for residency or residency and internship is an effective and inexpensive way of acquiring more physicians. Again, we cannot interpret these probabilities as marginal since we have not held other important factors constant. This policy also ignores consideration of whether there are any quality differentials between FMG's and American graduates. The latter is not an issue we consider in this paper.

MODEL

The present study relies heavily on the theoretical framework developed by Hadley (1975).[7] In essence, the theoretical structure is based on an economic theory of migration where physicians are assumed to be rational decision makers who consider some set of alternatives, estimate the present discounted utility associated with this set of alternative locations and choose the location which maximizes their net monetary and nonmonetary returns. The existence of search costs in such a model acts to limit the set of alternatives considered.

The specification of the model to be estimated is also similar to the one developed by Hadley (1975).[8] The location choices we try to predict are the probability of a Michigan trained physician staying in Michigan, of locating in the same SMSA as his residency, of locating in the same SMSA as his medical school, and of locating in a state which the physician had no contact with during his medical education. The dependent variable of each of the equations is a dichotomous variable which assumes the value of one if the physician made the choice specified in the equation, and a value of zero otherwise.

The mean values of the dependent variables are shown in Table 4. The probability of locating in Michigan is shown as being slightly smaller than the probability shown in Table 1 because, as is explained in the footnote to the table, some observations we initally considered were ineligible for

Table 4. Mean Values for Various Location Choices

	Mean Values
Probability of a Michigan-trained physician locating in Michigan	.42[a]
Probability of a Michigan-trained physician who lives in an SMSA locating in an SMSA he was in as a resident	.45
Probability of a Michigan-trained physician who lives in an SMSA locating in an SMSA he was in as a medical student	.16
Probability of a Michigan-trained physician locating in a state with no medical education contact	.45

[a] The reason that this figure is lower than the percentage shown in Table 1 is that it is based on a modestly different sample. Table 1 is based on all physicians who returned a questionnaire. The figure cited above is based on the observations used in the regression analysis. If there were any missing values for the variables used in the regression, a missing value coded was inserted and the observation was lost for the regression. This resulted in an 8 percent reduction in the sample.

inclusion in the regression. The probability of locating in an SMSA the physician had contact with as a resident or had contact with as a medical student is shown *only* for those physicians who practice in an SMSA. Since about 20 percent of the sample practices outside an SMSA, the probability of a physician in the whole sample locating in a residency SMSA is about 36 percent, and the probability of locating in a medical school SMSA is about 13 percent. The most interesting finding is that 45 percent of the sample located in a state they had not had contact with as a medical student or a resident. Although Weiskotten (1960), Held (1972), and Hadley (1975) all report sizable "no contact" populations,[9] 45 percent is substantially larger than the other findings. Part of the difference is probably due to the different type of sample concerned here. By definition the physicians in this sample must have had some medical contact with Michigan. This is therefore clearly not a representative sample of physicians. However, this is also a more recent sample of physicians. Most of the physicians in the sample did not complete their residency until after the late 1960s. It is thus not surprising that this sample might be more mobile than earlier samples.

We have three types of independent variables: variables which reflect the degree and type of contact the physician had with the particular location choice being considered, variables which reflect characteristics about the individual physician, and variables which reflect the characteristics of the location choice being considered relative to those same characteristics in an alternative site. The latter is the least obvious of the variable structures. It was necesary because of the unavailability of an estimating procedure which let us compare more than two choices at a time.[10]

The way we define the choice/alternative variables used to reflect relative characteristics of alternative locations being considered varied according to the equation being specified. Our basic procedure for identifying the relevant alternative to the location being specified is to consider the places the physician listed as being his second choice or the place where the physician is at if he isn't in the location we have specified. In cases where the physician didn't list a second choice, we went back through his medical education history and selected the most recent place of contact. This assumes that if we have no other information available, the physician's last place of contact was the alternative being considered.

Some examples of this procedure should clarify the variable construction process used. In estimating the probability of locating in Michigan, the value of the dependent variable for each observation is either one or zero, depending on whether the physician located in Michigan or didn't locate there. If the physician located in Michigan, then the independent variable, for example, population growth, would be equal to population growth in Michigan relative to population growth in the physician's sec-

ond choice of location. If the physician located outside of Michigan, the
same independent variable would be equal to population growth in Michigan relative to population growth in the state actually chosen. The logic is
thus to look at the value of the variable in the location we have specified
versus either the value of the variable in the physician's second choice or
the value of the variable in the place the physician actually chose. The
construction of the choice/alternative choice variable for the "no contact" equation is less obvious but the logic is similar.[11]

Since we assume that the physician chooses his location on the basis of
the expected net monetary and nonmonetary returns in alternative locations, we need to include variables which reflect monetary and nonmonetary returns and costs in these locations. The most direct monetary
return is expected income. We include mean income for physicians in the
relevant specialty for choice and alternative states as of 1965 as a measure
of expected income. Although we asked the physician to estimate his
expected income ten years from now, we could not use this variable since,
unfortunately, we had not asked him to estimate his income in his
second-choice location. Both because mean income experienced in the
past may not be a good approximation of expected income in the future
and because of the peculiar nature of the medical sector such as the
existence of third-party payments, uncertain outcomes, etc., we can't
assume that income differentials serve as normal market signals. We
therefore also include proxies for expected demand. Examples include
per capita income and urbanization.

Nonmonetary returns have been notoriously difficult to operationalize
although few have doubted their importance.[12] Net migration rates should
be a good proxy since this should reflect the basic attractiveness of the
area as a place to locate. The existing supply of physicians in the area may
also reflect its basic attractiveness for physicians, although this variable
could reflect an expected cost since it could also reflect potential competition for a new physician. Another measure is the distance from the coast.

Monetary and nonmonetary costs are also difficult to measure. The
supply of physicians and the supply of residents and interns could be
regarded as either a cost or a return. They reflect costs if they reflect
competition to the new physician. They reflect returns if, as indicated
above, they reflect the basic attractiveness of a location or if, in the case
of residents and interns, they reflect free inputs to the physician. Expected level of effort would be a good measure of expected costs, but we
do not have an estimate of this variable.

We have constructed several categorical variables which reflect the
number and/or mix of contact events which the physician has experienced. By including these variables in the estimation, we will be able to

measure the marginal contribution of these events on the physician's location decision.

The last set of variables include the relative importance with which physicians in our sample viewed factors which either characterized or would influence their location choice. These include the relative importance of having specialists in other areas or of having other physicians in his own area, the ability to obtain hospital privileges, expected income, recreational facilities, and so forth. Although it is not clear that this information will facilitate policymaking, it will at least enable us to better understand the kinds of physicians who make various types of location decisions.

The model was estimated as a linear probability function using ordinary least squares regression.[13] There are some well-known problems associated with using ordinary least squares regression in the analysis of dichotomous dependent variables.[14] We have not made any attempts to adjust the inefficient (although unbiased) estimators which result in such a case. For our purposes, the most noticeable effect of using regression with dichotomous dependent variables is that the R^2's are typically low. The value of model should therefore not be judged solely on the basis of the resulting R^2's.

RESULTS

The major purpose of this study is to explain the probability of a set of Michigan trained physicians locating in Michigan. The results of two regressions predicting the probability of locating in Michigan are presented in Tables 5 and 6. Table 5 shows the results of including contact variables, attitudinal variables, and measures of the expected returns and costs associated with locating in Michigan relative to locating in the physician's second choice or in the state actually chosen.[15] Table 6 shows the results of including primarily contact variables plus two shift variables which reflect the influence of being an FMG and of finishing a residency between 1968 and 1971, and after 1971 relative to finishing before 1968. As we would expect, the fuller model presented in Table 5 accounts for more of the variation in predicting the probability of locating in Michigan.

We selected what we thought were the major contact categories to include in the regression. Because the conditional probability tables indicated that FMG's and non-FMG's react differently to a residency-only contact, we allowed for an interaction between having only a residency in Michigan and being an FMG. The coefficients associated with the contact variables generally support expectations established by Yett and Sloan

Table 5. Regression Predicting the Probability of Michigan-
Trained Physicians Locating in Michigan

Variable	Regression Coefficient	T Statistic
Constant	.3983	
Residency-only non-FMG	.0282	.59
Residency-only FMG	.3145**	3.33
Medical school only	-.0958	1.68
Residency and medical school	.1863**	3.63
Residency, medical school, childhood and birth	.2419**	5.67
Specialty	-.0036	.15
Dollars of debt	.0000	1.03
FMG	-.0249	.27
Need more in your specialty	.0209	.67
Ability to get hospital privileges	.0756*	2.49
Cultural opportunities	-.0615	1.60
Expected income	.0214	.65
Recreational facilities	-.0187	.46
Employment for spouse	-.0251	.65
Climate	-.2335**	7.46
Proximity to friends and relatives	.2319**	7.93
Finished residency 1968 - 1971	-.0013	.03
Finished residency after 1971	-.0595	1.4
Relative physician income	.1329*	1.97
Relative population growth	-.0030	.67
Relative net migration	.0691**	2.73
Relative urbanization	.0419	.52
Relative per capita income	-.2381	1.61
Relative number of physicians	-.0011	.33

R^2 (adj) =   .24
F   = 12.974

*   Significant at .05 level
** Significant at .01 level

[a]   rounded to zero.

(1974). Experiencing medical school and residency in Michigan, experiencing birth, childhood, medical school, and residency in Michigan,
and experiencing only residency as an FMG are all significant and positively associated with locating in that state. Furthermore, experiencing
four contact events rather than two, other things being equal, increased

Table 6. Predicting the Probability of Locating in Michigan
Using Contact Variables

Variable	Regression Coefficient	T Statistic
Constant	.2930	
Residency only non-FMG	.0402	.79
Residency-only FMG	.2467*	2.43
Medical school only	-.1159	1.90
Residency and medical school	.2216**	4.06
Residency, medical school, childhood, birth	.3125**	6.94
FMG	.1136	1.14
Finished residency 1968 - 1971	-.0492	1.12
Finished residency after 1971	-.0890*	1.99

R^2 (adj) =   .11
F   = 12.26

* Significant at .05 level
** Significant at .01 level

the probability of locating in Michigan—a probability of .24 versus a probability of .19, respectively. What would not have been expected a priori is the very high probability associated with an FMG who has had a residency in Michigan. The negative but not significant coefficient associated with a medical school-only contact was not expected, although it is not difficult to understand. These physicians have had little attachment to Michigan and may either have other attachments elsewhere or else be a part of the mobile population which chooses a no-contact state. It should be recalled that the conditional probability of locating in Michigan was exactly the same for birth, childhood, and medical school group as for the medical school-only group, which means the coefficient for birth, childhood, and medical school only would also probably not be significant.

Three attitudinal variables were also significant with at least two clearly expected and with the expected signs. It is reasonable to assume that physicians who locate in Michigan would tend to regard climate as unimportant and that those who have experienced at least one medical education contact in Michigan and then locate in Michigan would regard the importance of being near family and friends. It is less obvious but not unreasonable that physicians who locate in a state they have had some medical contact with would think the ability to obtain hospital privileges is important. As we would expect, the magnitude of the response is much smaller for this variable than for the climate or proximity variables. Two of the variables reflecting expected returns—mean physician income and net migration rates—were also significant and with the expected signs. This finding provides some support that this sample of physicians chose their location according to expected monetary and nonmonetary returns.

There are several variables whose importance we might have expected that, in fact, were not. Being in a secondary specialty rather than a primary specialty, which is the way the specialty variable is defined, was not significantly associated with the probability of locating in Michigan.[16] Finishing a residency after 1968 was also not significant, although, as indicated earlier, the sign was negative indicating that more recently trained physicians tend to be more mobile. Finally, as we would expect, the R^2 is relatively low, but there are significant coefficients associated with some of each of the three types of independent variables included in our model and all with the expected signs.

Table 7 shows the result of regression equations which predict the probability of locating in an SMSA where the physician was a resident or in a SMSA where the physician was a medical student. This analysis is limited to those physicians whose practice is located in an SMSA. Our presumption was that this was intuitively a more reasonable analysis based on the assumption that physicians and others choose to locate in a particular area and not to locate in a state, per se. Unfortunately for the analysis, most of the physicians in the sample limited their specification of their second choice location to the state-level description. This meant that when we considered variables which reflected the relative advantage of being in the choice area rather than in the alternative, the alternative could only be defined in terms of the (next) most recent contact. For the residency equation this was defined as the SMSA of medical school. For the medical school equation this was defined as the residency SMSA or else the SMSA where the physician was an undergraduate, and so forth. In addition, several variables of interest were not available at the SMSA level. The most important of these is the mean physician income by specialty.

The most important finding is that the same variables tend to be significant in both equations. The significant variables also have the same sign and generally are about the same order of magnitude. Climate and proximity are important here, with the signs the same as in the state equation. For purposes of these equations, contact is defined in terms of the number of contacts, with an interaction allowed between number of contacts and FMG status.[17] The number of contacts the physician has had with the SMSA is shown to significantly affect his probability of locating there. As before, the impact of contact is especially strong for FMG's. The signs of the significant relative choice variables were not as obvious.

Table 7. Regression Predicting the Probability of Locating in a Medical School of Residency SMSA for Physicians Practicing in an SMSA

Variables	Residency SMSA Coefficient (T Statistic)		Medical School SMSA Coefficient (T Statistic)	
Constant	.124		.111	
FMG	-.1051	(1.54)	– – –	
Year finished residency	-.0008	(.28)	.0008	(.33)
Specialty	-.0009	(. 82)	.0030	(.10)
Need more in your specialty	-.0512	(1.32)	-.0381	(1.24)
Need others for consultation	-.0312	(.84)	-.0497	(1.75)
Cultural opportunities	.0054	(.11)	.0550	(1.39)
Expected income	-.0577	(1.38)	-.0258	(.82)
Recreational opportunities	.0365	(.71)	.0706	(1.78)
Climate	-.1479*	(3.79)	-.0983**	(3.13)
Proximity to friends and relatives	.1304**	(3.58)	.1214**	(4.31)
Number of contacts non-FMG's	.0662**	(5.02)	.1161**	(12.21)
Number of contacts FMG	.3170**	(5.71)	– – –	
Relative number of physicians	.0017	(.92)	.0008	(.41)
Relative population growth	-.0010	(.14)	-.0025	(.66)
Relative net migration	-.0071*	(2.47)	-.0028	(1.66)
Relative urbanization	.3603**	(2.97)	.2270*	(2.37)
Relative per capita income	-.1.1275**	7..83)	-.3814**	(3.55)
Relative number of interns and residents	-.0004**	(3.90)	-.0002*	(2.00)
R^2 (adj) =	.28		.36	
F =	13.42		16.40	

* Significant at the .05 level
** Significant at the .01 level

A higher rate of urbanization is associated with a higher probability of locating in the specified location as we would expect. However, a higher rate of net migration and a higher level of per capita income is associated with a lower probability of choosing the specified location. This is not what we would expect, although a negative sign on the per capita income variable has been reported before.[18] The only logical explanation for this finding is that areas with high migration rates and high levels of per capita income are difficult places to establish a practice because they are attractive to a lot of other people and, presumably, a lot of other physicians. This explanation is consistent with the significantly negative sign on the number of interns and residents available. High values for this variable are probably associated with medical centers which are not easy places for new physicians to begin a practice.

Since the two proxies for expected demand and/or intrinsic attractiveness of the area have negative coefficients, the impression we are left with is that when location decisions are viewed at a more micro level, physicians do not seem very responsive to expected economic returns. This conclusion must be viewed very cautiously, however, since we include neither a measure of physician income nor average weeks worked.

Table 8 shows the results of the regression predicting the probability of

Table 8. Regression Predicting the Probability of Locating in a State with No Medical Education Contact

Variable	Regression Coefficient	T Statistic
Constant	.470	
Specialty	.0299	.87
Dollars of debt	-.0000	1.10
FMG	-.0358	.70
Need more in your specialty	-.0111	.32
Ability to get hospital privileges	.0115	.34
Cultural opportunities	.0380	.93
Expected income	.0271	.75
Recreational facilities	-.0469	1.06
Employment for spouse	.0245	.58
Climate	.1819**	5.40
Proximity to friends and relatives	-.2552**	8.15
Finished residency 1968 - 1971	-.0247	.57
Finished residency after 1971	-.0131	.29
Relative physician income	.0480	1.68
Relative population growth	-.0053	.75
Relative net migration rate	.0012	.69
Relative urbanization	-.0639	1.24
Relative per capita income	-.0358	.67
Relative number of physicians	.0143*	2.10

R^2 = .11
F = 7.12

* Significant at the .05 level
** Significant at the .01 level

locating in a state that the physician had no contact with as a medical student or as a resident. The most striking finding is that we were much less successful in explaining this choice than in explaining other choices. In addition, only three variables were significant.

As we might expect, the importance of climate is positively associated with the choice of a no contact state and the importance of being near family and friends is negatively associated with a no-contact state, i.e., being near family and friends is not regarded as important to these physicians. The number of physicians also tends to be higher in no-contact states. This suggests that physicians who choose no-contact states go to states which are attractive to other physicians.

POLICY IMPLICATIONS

One of the policy issues which gave rise to this study is whether legislators should subsidize medical students and/or residents as a way of increasing the number of physicians who locate in their state. The findings of Yett and Sloan (1974) would suggest that increasing the number and recency of contacts with a state, whether by subsidization or by other means, should increase the likelihood of the physicians' locating in the state. Fein and Weber (1971) disagree with the causal relationship implied by Yett and Sloan. They believe that physicians choose the location of their residency on the basis of where they plan to practice. The findings of this study indicate that physicians with multiple contacts in Michigan and with contacts later in their training are more likely to locate in Michigan than other physicians. What was not clear earlier is that FMG's who do postgraduate training in a state—in this case Michigan—are more likely to locate in that state than any other group we have observed. This is not really surprising since the psychic costs associated with moving are likely to be greater for this group than for others.

The issue as to whether physicians pick the location of their residencies on the basis of where they plan to practice cannot be decided by reference to the conditional and marginal probabilities cited thus far. However, we do have information related to this issue which was collected as part of the survey. At the end of the questionnaire, we asked the physicians to indicate when in their career they chose their specialty and when they chose the location of their practice. There were two modal values regarding the timing of their specialty choice—the last half of medical school and internship, with 32 percent and 33 percent reporting in those periods, respectively. Almost 75 percent of the sample had chosen their specialty by the time of their internship. By way of contrast, only 10 percent of the sample had chosen their practice location by the time of their internship.

The implication of this finding is that specialty choice and location are not jointly determined, at least in a temporal sense, although the latter is partially constrained by the former; i.e., superspecialists cannot choose small rural areas as their practice sites.

The timing of the location choice for all physicians in the sample, for all physicians who practice in the same state as their residency, and for all physicians who practice in the same SMSA as their residency is shown in Table 9. The second and third groups are better approximations of the physicians relevant to the Fein and Weber (1971) hypothesis than the first group, but it is clear that the distribution of the timing of location choice is almost identical for all three of the groups of physicians shown in Table 9. It also seems clear that at least for this sample most of the physicians could not have chosen the location of their residency on the basis of where they intended to practice, since over 70 percent of the relevant group did not decide on the location of their practice until after beginning their residency. The only other group of any size are the physicians who made their location choice while in the armed forces. This could have been either before their residency or after some or all of their residency. If as many as half of the physicians who made their choice while in the armed forces were in the armed services after the beinning of their residency, the percentage of physicians who could not have chosen the site of their residency on the basis of where they intended to practice would be close to 80 percent. It thus appears that the Fein and Weber hypothesis is not supported by this sample.

However, it also appears that a high degree of personal attachment to the state may be causing the relationship between the number of contacts and the probability of locating in the state. This possibility was raised by Yett and Sloan (1974) and received some empirical support from Hadley (1975) although the direction of causation was still not clear. Here, the importance of being near family and friends was positively associated with the probability of staying in Michigan, with staying in the same SMSA as residency, and with staying in the same residency as medical school, and was negatively associated with going to a no-contact state. In all cases, the variable was highly significant. If this is true, it suggests that attempting to influence the place where a physician is a medical student and a resident is less likely to alter his location decision than would otherwise appear.

Because of the large percentage of our sample who located in a no-contact state and because of the possibility that strong psychic ties to a state causes the physician to have both multiple contacts with the state as well as to locate there, it may appear that subsidization of medical students and/or residents either directly or indirectly will not be very effective as a way of influencing their location decision. However, this may be

Table 9. Timing of Location Choice

When Location Chosen

	First Two Years Medical School	Last Two Years Medical School	Intern- ship (%)	Armed Forces	Beginning of Residency	End of Residency	Other
All physicians	2	2	6	18	5	62	5
Physicians practicing in same state as residency	3	2	6	12	7	67	4
Physicians practicing in same SMSA as residency	3	2	7	11	8	65	4

173

too strong a conclusion. First, it appears that any efforts which are made to induce FMG's to do their residency in a state are likely to have a high payoff. According to the results presented here, being an FMG and doing a residency in Michigan is associated with a 31 percent probability of locating in Michigan, other things being equal. Second, even if those who have had contact with Michigan and who locate in Michigan tend to feel that being near family and friends is important, causality remains unclear. It may be that, as the number of contacts with an area increases, the importance of being near family and friends also increases and the probability of remaining in the area therefore also increases. Third, according to our findings, being in medical school and a resident in Michigan rather than belonging to any of our other contact groups did, in fact, increase the probability of locating in Michigan. These three considerations, coupled with the realization that some states may not be able to depend on naturally high rates of net migration as a way of augmenting their physicians, may make preferential admissions policies and/or subsidization of medical training as effective a policy as is available to them. States which have experienced high migration rates have no need to subsidize medical students and/or residents. This, of course, means that as long as medical schools are primarily state-financed, some states will end up subsidizing other states. This type of logic has frequently been used to argue for Federal support of medical schools rather than state support.

There are, however, other mechanisms which can be used to influence the location decisions of physicians. Most of these policy tools have been discussed as a means of attempting to induce physicians to locate in scarcity areas.[19] These include policies which affect physicians' income, such as an adjusted fee schedule and a guaranteed minimum income, loan forgiveness, preferential admissions, and so forth. Subsidization and/or easier admissions policy for in-state students can be regarded as a form of preferential admissions policy. At least part of the assumption underlying such a policy is that these students are more likely to remain in the state than other students. As we have already observed, there is a relationship between contact with an area and the probability of locating there, but the direction of causality is somewhat obscure. Another form of such a policy is an easier admissions policy for individuals who indicate an interest in locating in areas of physician shortage.

Our sample can provide some estimate of the likely effectiveness of two other policies: policies that affect physicians' income and loan-forgiveness programs. As we indicated earlier, we would expect that the higher the physician income in an area, the greater the probability of locating in the area. Several studies have found this expected positive relationship, but the effect has usually been statistically and quantitatively insignificant.[20] We observed a positive relationship between relative physician income and the probability of locating in Michigan which was significant at the 5 percent level. The quantitative effect, however, appears to be small. The implied income elasticity is .36, indicating that physicians in this sample are not very responsive to different income levels between states, although the effect would be in the desired direction. To the extent that observed income levels in the past are not very well correlated with expected income, this may not be a very good measure of how responsive new physicians might be to different income levels. Given the uncertainty that exists about the effectiveness of differing income levels, guaranteed minimum income programs to induce physicians to locate in particular localities may be an appropriate area for social experimentation, provided that appropriate controls are established in the community or by a review committee to insure that the physicians continue to maintain an acceptable level of work effort.

A third way to influence location decisions is through a loan-forgiveness program. Recent evaluations of several loan-forgiveness programs which existed during the sixties indicate that service repayment rates have varied between 42 percent and 65 percent. It is not clear whether these rates should be regarded as successses or failures, but it is not very surprising that the service repayment rate was not very high since the amount of the loan rarely went above $6,000. Logically, it would seem that making substantially large loans available and increasing the pay-back interest rate for physicians who want to buy their way out would increase the service repayment rate. As part of our questionnaire, we asked our sample of physicians, if they had to pay a total tuition cost of $80,000—which was one study's estimate of the cost of training a physician—and had the choice of paying this amount with interest or serving in one of a list of designated underserved areas, whether their location choices would have been affected. They were also asked if they thought the location choices of new physicians would be affected. Of those who responded, 37 percent reported that this sort of policy would have affected their own location choices. This figure was almost identical across all specialties. The expected effect of this sort of policy regarding the location decisions that new physicians would make was even more impressive. Sixty-eight percent of the sample thought this policy would affect the location choices of new physicians. The figure for surgeons and surgical subspecialists was a little lower than the average for the entire group. What this suggests is that if states were to end the state and Federal subsidization of medical schools and charge full cost tuition, a policy choice such as the one indicated above may be an effective way of altering physicians' location decisions over what they would otherwise be.

One final area of interest is to look at the second choice of location for those physicians who did not locate in Michigan and to examine the responses as to whether there was something the community could have offered to induce the physician to locate in his second choice rather the first. Michigan was clearly a major alternative for the physicians who did not locate there. Of those who did not locate in Michigan and who responded to the question, almost one-third said that Michigan was their second choice. California was the only other place which was a focus of choice with 19 percent listing California. The response to the question whether there was anything the second choice community could have offered to make the physician locate there was not as encouraging. Almost one-half didn't respond and, of those who did, more than half said no. The only other responses of any importance related to personal factors such as recreation, school, culture, social climate, crime rates, etc., and professional factors such as better working conditions, higher-quality medical community, back-up coverage, presence of medical school, etc. In general, these are not areas which are subject to policy intervention. This suggests then that contact with Michigan is associated with Michigan's being a likely second choice for physicians who did not locate in Michigan but that there are not obvious measures available to a community which will alter the physicians' location decisions. Reliance will have to be placed on the types of policies reviewed above, such as preferential admissions and loan-forgiveness programs.

CONCLUSIONS

In this study we attempt to explain and understand the probability that a sample of Michigan-trained physicians will locate in Michigan, will locate in the SMSA of their residency or medical school, and will locate in a state with which they have had no medical education contact. We assumed a rational choice model in which physicians are expected to choose their locations according to their expected economic returns and according to their attitudes toward mobility and risk. The probability of locating in Michigan is found to vary according to the number and recency of contacts, with FMG's who have done their residency in Michigan especially likely to choose that state, to vary according to attitudes about climate and the importance of being near friends and family and according to several measures of expected returns such as relative physician income and net migration rates. All of these variables had plausible signs.

We expected that predicting the probability of locating in a residency or medical school SMSA would be of particular interest because of our assumption that physicians choose to locate in localized areas rather than in large geographical areas such as states. The predicted equations were very similar. Important predictors included climate, proximity to friends and family, number of contacts, and various measures of economic returns. Several economic variables did not have the expected sign and seemed to indicate that these physicians were not likely to locate in residency or medical school SMSA's that were intrinsically attractive, or which had high expected demand presumably because of the greater competitive pressures associated with such areas. Since several of the variables of interest were not available at the SMSA level, it is not clear whether these differences with the state equation are real or are due to measurement problems.

Variations in the probability of locating in a no-contact state were harder to explain but are important since they represent a very large group. Climate and proximity to friends and family were again important but, as expected, with opposite signs. It also appeared that these physicians were attracted to places which were attractive to other physicians and which have relatively high physician income, although the latter was significant only at the .10 level. The impression we are left with is that physicians who go to no-contact areas have a taste for mobility and are attracted to places with expected high monetary and nonmonetary returns.

The issue of causation with respect to the contact variable remains unsettled, although we are able to conclude that most physicians in our sample did not choose the location of their residency with the intention of practicing there. It is not clear, however, whether strong psychic ties to an area cause multiple contacts, whether multiple contacts result in strong psychic ties, or whether the two interact in producing the relationship between the number of contacts and the probability of location. Despite this uncertainty, it appears that providing incentives for individuals to undertake both medical school and residency in a state may be a reasonably effective policy provided that at least these two events occur in the same area. Subsidizing only medical school does not appear to be an effective policy. It was also observed that FMG's who had a residency in Michigan were more likely to locate in Michigan than any other group and thus represented another group which might be susceptible to an appropriate incentive program.

Two other policies were considered: income guarantees and a loan-forgiveness program. Income guarantees will probably not be very effective as a means of altering location decisions since physicians do not appear to be very responsive to differences in expected income. A loan-forgiveness program has the potential for being an effective policy, provided that the amount of money being loaned and the penalty interest rate for repayment are substantial. This could happen either with the adoption of a full cost tuition plan or it may happen more gradually as state legislatures and other groups cut back on their rates of general subsidization.

There are other programs which we have not considered here but which appear to be effective in influencing location decisions. These include Area Health Education Centers, which are designed to alleviate professional isolation in rural areas and the National Health Service Corps, which is a new Federal program aimed at providing health shortage areas with physicians and other personnel.

FOOTNOTES

1. This study was begun while the author was an associate research scientist, School of Public Health, and Visiting Assistant Professor of Economics, University of Michigan. Financial assistance was provided by the Office of Health and Medical Affairs, State of Michigan, and the Michigan Medical School Council of Deans. Computer support was provided by Marilyn Barron, DHEW. Jack Hadley, of The Urban Institute, contributed generously to the development, specification, and estimation of the model. The views expressed in the paper do not necessarily reflect the views of the above-named organizations.

2. Herman G. Weiskotten et al. (December 1960), p. 1086.

3. Fein and Weber (1971), p. 177.

4. Yett and Sloan (June 1974), pp. 126–130.

5. Philip J. Held (1972), p. 34.

6. Jack L. Hadley (1975), pp. 82–85, 276–277.

7. Hadley, ibid., pp. 72–80.

8. Hadley, ibid., pp. 82–105.

9. H. G. Weiskotten et al., op. cit., based on figures provided on p. 1088, cited in Hadley, ibid., p. 31; P. J. Held, op. cit., p. 53; and J. L. Hadley, ibid., p. 232.

10. A conditional logit model is the appropriate estimating procedure to use. Up to the present time, we have not been able to get such a model operational. We have located a model which is operational elsewhere and plan to re-estimate the equations at a later time. The present equations will provide a useful initial approximation and will also serve as a point of comparison with later results.

11. If the phsician is in a no-contact state, then the independent variable, for example population growth, is defined as the population growth in the state they are in relative to the population growth in their second choice, if that was a no-contact state or their state for residency. If the physician is not in a no-contact state, the variable would equal population growth in their second choice if that was a no-contact or in their undergraduate or childhood state relative to population growth where they are at. The logic is to look at the value of the variable in the location being specified versus the value in what was their second choice or where they are at, if they are not in the choice being specified. The difficulty here is in constructing a reasonable no-contact proxy if they are in a contact state.

12. Some of the variables which have been used to measure nonmonetary returns include square miles of park, public dollars spent on recreation, degree days, and so forth. Among other difficulties, preferences among physicians for these leisure-related activities can be expected to vary substantially. Held (1972) argues that intrinsic advantages of an area would

be reflected in the value of land and constructs a variable to measure this. He also argues for measures of distance from the coast and the use of net migration rates.

13. The basic form of the regression equation is:

$$P_i = a_o + b_i x_i \ldots b_n x_n + u$$

14. There are three problems with using least squares regression in the analysis of a dichotomous dependent variable. First, the estimated probabilities are not constrained between 0 and 1. Second, there is a problem relating to the linearity assumption. Third, the error term is heteroscedastic, which means that the estimates are inefficient, i.e., result in nonminimum variance. Although the degree of heteroscedasticity and the direction of bias varies with the particular distribution, there is some evidence that the t statistic computed with OLS is conservative. In addition, models where the mean probability is near .5 will be less heteroscedastic than other models. Three of the four equations estimated have mean values near .5. Our conclusion is that while it would be better to estimate the equations using a conditional logit model, we expect the general conclusions would be the same as they are here. See discussions by Abraham Haspal (1974), and James Morgan (1974), Appendix E, and Arthur Goldberger (1964), pp. 248–250.

15. The independent variables which show the expected returns of locating in Michigan relative to their second choice or their actual location could have been constructed either as first differences or as ratios. The use of first differences reflects the assumption that the internal rate of return to a location choice will depend on the difference in expected returns across locations. The use of ratios, which is the procedure used here, implies that the choice depends on the relative characteristics of the alternatives rather than the absolute differences between them. Hadley suggests this seems more consistent with the notion of diminishing marginal returns and with a behavioral model where physicians are assumed to maximize utility, with income and leisure as arguments in their utility functions. [See Hadley (1975), pp. 139–140.]

16. Primary specialists were defined to include general practitioners, internists, obstetrician/gynecologists, and pediatricians. All others are secondary specialists. We also estimated separate equations for primary and secondary specialists as well as single equations with all physicians to test the null hypothesis that specialty has no effect on location. This hypothesis is equivalent to the hypothesis that the parameters of the independent variables are the same for all physicians, irrespective of their specialty. With the use of separate equations, all parameters are allowed to vary with specialty. We used an F statistic based on the sum of squared residuals under the null and alternative hypotheses and were unable to reject the null hypothesis. We therefore estimate a single equation for all specialists.

17. Defining the variable as the number of contacts rather than as separate dummy variables for each contact could mean we are including part of the same variable on both sides of the equation if the choice of residency location is in part dependent on the location of medical school. The equations were estimated both ways and the results were similar. The major variable of importance in the alternative specification was having a residency in the same SMSA as the medical school in the medical school SMSA equation.

18. J. L. Hadley (1975), p. 226.

19. See, for example, Human Resources Research Center (1976), and Gail R. Wilensky (1976).

20. See, for example, Lee Benham, Alex Maurizi, and Melvin Reder (1968), p. 341; Frank A. Sloan, "Economic Models of Physician Supply," unpublished Ph.D. dissertation, Harvard University, 1968, p. 358; and Jack L. Hadley, op.cit., p. 235.

21. Consad Research Corporation (1973), and H. R. Mason (July 1971).

REFERENCES

Benham, Lee, Maurizi, A., and Reder, M. (August 1968), "Migration, Location and Remuneration of Medical Personnel: Physicians and Dentists," *The Review of Economics and Statistics* 50.

Consad Research Corporation (January 31, 1973), *An Evalutaion of the Effectiveness of Loan Forgiveness as an Incentive for Health Practitioners to Locate in Medically Underserved Areas*, funded under contract from DHEW, Publication No. DHEW-OS-73-03

Fein, Rashi and Sloan, F. A. (1971), *Financing Medical Education: An Analysis of Alternative Policies and Mechanisms*, New York: McGraw-Hill.

Goldberger, Arthur (1964), *Econometric Theory*, New York: Wiley.

Hadley, Jack L. (1975), "Models of Physicians Specialty and Location Decisions," No. 6, Technical Paper Series, National Center for Health Services Research.

Haspal, Abraham (1974), "Occupational Decision Making," unpublished Ph. D. dissertation, University of Pennsylvania.

Held, Philip J. (1972), "The Migration of the 1955-1965 Graduates of American Medical Schools," Ph. D. dissertation, University of California, Berkeley.

Human Resources Research Center (August 1976), "Policies to Influence Physicians to Locate in Scarcity Areas," prepared for the Robert Wood Johnson Foundation, University of Southern California.

Mason, H. R. (July 1971), Effectiveness of Student Aid Programs Tied to a Service Commitment," *Journal of Medical Education* 48.

Morgan, James (1974), *500 American Families*, Vol I, Institute for Social Research, Ann Arbor: University of Michigan.

Sloan, F. A. (1968), "Economic Models of Physican Supply," unpublished Ph. D. dissertation, Harvard University.

Weiskotten, Herman G. et al. (December 1960), "An Analysis of the Distributional Characteristics of Medical College Graduates, 1915-50," *The Journal of Medical Education* 35.

Wilensky, Gail R. (August 1976), "Policy Options for Attracting Physicians to Rural Locations," mimeo.

Yett, Donald and Sloan, F. A. (June 1974), "Migration Patterns of Recent Medical School Graduates," *Inquiry* XI.

Appendix 1

Doctor's Name:. . . . .
                              Last   First   Middle

We are interested in how physicians decide where to practice. In addition to questions about how you made your decision, we also need some demographic information about you and your background. In the following questions, please indicate the CITY, STATE, (COUNTRY if not U.S.) and HOSPITAL AFFILIATION where appropriate.

1. Where do you practice now? . . . .
2. Where did you *first* go into practice (if different from Q. 1)?
   . . . .
3. Where did you do your service in the Armed Forces? . . . .
4. Where did you do your residency? . . . .
5. Where did you do your internship? . . . .
6. Where did you go to medical school?. . . . .
   school   state
7. Where did you go to college? . . . .
   school   state
8. Where did you grow up (spend majority of time before age 16)?. . . . .
   . . . .
9. Where were you born? . . . .
10. *When* did you finish your residency?. . . . . Month . . . . . Year . . . . .
11. In what specialty was your residency? . . . .
12. Are you board certified in your specialty?   ☐ Yes   ☐ No
13. Were you married at the time you finished your residency? ☐ Yes ☐ No
14. Are you married now?   ☐ Yes   ☐ No
15. What *type* of practice do you have? ☐ Solo ☐ Group ☐ Hospital-based
    ☐ Prepaid   ☐ Academic   ☐ Military ☐ Other (Specify). . . . .
16. When you finished your residency, how much were you in *debt*? . . . .
    (dollars)
17. What was/is/will be your approximate net income?

	When you started practice	Now?	Expected ten years from now?
Less than $15,000	☐	☐	☐
$15,000 – 25,000	☐	☐	☐
$25,000 – 50,000	☐	☐	☐
$50,000 – 75,000	☐	☐	☐
$75,000 – 100,000	☐	☐	☐
$100,000 – 200,000	☐	☐	☐
More than $200,000	☐	☐	☐

18. When you were deciding where to practice did you have minimum require-
    ments that had to be satisfied before you would consider a particular
    location   Yes   No → Go to Q. 19
    ↓

    18a. What were your minimum requirements?. . . . .
    . . . .
    . . . .

19. Indicate the degree of importance for each of the following (at the time you were deciding where to practice).

		Very important	Somewhat important	Not very important	Not at all important
a.	Adequacy of specialists in other area?	☐	☐	☐	☐
b.	Need for more people in your specialty?	☐	☐	☐	☐
c.	Need for others in your specialty for consultation?	☐	☐	☐	☐
d.	Size of city?	☐	☐	☐	☐
e.	Ability to obtain hospital privileges?	☐	☐	☐	☐
f.	Cultural opportunities?	☐	☐	☐	☐
g.	Expected income?	☐	☐	☐	☐
h.	Recreational facilities and opportunities?	☐	☐	☐	☐
i.	Employment opportunities for your spouse?	☐	☐	☐	☐
j.	Climate?	☐	☐	☐	☐
k.	Proximity to friends or relatives?	☐	☐	☐	☐

20. Was there one crucial factor that made the difference in your decision about where to locate?   ☐ Yes   ☐ No → Go to Q. 21

    20a. What was the crucial factor?

    . . . .
    . . . .

21. Was the place you chose your first choice?
              ☐ Yes → Go to Q. 22.   ☐ No → Go to Q. 21a.

    21a. What was your first choice? . . . .
    21b. Why didn't you go there? . . . . . . , ...
    . . . .

22. Thinking now of your second choice of location – where was it? . . . .
23. Is there anything the community could have offered you to make you locate in their community rather than where you did?

    . . . .
    . . . .

24. How *many* places, other than the one you chose, did you seriously consider? . . . .
    24a. What were some of the other places? . . . .
    . . . .

25. Did you consider locating in any places that were "underserved" by physicians? □ Yes □ No → Got to Q. 26

    25a. What led you to decide against them? . . . .
    . . . .
    . . . .

26. A recent study estimates the total cost of turning out an M.D. to be approximately $80,000. Medical school tuition for four years amounts to $6,400 ($12,800 for nonresidents) at the University of Michigan and $5,180 ($10,600 for nonresidents) at Wayne State. There is a proposal to consider the state subsidy for medical education as a loan, to be repaid with interest unless the doctor serves in one of a list of designated underserved areas in the state. Would that policy have affected your choice of location?

    □ Yes □ No

    26a. If some states did not have this policy, would you still have chosen to go to medical school in Michigan? □ Yes □ No

    26b. Do you think this policy would affect the location choices new doctors make? □ Yes □ No

27. *When* did you choose your specialty? □ 1-2 year Med School □ 3-4 year Med School □ Internship □ Armed Forces □ Beginning of residency

28. *When* did you chose the location of your practice? 1-2 year Med School □ 3-4 year Med School □ Internship □ Armed Forces □ Beginning of residency □ End of residency

29. Is there anything else you would like to tell us to help us understand how physicians make their locational decisions?

    . . . .
    . . . .

A MODEL OF PHYSICIAN LOCATION AND PRICING BEHAVIOR*

Roger Feldman, UNIVERSITY OF MINNESOTA

This study develops and empirically estimates a model of the physicians' services market. The common mode of private medical practice is to have hospital admitting privileges and to make both hospital and office visits,[1] so section I explains the individual physician's allocation of production between hospital and office. Since the hospital staff share common facilities, the model requires a theory of hospital organization. Administrators run the hospital in my model. Their decisions to build beds and hire interns and residents influence the allocation of production and the distribution of physicians across markets.

Section II estimates the model with a cross section of state observations

Research in Health Economics, Vol. 1, pp 185–215.
Copyright © 1979 by JAI Press, Inc.
All rights of reproduction in any form reserved.
ISBN 0-89232-042-7.

for 1971. Hospital beds depend directly on hospital insurance coverage and inversely on net white immigration. More interns and residents are found in states with large teaching and research establishments. Physicians are attracted to states with high per capita incomes, more research physicians, and more teaching hospital approvals. Supplies of hospital and office visits, for both the individual physician and the state market area, depend on the relative attractiveness of each production site, confirming the theory of physician's behavior.

Section III briefly contrasts several models and shows that only the present one provides a unified view of patients, physicians, and hospitals.

I. THEORY

Most physicians produce both hospital and office care. Enterline (1973) found that the allocation of production between hospital and office responds to economic influences. He studied the Canadian experience with Medicare, a universal compulsory health insurance program. Medicare covers both hospital and office care, and in Quebec, where it was superimpossed on a system which already included hospitalization insurance, the program increased the relative demand for office care. Office patient contacts by active physicians in Montreal rose 32.5 percent from pre-Medicare levels, and hospital contacts fell 16 percent.

This section theoretically explains the behavior noted by Enterline. I assume that each physician has admitting privileges at a nonprofit hospital. Hospital administrators purchase inputs (H), offer them to staff physicians in fixed-proportion bundles (h), and bill the average cost to patients. Since the benefits of hospital inputs accrue to individual physicians, whereas costs are spread over all patients, physicians overutilize hospital inputs unless they are rationed.

The traditional hospital literature has long been concerned with noncooperative behavior among the hospital staff. "The distinctive feature of the Anglo-American voluntary hospital has been its use by private physicians for private patients with little or no accompanying financial or administrative responsibility" Somers (1961). In return the physician was supposed to provide charity care for the sick poor who constituted the majority of patients. But patients now have high incomes and insurance to pay for admissions. Technological change has also transformed the hospital into an "indispensable workshop" for the modern M.D. The use of hospital resources without responsibilities makes the relation of the staff to the hospital "increasingly contradictory," and at one point the Somerses even describe the modern voluntary hospital as an "organizational anomaly" (1967).

Compensatory organizational controls may take over resource allocation in this price-free environment. Roemer and Friedman (1971) find that surgical privileges of general practitioners are more carefully stipulated in hospitals where staff memberships are easily obtained. Clarkson (1972) reports that nonstaff members are more often denied practice in proprietary hospitals, but restrictions on staff surgical privileges are more common in nonprofit hospitals. This again implies a compensatory system: private owners want to, and can, keep nonmembers out; this is less easily done in a nonprofit hospital, so other restrictions are practiced.

May (1969) has suggested that hospital inputs are sold to physician-entrepreneurs who organize the production process. This transaction involves a labor payment by the physician to the hospital, so May's argument implies that each physician's hospital care output (x) is proportionate to his own hospital practice hours (m):

$$x = \alpha \cdot m.^2 \qquad (1)$$

Evidence that this implicit market exists is found in the practice of awarding preferred staff privileges to physicians with stronger hospital commitment Letourneau (1964), Roemer and Friedman (1971). Commitment usually means primary affiliation to that particular hospital, participation in the departmental affairs and committees of the medical staff, or acceptance of teaching responsibilities in a hospital with training programs. Each of these requirements indicates a labor payment by the physician to the hospital, and in return the physician gets preferential admitting privileges.

For each unit of hospital care the physician receives p dollars, a constant price outside the individual's control. This choice differentiates the model from Sloan's, where the physician is a price-setting monopolist (1974, 1976). Physicians bear no financial responsibility for hospital inputs, so gross and net income from hospital practice equals $p \cdot x$.

Office care (v) is produced by office hours (w) and other inputs (z). A Cobb-Douglas[3] production function is chosen:

$$v = w^{\gamma} z^{\tau}, \gamma + \tau < 1. \qquad (2)$$

For each unit of office care the physician receives a given fee of f dollars. Gross and net revenue from office practice differ because of office costs. Let office inputs be hired a c dollars per unit. Therefore, net office income is $f \cdot v - c \cdot z$. Total net income is

$$y = p \cdot x + f \cdot v - c \cdot z. \qquad (3)$$

The physician's utility function includes net income (y) and total hours worked ($l = m + w$):

$$u = u(y,l), \tag{4}$$

where $u_1 > 0$, $u_2 < 0$, and $u_{12} < 0$. Utility is maximized subject to the income constraint and the production functions for hospital and office care. From the Lagrangean,

$$L = u(p \cdot x + f \cdot v - c \cdot z, m + w) + \mu(x - \alpha \cdot m) + \delta(v - w^{\gamma} z^{\tau}), \tag{5}$$

first-order conditions are

$$-u_2/u_1 = p \cdot \alpha = f \cdot \gamma \cdot w^{\gamma-1} z^{\tau} \tag{6}$$

$$c = f \cdot \tau \cdot w^{\gamma} z^{\tau-1} \tag{7}$$

subject to $\partial L/\partial \mu$ and $\partial L/\partial \delta$ equal zero. Equation (6) states that the marginal rate of substitution of work time for income equals the marginal revenue product of work in either hospital or office. And equation (7) shows that prices of physician-purchased inputs equal their marginal revenue products.

Information about the utility function or a constraint on total hours worked is required to solve these equations for hospital and office work time. However, the essential features of the physician's time allocation are revealed by Figure 1.

Hours worked and net income in hospital and office practice are related by functions $\pi(m)$ and $\chi(w)$. Hospital $\pi(m)$ is a straight line,

$$\pi(m) = p \cdot \alpha \cdot m, \tag{8}$$

with the slope controlled by p and α. The slope of office $\chi(w)$ falls as office practice hours rise because of diminishing returns to scale in production. By first-order condition (6) the physician works in office practice up to w^* where the slopes of $\pi(m)$ and $\chi(w)$ are equal. He then extends hospital practice from w^* to l^* where $\pi(m)$ is tangent to indifference curve uu.

The comparative statics of the model can be demonstrated by differentiating the equilibrium conditions or manipulating Figure 1. An increase in f, or a decrease in c, raises both $\chi(w)$ and its derivative at any w, causing substitution from hospital to office practice. An increase in p or α reduces office hours and, although offsetting income and substitution effects influence hospital hours, empirical evidence suggests that hospital hours rise.[4]

Labor supply responses are converted into individual physician's product supply curves by the hospital and office production functions. Equations (9) and (10) are the individual supply curves of hospital and office care, and Table 1 shows the predicted signs of individual supply elasticities:

$$x^s = x^s(p, f, c, H/POP, DOCS/POP, SS) \tag{9}$$

$$v^s = v^s(p, f, c, H/POP, DOCS/POP, SS).[5] \tag{10}$$

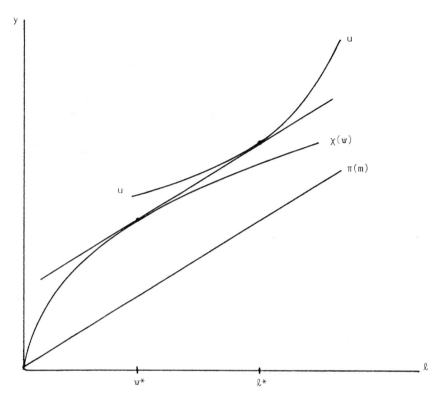

Figure 1.   Physician's Time Allocation Between Hospital and Office

Table 1. Predicted Signs of Individual Supply Elasticities

Variable	Elasticity in Hospital Supply Equation	Elasticity in Office Supply Equation
p	+	−
f	−	+
c	+	−
H/POP	+	−
DOCS/POP	−	0

H replaces α as an observable shift parameter in the supply functions because, as H increases, physicians perceive a higher value of α and reallocate supply toward the hospital. As the number of physicians (DOCS) in the market area increases, *ceteris paribus,* the demand for H increases. Each physician receives less H and produces less hospital care. On the other hand, DOCS will not affect the individual's office output unless the supply of office factors is inelastic to the industry. No empirical evidence suggests a rising office factor supply price. The final variable is a vector of supply shift parameters (SS) which may differ between the two functions. The composition of SS depends on special features of the markets which will be explained in section II.

The distribution of physicians is an endogenous variable in the model. Physicians will move between markets until the attainable utility in each location is equal.[6] Variables which raise π(m) or χ(w) increase utility. Therefore, DOCS is explained by the equation,

$$DOCS/POP = DOCS(p,f,c,H/POP, SS) \tag{11}$$

Physicians should be attracted to a state where fees and hospital visit prices are high, office input costs are low, and hospital inputs are plentiful. Two hospital inputs which may attract physicians are interns and residents (HBMD) and (BEDS). In 1971 there were 48,000 hospital-based interns and residents in the United States [American Medical Association (1971)]. Rosett (1974) argues that HBMD substitute for physicians' labor in caring for hospitalized patients.[7] HBMD, therefore, should attract physicians to a state.

The role of hospital beds is unclear. Feldstein (1967) found that beds increase output in a Cobb-Douglas production function. This would attract physicians. However, Vladeck (1976) argues that beds merely increase capacity unless accompanied by a proportionate addition to labor. Rosett even suggests that beds lower output by "diluting" HBMD.[8] This would drive physicians away. These hypotheses can be tested by including HBMD and BEDS in the estimated distribution of physicians equation.

Individual supplies are multiplied by the distribution of physicians to produce aggregate supplies of hospital (X) and office (V) care. Since individual supplies and DOCS depend on the same variables, aggregate supplies are also functions of those variables:

$$X^s/POP = x^s \cdot DOCS/POP = X^s(p, f, c, H/POP, SS) \tag{12}$$

$$V^s/POP = v^s \cdot DOCS/POP = V^s(p, f, c, H/POP, SS). \tag{13}$$

Hospital inputs are exogenous to physicians but not to administrators. To explain how H is chosen, the demand side of the model must be introduced. Assume for now that there is no insurance, so consumer demands for hospital and office care depend on gross prices. Hospital price is the sum of the physician's price and the hospital's bill (t). Demands also depend on per capita income (Y) and a vector of demographic variables (DEM):

$$X^d/POP = X^d(p+t, f, Y, DEM) \tag{14}$$

$$V^d/POP = V^d(p+t, f, Y, DEM). \tag{15}$$

The administrators' choice of H obeys a budget constraint. Since charitable contributions are relatively small, average revenue equals average cost:

$$X \cdot t = b \cdot H, \tag{16}$$

where b is the market price of hospital inputs. As X rises the average bill required to break even falls, and when inputs are given, the relation between t and X is a rectangular hyperbola.

Altogether the administrators face equations (12) through (16)—i.e., supplies, demands, and the budget constraint. These five equations solve for five endogenous variables—p, t, f, X, and V—in terms of H and exogenous variables:

$$X = X(H, Y, DEM, b, c, SS). \tag{17}$$

Assume that the administrators maximize a utility function which includes output and hospital inputs:

$$U = U(H,X).^9 \tag{18}$$

The first-order condition for a maximum,

$$\partial U/\partial H = U_1 + U_2 X_H = 0, \tag{19}$$

implies that output is falling at equilibrium. The second-order condition,

$$\partial^2 U/\partial H^2 = U_{11} + 2 \cdot U_{12}X_H + U_2 X_{HH} + U_{22}X_H^2 < 0, \tag{20}$$

is met if X_{HH} is not too positive. Equilibrium H* is illustrated in Figure 2 where an indifference curve, UU, is tangent to X(H).

A change in a variable exogenous to both physicians and administrators shifts the opportunity locus in Figure 2. But the direction of the shift is ambiguous due to cross-price elasticities of demand and supply in the five-equation model. To simplify the problem I assume that cross elasticities are zero, so changes are confined to the market in which they originate. Administrators now face only (12), (14), and (16). The Appendix shows that the opportunity locus shifts outward when 1) the demand curve for hospital care shifts to the right, 2) the supply curve shifts to the

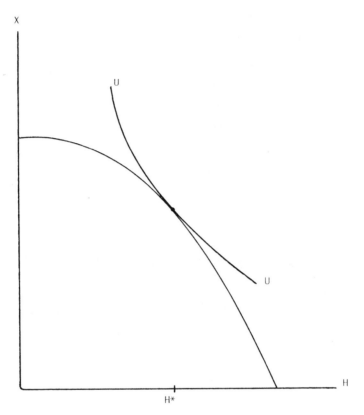

Figure 2. Hospital Administrators' Choice of Inputs

right, or 3) hospital input prices fall. If inputs are normal goods, more will be hired. Therefore, the system is closed with

$$H/POP = H(Y, SS, b), \tag{21}$$

and the predictions that $H_1 > 0$, $H_2 > 0$ for those elements of SS that increase supply, and $H_3 < 0$.

In summary, this section explained how physicians allocate production between hospital and office depending on the relative attractiveness of each production site. Physicians also migrate to areas where attainable utility is higher. The behavior of physicians and consumers constrains hospital administrators, who will hire more inputs when the supply or demand for hospital care increases and input prices fall. In the next section I will test these hypotheses.

II. ESTIMATION

The model is estimated with state mean data for 49 states and the District of Columbia for 1971, or a year as close to 1971 as sources permit. Table 2 summarizes the data.

First, I estimate the distributions of hospital beds (BEDS) and interns and residents (HBMD). The location of hospital beds depends on con-

Table 2. Variables in the Model of Supply of
Physicians' Hospital and Office Visits

Variable Name	Description
Exogenous variables	
DIS	Deaths per 100,000 from certain diseases of early infancy
INS	Proportion of under-65 population with hospital insurance
Y	Real income per capita
CTH	Council of Teaching Hospital approvals
CON	Hospital bed control program (1 if absent, e^1 if present)
CONSWG	Annual real wage of construction workers
HILBUR	Real Hill-Burton allocations per capita, fiscal 1960 - 1970
MDRES	Research physicians
MDTCH	Teaching physicians
MIG	One plus the proportion of 1970 population due to net white immigration from 1960 - 1970
WG	Index of real weekly wages of office labor
Endogenous variables	
BEDS	Community hospital beds
DOCS	Non-Federal physicians in office based practice
f	Fee for quality-adjusted office visit[a]
HBMD	Interns and residents in nonfederal hospitals
p	Price for quality-adjusted hospital visit paid to physician
(p + t)	Total price for quality-adjusted hospital visit
x	Quality-adjusted hospital visits per physician
V	Quality-adjusted office visits
v	Quality-adjusted office visits per physician
X	Quality-adjusted hospital visits
DD	Dentists

[a] Prices and quantities are adjusted for quality differences between states by a method described in Feldman (1976).

sumer demand, hospital construction costs, and regulatory or institutional features of the market for funds. Steinwald and Neuhauser (1970) found that proprietary hospitals concentrate in states where population is rapidly increasing. They argue that the philanthropic tradition and capital markets necessary to support nonprofit hospitals have not developed in these states. Smaller, more adaptable proprietaries fill some of the gap. If, as Steinwald and Neuhauser suggest, the institutions necessary to support the normally dominant form of hospital are not present, we should observe fewer total beds in rapidly growing states. This will also be true if hospitals respond to population growth with a simple construction lag. In either case I hypothesize a negative relation between population growth and hospital beds per capita. Population growth is measured by MIG, which is one plus the proportion of 1970 population due to net white immigration from 1960 to 1970.[10]

Real per capita income (Y) and hospital insurance coverage (INS) increase the demand for hospital visits. In Section I, I showed that an increase in demand shifts the hospital administrators' opportunity locus outward, and I predicted that beds should increase.

In 1973, twenty-two states had "certificate of need" laws regulating investment in hospital facilities.[11] Certificate of need, sometimes called "bed control," is a franchise where hospitals apply to a regulatory body for approval of investment projects. Although laws vary by state, they are often invoked to limit bed expansion. Five states had certificate of need laws for more than half of the period from 1968 through 1972.[12] These states, indicated by dummy variable CON, should have fewer hospital beds per capita.

The Federal government has subsidized the construction of hospital facilities through the Hill-Burton program since 1948. Funds were originally allocated by a formula that favored rural areas within a state, and also states with lower per capita income. However, as the program progressed, aid has gone to states with more beds per capita (1973). The effect of this program is measured by variable HILBUR, which is the real per capita value of Hill-Burton allocations from fiscal year 1960 through 1970.[13] States where HILBUR is high should have more beds per capita.

Construction costs are a major part of hospital investments. Construction wages are measured by CONSWG, the average annual real wage rate of construction workers in 1970.[14] Higher construction wages shift the hospital administrator's opportunity locus inward, thereby lowering BEDS.

The complete equation for the distribution of hospital beds is

$$\text{BEDS/POP} = \text{BEDS(MIG, Y, INS, CON, HILBUR, CONSWG)}. \quad (22)$$

Table 3. Determinants of the Distribution of Hospital Beds

Variable	Short Description	Equation					
		(1)	(2)	(3)	(4)	(5)	(6)
	Dependent variable – hospital beds per capita						
MIG	Migration	-1.61 (-5.01)[a]	-1.41 (-5.04)	-1.33 (-4.82)	-1.36 (-5.22)	-1.12 (-4.29)	-1.11 (-4.2)
INS	Hospital Insurance		.905 (4.25)	.96 (4.59)	.797 (3.85)	.949 (4.68)	.94 (4.46)
CON	Hospital bed control program			-.14 (-1.94)	-.186 (-2.64)	-.0917 (-1.22)	.0965 (-1.21)
Y	Per capita income				.495 (2.59)	.834 (3.76)	.841 (3.71)
HILBUR	Hill-Burton Allocations per capita					.21 (2.62)	.2 (2.15)
CONSWG	Construction wage						-.0373 (.205)
R²		.343	.525	.561	.618	.67	.67

[a] Numbers in parentheses below the coefficient are t-values.

195

Ordinary least squares estimates of the equation, specified in double log form, are shown in Table 3. Six versions of the equation illustrate how the results change as variables are added. Variables are added in stepwise order, so the R^2 difference between equations measures the contribution of each new variable to the explanatory power of the regression. All variables have the predicted signs, and all but CONSWG and CON are significant at the .025 level of confidence or better (in a one-tailed t-test). Migration is the best predictor of fewer beds per capita. Hospital insurance coverage adds another .182 to R^2, so the two variables together explain .525 of the variance in beds per capita.

The location of interns and residents depends on training opportunities, demand factors, and anticipated future practice income (since many interns and residents practice in their training state). Training opportunities are represented by MDTCH, MDRES, and CTH. The first two variables are non-Federal physicians engaged in teaching and research. CTH is the number of member hospitals of the Council of Teaching Hospitals.[15] Office visit fees measure demand for office care, and INS represents demand for hospital care. Better hospital insurance coverage should strongly attract interns and residents, because it increases both their future opportunities in private practice and the derived hospital demand for their services.[16]

Hadley (1975), in his microeconomic location study of new physician cohorts, found a propensity to locate in states where in-migration is high. Migration should also attract HBMD. Migration signals high future demand and practice income. And interns and residents, like other Americans, may prefer the South to the North and the coasts to the interior of the country. For either reason, I hypothesize a positive relation between HBMD and MIG.

The complete equation for the distribution of interns and residents is

$$\text{HBMD/POP} = \text{HBMD(MDTCH/POP, INS, MIG, CTH/POP, f, MDRES/POP).}^{17} \qquad (23)$$

Stepwise two-stage least squares estimates of the equation, specified in double log form, are presented in Table 4. All variables have the expected signs and all but research physicians per capita have t-statistics greater than one. The best predictor of more HBMD per capita is teaching physicians. Hospital insurance coverage is the next best predictor. The large numerical elasticity, 3.57, supports the Rosett-Berg conjecture that insurance is important in the bidding for interns and residents. The coefficient of office fees shows that demand conditions attract HBMD, and the predicted relation between HBMD and MIG is confirmed.

The distribution of physicians should depend on present and expected future demand conditions, office practice costs, and the supply of hospital

Table 4. Determinants of the Distribution of Interns and Residents

Variable	Short Description	Equation					
		(1)	(2)	(3)	(4)	(5)	(6)
Dependent variable – interns and residents per capita							
MDTCH/POP	Teaching physicians per capita	1.53 (11.7)[a]	1.26 (9.4)	1.26 (10.1)	1.11 (7.63)	.994 (6.00)	.949 (5.09)
INS	Hospital insurance		3.67 (3.83)	4.04 (4.5)	3.89 (4.45)	3.80 (4.37)	3.57 (3.67)
MIG	Migration			2.97 (2.92)	3.44 (3.38)	2.98 (2.81)	2.64 (2.13)
CTH/POP	Approvals per capita				1.29E5 (1.93)	1.42E5 (2.11)	1.23E5 (1.63)
$\hat{f}$	Physician's fee for quality-adjusted office visit					.211 (1.38)	.188 (1.17)
MDRES/POP	Research physicians per capita						.097 (.542)
R^2		.741	.802	.833	.846	.853	.854

[a] Numbers in parentheses below the coefficients are t-values.

inputs. For professional or personal reasons, physicians may also prefer states that offer superior teaching, learning and research opportunities. Real per capita income (Y) represents the demand for both office and hospital care. Migration is a proxy for expected future demand (or location preferences). Research physicians and CTH approvals per capita measure the scope of the state's medical education facilities.

Physicians surveyed by the AMA often employed secretaries and registered nurses, so office input costs are measured by wages of nurses and secretaries (WG).

The hospital inputs emphasized in this study are HBMD and BEDS. Physicians should be directly related to HBMD if interns and residents substitute for physicians' labor. If, as Rosett suggests, hospital beds dilute HBMD, then an increase in beds should reduce DOCS/POP. Therefore, this equation can provide insight into the role of hospital inputs in the physicians' services market.

The full equation for the distribution of office-based private practitioners is:

$$DOCS/POP = DOCS(MDRES/POP, Y, CTH/POP, HBMD/POP, WG, MIG, BEDS/POP). \qquad (24)$$

Stepwise two-stage least squares estimates of the double log equation are shown in Table 5. The number of research physicians per capita is the best predictor for the distribution of physicians in private practice. Per capita income is also a good predictor, and the magnitude of the coefficient indicates that a 1 percent increase in Y is associated with a .77 percent increase in DOCS/POP. The coefficients of CTH approvals and office input wages also have the expected signs.

The coefficient of MIG is positive, as expected, but it is small and statistically insignificant. This offers an interesting comparison to the large significant effect of MIG on the location of interns and residents. The cost of relocation is higher for established physicians, causing them to lag behind changes in exogenous variables (as found by Benham et al. (1968). Also, the discounted returns from moving should be higher for young physicians. Therefore, both the costs and benefits of relocation explain the low migration elasticity of DOCS.

The effects of HBMD and BEDS are surprising. Interns and residents are inversely related to private practitioners with a t-statistic greater than one in absolute value. Beds are directly and insignificantly related to private practitioners. Therefore, this equation confirms neither the attraction of HBMD to DOCS, nor Rosett's hypothesis that BEDS dilute HBMD.

These unexpected results are due to different migration responses for each specialty. I regressed private practitioners per capita in four special-

Table 5. Determinants of the Distribution of Physicians in Office-Based Private Practice

Variable	Short Description		Equation					
		(1)	(2)	(3)	(4)	(5)	(6)	(7)
Dependent variable – physicians per capita in office-based private practice								
MDRES/POP	Research physicians per capita	.148 (6.11)[a]	.112 (5.02)	.083 (3.19)	.146 (3.59)	.133 (3.17)	.121 (2.76)	.122 (2.74)
Y	Per capita income		.779 (4.29)	.699 (3.89)	.675 (3.86)	.745 (4.03)	.730 (3.93)	.711 (3.46)
CTH/POP	Approvals per capita			3.23E4 (2.05)	4.29E4 (2.65)	3.82E4 (2.29)	4.62E4 (2.47)	4.74E4 (2.41)
HBMD/POP	Interns and residents per capita				-.0623 (-1.97)	-.0482 (-1.14)	-.0480 (-1.42)	-.0499 (-1.41)
WG	Office input wages					-313 (-1.14)	-.286 (-1.04)	-.294 (-1.05)
MIG	Migration						.253 (.953)	.310 (.835)
BEDS/POP	Hospital beds per capita							.0311 (.0004)
R^2		.437	.596	.630	.630	.669	.676	.676

[a] Numbers in parentheses below the coefficients are t-values.

ties[18] on the same exogenous variables and instruments. The results of the 2SLS double log specification are shown in Table 6. Each column headed by a specialty represents a different equation, and each row shows the migration effect of an independent variable or instrument.

Only general practitioners are not attracted to states with more research physicians and CTH approvals. This difference suggests that reasearch, teaching, and training opportunities are unimportant for GP's.

General practitioners are only weakly attracted by high per capita incomes, whereas the coefficients for all other specialties are positive and significant at the .05 level of confidence in a one-tailed t-test. The elasticity is also larger for other specialties (a 1 percent rise in Y is associated with a .958 percent increase in medical specialists and a 1.46 percent increase in other specialists). Consumer demand must switch from general practitioners toward specialists as per capita income rises.

All specialties are weakly and positively associated with migration. All but surgical specialties are negatively associated with office input wages. This difference is consistent with the fact that surgeons derive a large, proportion of their net income from hospital practice [American Medical Association (1971)]. Therefore, they should be less sensitive to office practice costs.[19]

More GP's are found in states with more beds. Because general practitioners' hospital staff privileges are often restricted, more beds may make it easier for GP's to obtain hospital admitting privileges. Beds may also be more productive in the kinds of hospital cases usually treated by GP's. Different hospital inputs (such as capital equipment or surgical facilities) may be more important for other specialties.

Although these equations illuminate the role of hospital beds in the physicians' services market, they confirm the negative relations between HBMD and physicians for all specialties. This may be due to the medical education variables that influence the distribution of both HBMD and physicians. Table 7 presents an experiment in which private practitioners are regressed on HBMD alone. Then other variables are added, and as MDRES is introduced, the coefficient of HBMD suddenly turns from positive and significant to negative. The coefficient remains negative when CTH is added. Student physicians trained without institutional and educational support apparently decrease the productivity of staff physicians, causing them to leave the area.

Let us turn to the individual supply equations. The output units for these equations are hospital and office visits. Signs of supply-determining variables predicted in section I indicate that higher office visit fees increase the supply of office visits per physician. The opposite effect should occur when office input prices or hospital visit fees rise. Individual office visit supply is not affected by physician density, but more physicians per

Table 6. Determinants of the Distribution of Physicians in Office-Based Private Practice by Specialty

Variable	Short Description	Dependent Variable			
		GP's per capita	Medical Specs. per capita	Surgical Specs. per capita	Other Specs. per capita
MDRES/POP[a]	Research physicians per capita	.0167 (.296)[b]	.191 (2.71)	.130 (2.62)	.231 (4.01)
Y	Per capita income	.205 (.781)	.958 (2.93)	.463 (2.00)	1.26 (4.71)
CTH/POP	Approvals per capita	-3.82E4 (-1.52)	7.83E4 (2.50)	6.32E4 (2.85)	6.64E4 (2.60)
$\widehat{\text{HBMD}}$/POP	Interns and residents per capita	-.042 (-.933)	-.00835 (-.149)	-.0647 (-1.63)	-.719 (-1.57)
WG	Office input wages	-.214 (-.598)	-.812 (-1.82)	.023 (.073)	-.133 (-.364)
MIG	Migration	.152 (.322)	.312 (.528)	.464 (1.11)	.335 (.696)
$\widehat{\text{BEDS}}$/POP	Hospital beds per capita	.371 (2.08)	-.25 (-1.12)	-.0715 (-.455)	-.83 (-.458)
R^2		.287	.742	.609	.796

a Variables are not entered in stepwise order

b Numbers in parentheses below the coefficients are t-values.

Table 7. Determinants of the Distribution of Physicians in Office-based Private Practice, as a Function of HBMD/POP and Other Variables

Variable	Short Description	Equation						
		(1)	(2)	(3)	(4)	(5)	(6)	(7)
Dependent variable – physicians per capita in office-based private practice								
HBMD/POP[a]	Interns & residents per capita	.0889 (4.3)[b]	.0887 (4.18)	.0636 (3.46)	.0682 (3.83)	.0683 (3.76)	-.017 (-.495)	-.0499 (-1.41)
BEDS/POP	Hospital beds per capita		.00506 (.0392)	-.144 (-1.29)	-.0061 (-.878)	-.101 (-.664)	-.064 (-.45)	.0311 (.00038)
Y	Per capita income			.976 (4.75)	1.05 (5.24)	1.05 (5.05)	.897 (4.46)	.711 (3.46)
WG	Office input wages				.643 (2.17)	-.641 (-2.12)	-.414 (-1.53)	-.294 (-1.05)
MIG	Migration					-.016 (-.044)	-.143 (-.423)	.310 (.835)
MDRES/POP	Research physicians per capita						.133 (2.85)	.122 (2.74)
CTH/POP	Approvals per capita							4.74E4 (2.41)
R^2		.278	.278	.516	.562	.562	.631	.676

[a] Variables are not entered in stepwise order.
[b] Numbers in parentheses below the coefficients are t-values.

capita should reduce hospital supply when hospital inputs are held constant.

The migration variable (MIG) reflects institutional features of the market. Overall, there is a moderate relation between migration and the location of physicians, and Hadley's (1975) study reveals a strong association between migration and location by newly graduated physicians. Physicians may find it easier to reestablish or build up practices by joining hospital staffs. Therefore, migrations should increase the supply of hospital visits and reduce the supply of office visits per physician.

The elasticities of supply with respect to hospital beds and HBMD provide clues to the nature of the hospital visit production function. If the Cobb-Douglas function featured in section I is correct, then both inputs will increase hospital visits and reduce office visits. HBMD may decrease hospital supply per physician if they substitute for staff labor, since the staff can care for patients with fewer of their own visits. And if beds are nonproductive (or counterproductive) they will not affect (or lower) hospital visits per physician.

Physicians may work harder, due to a "keeping up with the Joneses" effect, in areas with more high income professional people. Since dentists and physicians have similar incomes, and dentists also provide a health service, dentists may be a good reference income group for physicians.[20] Each physician will supply more hospital and office care in areas with more dentists. Therefore, an instrumental variable for the distribution of dentists (DD) is included in the supply equations.

A double log specification of the supply equations is shown in Table 8.[21] The hospital visit supply equation is generally satisfactory, with the exception of the insignificant negative own-price elasticity. Higher office fees cause physicians to reallocate production away from hospital care. Higher office input wages cause the opposite effect. More physicians per capita significantly reduce hospital visits per physician when hospital inputs are held constant, as predicted by section I. Of the two hospital inputs, only beds has a noticable effect on production; in fact, the coefficient indicates that a one percent increase in beds is associated with approximately a 1 percent increase in hospital visits. The predicted positive association of hospital visits with migration and dentists is confirmed, although both coefficients are statistically insignificant.

The existence of an upward-sloping supply curve for office visits, as well as the negative shift effect of hospital visit price, is strongly confirmed. More HBMD per capita appear to allow the allocation of production toward office care. Migration has the predicted negative effect and dentists is positive, although neither coefficient is significant. The coefficient of physicians per capita is numerically small ($-.1888$) and statistically insignificant, implying that expansion of the office visit industry

Table 8. The Supply per Physician of Hospital and Office Visits

Independent Variable	Short Description	Dependent Variable	
		Quality-adjusted Hospital Visits per Capita	Quality-adjusted Office Visits per Capita
$\hat{r}$[a]	Physician's fee for quality-adjusted office visit	-1.32 (-1.12)	.961 (2.7)
$\hat{p}$	Physician's price for quality-adjusted hospital visit	-.106 (-.497)	-.14 (-2.7)
WG	Office input wages	2.63 (1.95)	.169 (.414)
DÔCS/POP	Physicians per capita in office-based private practice	-2.39 (-2.53)	-.188 (-.653)
MIG	Migration	.896 (.951)	-.235 (-.831)
HBMD/POP	Interns and residents per capita	-.0428 (-.466)	.0316 (1.13)
BÊDS/POP	Hospital beds per capita	1.03 (1.88)	.0554 (.335)
DD/POP	Dentists per capita	.548 (.535)	.297 (.952)
R^{2c}		.741	.954

[a] Variables are not entered in stepwise order.

[b] Numbers in parentheses below the coefficients are t-values.

[c] R^2 statistics, artificially increased by the weighting procedure, indicate relative goodness of fit.

occurs through entry of optimal-sized firms. The only unsatisfactory coefficient is that of office input wages which ought to be negative but is insignificantly positive.

Table 9 shows the supply of office and hospital care per capita. The own-price elasticity of hospital visits is now positive as predicted. For office visits the WG coefficient also has the right sign. In both equations the effect of HBMD is more noticeable— interns and residents appear to cause substitution away from hospital visit production toward office visits.

In summary, the supply of hospital and office visits can be predicted with an economic model. Supply equations, with the exception of one negative price elasticity, confirm my theory of the allocation of production between hospital and office.

III. RELATION TO OTHER MODELS

My theory is related to the hospital models of Feldstein (1971), Pauly and Redisch (1973), and Rosett (1974). This section contrasts the models and shows that only the present one provides a unified view of patients, physicians, and hospitals.

Feldstein (1971) argues that administrators control hospitals. He includes patient days and quality of care in the administrators' utility function. Their problem is to maximize utility subject to production functions, consumer demand, and the budget constraint that average revenue equals average cost. These constraints define an opportunity locus between patient days and quality, and equilibrium occurs where the opportunity locus is tangent to an administrator indifference curve.

In contrast to Feldstein (1971), Pauly and Redisch (1973) emphasize the preferences of the physician staff members. In the short run the number of physicians with admitting privileges is fixed, and income per man is maximized by hiring nonphysician inputs according to the standard conditions that marginal revenue products equal marginal factor costs. In the intermediate run staff size can vary. The *closed-staff* hospital maximizes the money incomes of all members by adding staff only if it raises everyone's income—i.e., if the marginal revenue product of hospital staff is greater than the net average revenue product. A physician, on the other hand, wants to join the staff if his income exceeds the amount he could earn at another hospital or in office practice. In the long run with free entry, new hospitals will be built. Average revenue falls and the supply price rises until staff physicians' incomes equal their foregone opportunities.

The Pauly-Redisch (1973) model casts the staffing decision as an

Table 9. The Supply per Capita of Hospital and Office Visits

Independent Variable	Short Description	Dependent Variable	
		Quality-adjusted Hospital Visits per Capita	Quality-adjusted Office Visits per Capita
$\hat{f}$[a]	Physician's fee for quality-adjusted office visit	-1.92 (-1.65)	1.15 (2.24)
$\hat{p}$	Physician's price for quality-adjusted hospital visit	.0618 (.295)	-.128 (-1.57)
WG	Office input wages	.268 (1.96)	-.411 (-.771)
MIG	Migration	.337 (.348)	-.485 (-1.29)
HBMD/POP	Interns and residents per capita	-.0795 (-.904)	.0772 (2.26)
BEDS/POP	Hospital beds per capita	1.11 (2.03)	-.156 (-.732)
DD/POP	Dentists per capita	-.892 (-1.6)	.89 (4.11)
R^{2c}		.716	.936

[a] Variables are not entered in stepwise order.
[b] Numbers in parentheses below the coefficients are t-values.
[c] R^2 statistics, artificially increased by the weighting procedure, indicate relative goodness of fit.

economic problem. Nevertheless, it is highly artificial because each physician works a constant number of hours and specializes in either hospital or office practice. Another problem is the assumption of perfect cooperation implied by the average revenue maximization hypothesis. The self-interest of an individual physician suggests balancing the benefits of a hired input against his fractional share of the cost. If the problems of policing noncooperative behavior increase with staff size, physicians in large hospitals will not behave in the altruistic manner ascribed to them by Pauly and Redisch.

One typology (1974) classifies both the Feldstein (1971) and Pauly-Redisch (1973) approaches as "organism" models which imagine a single decision maker, either "the administrator" or "the medical staff." Organism models are criticized because they contain little institutional information and do not recognize that different groups within the hospital interact to pursue different goals. The distinction between organism and interactive theories provides a framework for introducing Rosett's hospital model. He argues that physicians, choosing a city in which to practice, assess its location, climate, and municipal resources that enhance the quality of life. They also calculate profit, which depends on the fee structure determined by supply and demand. Quality and profit interact, because physicians are attracted to a pleasant city, increasing the supply of services and lowering fees.

Rosett (1974) emphasizes the role of physicians in the hospital. He says, "In an important sense, the physician is the natural proprietor of the hospital to which he admits his patient." The physician prescribes treatment, and hospital resources are placed under his control since the hospital must assume responsibility for supervision of patients (including immediate response to emergencies) in his absence. Hospital-based physicians assist in caring for patients. An exogenous increase in HBMD leads to inmigration and lower profits, since supply increases while demand is unchanged. On the other hand, an exogenous increase in hospital beds dilutes HBMD and causes an exodus of physicians.

Rosett's theory appears to be a "physician's control" organism model. This interpretation is deceptively incorrect. The two important hospital inputs—HBMD and beds—are given exogenously to individual physicians. And Rosett, unlike Pauly and Redisch, does not argue that physicians collectively choose hospital inputs to maximize utility. Some group, of course, must purchase HBMD and beds. This group will be the administrators who share control with physicians.

To test his theory, Rosett examined the distribution of physicians among 27 metropolitan areas in 1970. He found more physicians in areas with more HBMD and fewer where there were more beds. He also used dentists per thousand population (DD) as a proxy for quality of life. Since dentists rarely admit patients to the hospital, he assumed that DD, HBMD, and BEDS are uncorrelated. But dentists and doctors have similar education and income, and if their tastes are similar, dentists should measure the qualities that attract physicians. Rosett found the predicted positive relation between dentists and physicians.

The causal relation between dentists and physicians overlooks consumer demand. If dentists' and physicians' services are both superior goods, both professions will concentrate in high-income areas. Rosett also does not pursue the relation between hospital staff and administrators. Beds and HBMD are exogenous to the staff, but they are endogenous in the complete model. Therefore, the distribution of physicians must be estimated by the two-stage procedure used in section II.

Table 10 shows that per capita income is the best predictor of the distribution of dentists. We also find fewer dentists in states where high wages increase dental practice costs. Dentists are unrelated to beds as Rosett predicted, but for some unknown reason they are positively related to HBMD. The location coefficient of DIS shows, not surprisingly, that a state with more childhood deaths is an unattractive location.[22]

The next regressions in Table 10 use dentists to predict the distribution of physicians. Rosett's argument is strongly supported when the equation includes dentists, income, HBMD, and beds. Adding WG and MIG does not lower the attractiveness of HBMD to physicians. But when MDRES and CTH are included, HBMD and beds become statistically insignificant. So Rosett's equation is like my result: an increase in HBMD, holding research physicians and approvals constant, does not attract physicians.

My model is synthesized from Feldstein's (1971), Pauly and Redisch's (1973), and Rosett's (1974). A common feature is the rather passive role of consumer demand. Hardly mentioned by Pauly-Redisch and Rosett, the demand equations in the other two models are mainly constraints on the discretion of hospital administrators.

All the models but the present one are limited to the hospital. Feldstein asserted that administrators run the hospital, and his major contribution was to derive an opportunity locus from consumer demand and the budget constraint. His shortcoming was to ignore the constraint imposed by physicians. Pauly and Redisch corrected this oversight but, by ignoring the administrator, went too far in the other direction.

Rosett (1974) had an intuitive interactive model. I extend his analysis by making hospital inputs endogenous and, more important, by letting physicians determine the allocation of production between hospital and office. Thus, I can estimate supply curves for both types of visits. The combination of patients, physicians, and hospitals in a single model provides a unified view of the physicians' services market.

Table 10. Determinants of the Distribution of Dentists and of Physicians in Office-Based Private Practice

Variable	Short Description	Dentists per Capita	Physicians per Capita	Physicians per Capita	Physicians per Capita
Y^a	Per capita income	1.47 (5.78)[b]	.448 (2.06)	.534 (2.32)	.483 (1.94)
DIS	Disease	-.375 (-2.69)			
$\widehat{HBMD}/POP$	Interns and residents per capita	.0541 (2.44)	.0424 (2.56)	.0469 (2.76)	.0198 (-.390)
WG	Office input wages	-.756 (-2.03)		-.433 (-1.6)	-.241 (-.814)
MIG	Migration	.157 (-.356)		.0469 (.148)	.389 (1.07)
$\widehat{BEDS}/POP$	Hospital beds per capita	.0135 (.0720)	-.251 (-2.53)	-.197 (-1.45)	-.0606 (-.403)
$\widehat{DD}/POP$	Dentists per capita		.603 (4.14)	.554 (3.73)	.338 (1.30)
CTH/POP	Approvals per capita				4.73E4 (2.00)
MDRES/POP	Research physicians per capita				.0537 (.757)
R^2		.607	.649	.669	.706

[a] Variables are not entered in stepwise order.
[b] Numbers in parentheses below the coefficients are t-values.

209

DATA

DD: American Dental Association, *Distribution of Dentists in the United States by State, Region, District, and County, 1970,* ADA, Chicago.

DIS, MIG: *Statistical Abstract of the United States,* 1974, Tables 87 and 29.

INS: Enrollments from Health Insurance Institute, *Source Book of Health Insurance Data,* 1974-75, Health Insurance Institute, New York, Under -65 population from U.S. Department of Commerce, "Estimates of the Population of States, by Age: July 1, 1973 and 1974," *Current Population Reports,* Series P-25, No. 539.

Y: American Medical Association, *Distribution of Physicians, Hospitals, and Hospital Beds in the U.S., 1972,* vol. 1, AMA Center for Health Services Research and Development, Chicago.

POP: *Statistical Abstract of the United States,* 1973, Table 13.

CTH, BEDS: American Hospital Association, *Hospital Statistics, 1971,* American Hospital Association, Chicago.

CON, CONSWG, HILBUR: Data developed by Professor David Salkever, Johns Hopkins University School of Hygiene and Public Health. CONSWG was taken from *County Business Patterns,* 1970 (general construction employees and taxable payroll).

MDRES, MDTCH, HBMD, DOCS: American Medical Association, *Distribution of Physicians in the U.S., 1971,* AMA Center for Health Services Research and Development, Chicago.

WG: U.S. Department of Labor, *Area Wage Surveys: Selected Metropolitan Areas 1970-71,* Bureau of Labor Statistics Bulletin 1685-91, Tables A-3 (secretaries) and A-5 (nurses). An average was formed using the national employments of secretaries and nurses per physician as weights.

f, p, v, x: American Medical Association, Seventh Periodic Survey of Physicians, AMA Center for Health Services Research and Development, Chicago, 1971.

Living costs from U.S. Department of Labor, *Autumn 1971 Urban Family Budgets and Geographical Comparative Indices,* Bureau of Labor Statistics Bulletin 1570-5 (supplement).

FOOTNOTES

*This study was partially supported by grant No. HS 01971 from the National Center for Health Services Research, HRA.

1. Ninety-six percent of physicians surveyed by the American Medical Association (1971) had at least one full staff privilege. Only 4.5 percent made no hospital visits during their last complete week of practice, and all indicated some office visits.

2. Assume a linear homogenous production function, $x = m^p h^{1-p}$. Let the hospital sell inputs at the price, in terms of labor per h, of $1/\beta$. Output becomes proportionate to the physician's own labor when h is substituted into the production function: $x = m^p (\beta m)^{1-p} = \alpha \cdot m$, $\alpha \equiv \beta^{-p}$

3. The Cobb-Douglas is a degenerate form of the translog production function for the physician who uses only essential inputs such as his own labor. See Feldman (1976) for empirical confirmation of diminishing returns to scale.

4. Recall that total labor l is the sum of m and w. When p changes, both m and w change. The supply elasticity of variable i with respect to a change in variable j is conveniently expressed as e_{ij}. In this case $e_{lp} = e_{mp} \cdot m/l + e_{wp} \cdot w/l$. Sloan (1973, 1974, 1976) estimates that e_{lp} is a small positive number between .03 and .25. Feldstein (1970) finds a negative

elasticity in time series data and infers that the long run supply curve is backward-bending. Certainly, minus one is a lower bound on e_{lp}, since physicians' incomes have risen dramatically in recent years. We can use this information to sign e_{mp}. First, solve the elasticity equation for $e_{mp} = (e_{lp} - e_{wp} \cdot w/l) \, l/m$. Next, solve (6) and (7) for w:

$$w = p^{\lambda} \alpha^{\lambda} \gamma^{-\lambda} f^{-\lambda/(1-\tau)} c^{\tau \cdot \lambda/(i-\tau)} \tau^{-\tau \cdot \lambda/(i-\tau)}, \; \gamma \equiv e_{wp} \equiv \left(\frac{1-\tau}{\gamma + \tau - 1} \right).$$

My estimate of the production function (1976) suggests that $\gamma = .35$ and the sum of the other elasticities is .22, so $e_{wp} = .78/-.43 = -1.8$. The ratio w/l is .62 for the average physician [American Medical Association (1971)]. We know that e_{mp} is positive unless $e_{lp} - e_{wp} \cdot$ w/l is negative. This requires $e_{lp}<(-1.8)(.62) = -1.12$. In other words e_{mp} is positive unless physicians cut back labor in greater proportion than price increases. This is out of the question, because it implies falling physician incomes. Therefore, hospital labor rises as p rises.

5. H and DOCS are deflated by the market area population (POP) to control for different market sizes.

6. Although only 2 percent of established physicians move each year, the velocities of migration and exogenous variables are approximately equal. For example, per capita incomes rise by about 2.5 percent each year. Hospital inputs take large discrete jumps when a new hospital is constructed but normally change slowly over time. And subjective factors, such as local quality of life, may be even slower to change. Therefore, relatively small flows of physicians can equilibrate the model. Also, physicians need not react instantly to disequilibrium conditions. Benham, Maurizi, and Reder (1968) found that changes in physicians per capita during decade-long periods were not affected by contemporaneous changes in exogenous variables. However, physicians responded to initial disequilibrium conditions. They moved to states that had high per capita income and more medical school places at the beginning of the decade.

7. Empirical evidence that HBMD substitute for staff labor was collected by Kieferle and Fish (1971). Although medical administrators emphasize the training opportunities provided by internship and residency programs (Canadian hospitals report students' salaries as "medical education" expenses), Kieferle and Fish point out that learning is maximized when the student performs services consistent with his professional qualifications and experience. In a sample of U.S. and Canadian hospitals, residents spent 50 hours per week, three-quarters of their duty time, on patient care.

8. On the face of it, this argument is difficult to support. Perhaps HBMD are assigned to wards, where if beds are increased without a corresponding increase in patients, they sit around idly. However, this interpretation is inconsistent with physicians' maximizing behavior, since although unfilled beds may be a useful inventory against emergencies, HBMD can work more intensively when occupancy falls.

9. If administrators value staff labor, an aggregate labor supply equation is included in the utility function.

10. The proportion is transformed so that it is always positive. Otherwise, MIG would be negative for states with white emigration, and logarithms of negative numbers do not exist.

11. I wish to thank Professor David Salkever for his generous permission to use data—CON, HILBUR, and CONSWG—from his ongoing research.

12. The states were California, Connecticut, Maryland, New York, and Rhode Island. In 1972 there was no Federal legislation encouraging certificate of need laws (all states must now have the program). Therefore, the original group of five was self-selecting, and certificate of need and hospital beds may not be related for the entire country after 1973.

13. Data were unavailable for earlier years. The real value is found by dividing allocations by a cost of living index for 1971 described in Feldman (1976). A single deflator can be used

for all years if cost of living ratios between states were fairly stable over the 1960 decade.

14. CONSWG is found by dividing the number of workers into total wage payments. It avoids the overstatement built into weekly wage rates by unemployment.

15. The Council of Teaching Hospitals (CTH) is an institutional interest group within the Association of American Medical Colleges (AAMC). Although not an accrediting body, CTH makes recommendations on medical education to the Joint Commission on Accreditation of Hospitals (JCAH). Each approved medical school designates one primary affiliated hospital for CTH membership. Other CTH members are nonaffiliated hospitals with certain prerequisite internship and residency programs. The 400 member hospitals in 1971 represent the medical training establishment, both within and outside medical schools [American Hospital Association (1971)].

16. Rosett and Berg (1973) speculate that increased competition between hospitals, made possible by insurance coverage, bids up wages for HBMD. This lowers the cost of training and aggrevates the shift of physicians away from primary care toward specialities that require postgraduate training.

17. A circumflex sign ($\hat{}$) over a variable signifies an instrument estimated from the exogenous variables in Table 2 plus four other variables which may influence the demand for medical care: the proportion of the population over 65, real Medicaid payments per capita, the proportion of the under-65 population with major medical insurance, and median education of persons over 18. Office fees are endogenous, so $\hat{f}$ is an instrument. Equations like (23) are neither recursive nor "pure" reduced forms, since they may include endogenous variables from other equations of the model as well as shift variables from the factor supply and demand equations. For another example of this specification, see Fuchs and Kramer (1972), where an instrumental price variable is included in a distribution-of-physicians equation.

18. General practitioners, medical specialists (pediatricians, internists, other medical specialists), surgeons (general surgeons, other surgeons, obstetricians), and other specialists (mainly psychiatrists).

19. Office input wages are often higher in high-income states. The positive coefficient here may reflect loading of some of the income effect onto the wage rate variable.

20. Feldstein (1970) used an income measure of the reference group. His choice of the income corresponding to the 95th percentile of the income distribution was unwise, because this measure is almost perfectly correlated with per capita income, another variable in his model.

21. Quantities demanded are quality-adjusted and demographically weighted by an index described in Feldstein (1971). Prices are instruments for real-quality adjusted prices. All variables have been weighted by the square root of the state sample size to correct for heteroscedasticity.

22. DIS may be a good quality of life proxy for a profession whose services are unrelated to disease.

APPENDIX

The Comparative Statics of the Hospital Market

Hospital administrators face aggregate demand, supply, and budget constraints. Without the cumbersome per capita notation, these equations are:

$$X - D(p+t, Y) = 0 \qquad (A-1)$$
$$X - S(p, MIG) = 0 \qquad (A-2)$$
$$b \cdot H - X \cdot t = 0. \qquad (A-3)$$

For simplicity, only two shift variables are shown: an increase in per capita income (Y) shifts demand to the right; an increase in the proportion of population due to net white immigration (MIG) shifts the supply curve to the right.

The total differential of the system is

$$dX - D_1 dp - D_1 dt = D_Y dY \qquad (A-4)$$

$$dX - S_p dp \qquad\qquad = \qquad S_{MIG} dMIG$$

$$- t \cdot dX \qquad\qquad - X \cdot dt = \qquad - H \cdot db.$$

We first solve for the derivative $\dfrac{dX}{dMIG}$:

$$\frac{dX}{dMIG} = \frac{-X \cdot S_{MIG} D_1}{t \cdot S_p D_1 + X \cdot S_p - X \cdot D_1}. \qquad (A-5)$$

Since it is easier to work with elasticities, this is rewritten:

$$\frac{dX \cdot MIG}{dMIG \cdot X} = \frac{-e_{XMIG} n_{p+t}}{\dfrac{t}{p} \cdot e_{Xp} n_{p+t} + \dfrac{(p+t)}{p} \cdot e_{Xp} - n_{p+t}}. \qquad (A-6)$$

The supply elasticity of variable i with respect to variable j is written e_{ij}. Elasticity of demand with respect to total price is n_{p+t}; with respect to income, n_Y. The numerator of (A-6) is clearly positive. The denominator, "Δ", can be simplified:

$$\Delta = e_{XP} \left(1 + \frac{t}{p} (1 + n_{p+t})\right) - n_{p+t}. \qquad (A-7)$$

Δ is clearly positive if $|n_{p+t}| < 1$. My estimate in Section II indicates that $|n_{p+t}|$ is slightly greater than one. However, for the average value of t/p in the sample, 2.88, the terms in parentheses are still positive. Therefore, Δ is positive, and (A-6) is positive—X rises as MIG increases.

We can also show that the physician's price falls as supply shifts to the right. The elasticity is

$$\frac{dp \cdot MIG}{dMIG \cdot p} = \frac{\dfrac{-(p+t)e_{XMIG}}{p} - \dfrac{t}{p} n^{p+t} e_{XMIG}}{\Delta}. \qquad (A-8)$$

The numerator is rewritten and signed:

$$- e_{XMIG}(1 + \frac{t}{p}(1 + n_{p+t})) < 0. \tag{A-9}$$

Therefore, the elasticity is negative.

The demand curve shifts to the right as Y increases, and quantity and physician's price both rise:

$$\frac{dX \cdot Y}{dY \cdot X} = \frac{n_Y e_{Xp} \frac{(p+t)}{p}}{\Delta} > 0. \tag{A-10}$$

$$\frac{dp \cdot Y}{dY \cdot p} = \frac{n_Y \frac{(p+t)}{p}}{\Delta} > 0. \tag{A-11}$$

When the price of hospital inputs rises, quantity and physician's price fall:

$$\frac{dX \cdot b}{db \cdot X} = \frac{t \cdot e_{Xp} n_{p+t}}{\Delta} < 0. \tag{A-12}$$

$$\frac{dp \cdot X}{db \cdot p} = \frac{t \cdot n_{p+t}}{\Delta} < 0. \tag{A-13}$$

REFERENCES

American Hospital Association (1971), *Hospital Statistics*, American Hospital Association, Chicago.
———— (1971), *Distribution of Physicians in the U.S.*, AMA Center for Health Services Research and Development, Chicago.
———— (1971), *Seventh Periodic Survey of Physicians*, AMA Center for Health Services Research and Development, Chicago.
Benham, L., Maurizi, A., and Reder, M. W. (August 1968), "Migration, Location and Remuneration of Medical Personnel: Physicians and Dentists," *Review of Economics and Statistics* 50: 332-347.
Clark, Lawrence and Koontz, Theodore (1973), *Impact of Hill-Burton Subsidized Construction on Interstate Distributions of General Hospital Beds and Physicians, 1950 to 1970*, Department of Medical Care Organization, School of Public Health, University of Michigan.
Clarkson, Kenneth W. (October 1972), "Some Implications of Property Rights in Hospital Management," *Journal of Law and Economics* 15: 363–384.
Enterline, Philip E. et al. (February 1973), "Physician's Working Hours and Patients Seen Before and After National Health Insurance: 'Free' Medical Care and Medical Practice," *Medical Care* 13.
Feldman, Roger (1976), *The Supply and Demand for Physicians' Hospital and Office Visits*, University of Rochester Ph.D. thesis.

Feldstein, Martin S. (1967), *Economic Analysis for Health Service Efficiency: Econometric Studies of the British National Health Service*. Amsterdam: North-Holland.

―――― (May 1970), "The Rising Price of Physicians' Services," *Review of Economics and Statistics* 52: 121–133.

―――― (December 1971), "Hospital Cost Inflation: A Study of Nonprofit Price Dynamics," *American Economic Review* 61: 853–872.

Fuchs, Victor R. and Kramer, Marcia J. (December 1972), *Determinants of Expenditures for Physicians' Services 1948-68*, Washington D.C.: U.S. Department of Health, Education, and Welfare, DHEW Publication No. (HSM) 73-3013.

Hadley, Jack (1975), "Models of Physicians' Specialty and Location Choices," National Center for Health Services Research, USDHEW, Technical Paper Series No. 6.

Jacobs, Philip (June, 1974), "A Survey of Economic Models of Hospitals," *Inquiry* 11: pp. 83–97.

Kieferle, Hans J. and Fish, David G. (1971), "Interns and Residents: The Cost of Their Training and the Supply of Physicians' Services," *International Hospital Federation Newsletter No. 10*, University of British Columbia, pp. 6–18.

Letourneau, Charles U. (1964), *The Hospital Medical Staff*, Chicago: Sterling Publications.

May, J. Joel (September 1969), "Physician Productivity and the Hospital," introduction to a symposium, *Inquiry* 6: 57–58.

Pauly, Mark and Redisch, Michael (March 1973), "The Not-For-Profit Hospital as a Physicians' Cooperative," *American Economic Review* 63: 87–99.

Pearlman, Mark, ed. (1974), *The Economics of Health and Medical Care*, New York: John Wiley & Sons.

Roemer, Milton I. and Friedman, Jay W. (1971), *Doctors in Hospitals: Medical Staff Organization and Hospital Performance*, Baltimore: The Johns Hopkins University Press.

Rosett, Richard N. (1974), "Proprietary Hospitals in the United States," in Perlman, op. cit., pp. 57–65.

―――――, and Berg, Robert L. (February/March 1973), "Health Insurance: The High Cost of Violating Sound Principles," *Private Practice:* 10–14f and 37f.

Sloan, Frank A. (March 1973), *Supply Responses of Young Physicians: An Analysis of Physicians in Residency Programs*, The Rand Corporation, R-1131-OEO.

―――― (1974), "A Microanalysis of Physicians' Hours of Work Decisions," in Perlman, op. cit., pp 302–325.

―――― (1976), "Physician Fee Inflation: Evidence From the Late 1960s," in Richard N. Rosett, ed., *The Role of Health Insurance in the Health Services Sector*, New York: National Bureau of Economic Research.

―――― (January 1975), "Physician Supply Behavior in the Short Run," *Industrial and Labor Relations Review* 28: 549–569.

―――――, and Steinwald, Bruce (October 1974), "Determinants of Physicians' Fees," *Journal of Business*.

Somers, Herman M., and Somers, Anne R. (1961), *Doctors, Patients, and Health Insurance*, Washington, D.C.: The Brookings Institution, p. 68

―――― (1967), *Medicare and the Hospitals: Issues and Prospects*, Washington, D.C.: The Brookings Institution, pp. 51–55.

Steinwald, Bruce, and Neuhauser, Duncan (1970), "The Role of the Proprietary Hospital," *Law and Contemporary Problems*.

Vladeck, Bruce C. (Winter 1976), "Why Nonprofits Go Broke," *The Public Interest* 42: 86–101.

DETERMINANTS OF PROFESSIONAL NURSES' WAGES*

Frank A. Sloan, VANDERBILT UNIVERSITY

Richard A. Elnicki, UNIVERSITY OF FLORIDA

I. INTRODUCTION

The containment of rapidly increasing health-care costs has become an important public policy objective at all levels of government. Within the health-care field, inflation has been most pronounced in the hospital sector. Over a period extending beyond the past decade, hospital expenses per patient day have risen at an annual rate exceeding 10 percent. Most empirical research on hospital costs has described changes in the components of hospital costs or has assessed the extent of economies of scale in hospitals. Few studies have analyzed the behavioral forces underlying changes in the quantities of inputs used to produce hospital services

Research in Health Economics, Vol. 1, pp 217–254.
Copyright © 1979 by JAI Press, Inc.
ISBN 0-89232-042-7.

and/or in input prices. A prerequisite for the formulation of effective hospital cost control policies is an understanding of the nature of these behavioral forces. Potential sources of inflation include changes in exogenous product demand, factor supply, and regulatory influences. The hospital and the market for professional nurses are closely linked. As of 1972, 66 percent of all employed professional nurses were employed by hospitals. The next largest type of employer, nursing homes, employed a much smaller proportion.[1]

This study isolates the effects of various types of factors on professional nurses' wages using data from a 1973 cross section of hospitals. The list of potential sources of wage variation is quite lengthy, and it would be impossible within the context of a single paper to adequately specify the role of each factor and then in turn fully evaluate empirical findings pertinent to each potential wage determinant. Therefore, although the multivariate analysis includes a large number of explanatory variables, we have chosen for purposes of this chapter to emphasize the roles of these variables as sources of wage variation: monopsony power, collective bargaining, nonwage benefits including fringe benefits, working conditions, amenities associated with the hospital's location, and "philanthropic wage effects." A more extensive specification of the other wage determinants may be found in Sloan and Elnicki (1976).

It has been alleged by Donald Yett (1970) and others that hospitals exercise monopsony power in the market for professional nurses' services. First, it has been noted that nurses are frequently "secondary wage earners," a factor tending to limit nurse geographic mobility. Second, because nursing is a skilled occupation, and because of the existence of state licensure laws, possibilities for substituting other types of personnel for nurses are somewhat limited, though clearly not impossible. Third, over 70 percent of U.S. hospitals are located in one-hospital communities [Baird (1969)]. As the dominant employers of nurses in their respective communities, and considering the other two factors, it would not be at all surprising if at least these hospitals possessed a degree of monopoly power in the market for nurses. As seen in the following section, there has been some recent research on the monopsony issue as it relates to nursing, but there is certainly room for additional evidence.

Rather dramatic changes have been occurring with regard to collective bargaining in the health-care field. Data on collective bargaining of nurses are very fragmentary. However, the American Nurses' Association, which is the dominant organizer in the nursing field, estimates that, through its affiliates, it represented almost 100,000 professional nurses as of year-end 1976.[2] Judging from statements in the trade literature, it would appear that recently enacted state legislation requiring public employers to recognize and negotiate with collective bargaining units representing public employees, and the 1974 change in the Taft-Hartley law requiring nonprofit health sector employers to do likewise, these statements are at least partly responsible for recent growth in collective bargaining in hospitals in general and among professional nurses in particular.[3] To the extent that collective bargaining is to be an important force, it is useful to gauge its potential effects.

Jobs in nursing may be expected to differ substantially in terms of various kinds of fringe benefit offerings, working conditions, and amenities associated with the employer's location. In equilibrium, one expects to observe compensating wage differentials that reflect features of employment which nurses find particularly attractive or unattractive. Economists are frequently subject to criticism by noneconomists on grounds that they supposedly emphasize responses to financial incentives when many nonfinancial factors also matter. The "hedonic" method allows one to assess the amounts nurses are willing to pay in terms of reduced earnings to "purchase" attributes of jobs they find attractive.[4]

Martin Feldstein (1971) has argued that not-for-profit hospitals pay wages in excess of the level required to obtain the number of employees they desire. Rather than exploit employees, as the monopsony hypothesis implies, Feldstein's "philanthropic wage hypothesis" asserts that hospitals pay more than their employees' opportunity wages. To the extent that hospital employers are "charitable," this would be of interest to third party payors, both private and public, who offer cost-based reimbursement and would foot the bill for hospitals' generosity (if in fact hospitals are generous in this regard).

Section II provides a brief review of literature pertinent to this study. Section III, the first section presenting our original research, describes our overall conceptual framework. Empirical specification and our data base are described in section IV. The next three sections present empirical results. In section V, regressions using the "basic" model are presented. Section VI specifically examines the effects of selected fringe benefits and working conditions variables on nurses' wages. Section VII considers the impact of collective bargaining in a two-equation framework in which both nurses' wages and nurse collective bargaining are endogenous variables. Section VIII concludes the study.

II. PERTINENT LITERATURE

This section begins with a discussion of theory and empirical evidence on the monopsony issue. We then consider previous research of the effects of unionization on wages, emphasizing research in which unionization and wages are jointly determined. This discussion is followed by a few comments on the "philanthropic wage hypothesis."

Monopsony

There are essentially two origins of monopsony power, contrived and natural. In the case of a contrived monopsony, employers of specific specialized types of labor make an agreement to purchase personnel on specific terms, promise not to undercut one another, and presumably establish effective means for discouraging "chiseling" on the agreement. Examples of *national* contrived monopsonies are found in professional athletics. By contrast, a principal source of natural monopsonies is the immobility of a factor of production in the face of a dominant employer of that factor.

In the present application, the potential source of monopsony power is the professional nurse's immobility and the large number of situations in which a single hospital is a dominant employer. Contrived monopsonies cannot be ruled out in nursing in cases where hospital employers in a locality form an association to serve their "mutual interests."[5] Such *local* employers' associations, however, could not succeed were it not for the geographic immobility of nurses, as there are certainly no national associations as in athletics. Before concluding that monopsony situations must be prevalent in nursing, particularly in view of empirical evidence suggesting that a high proportion of nurses are immobile, it is essential to consider the following factors.[6]

First, it is *not* necessary for all persons in a labor market to be geographically mobile for the market to be competitive rather than monopsonistic. It is only necessary that some prospective employees be mobile. For this reason, it is very difficult to establish the existence of monopsony power per se from data on mobility rates. On the other hand, if nurses move with their spouses to take advantage of the spouses' earnings opportunities and do *not* move to improve their own earnings, as evidence presented in Sloan (1976a) indicates, nurse mobility rates may overstate the proportion of nurses who purposefully seek out job opportunities in other locations.

Second, employers are more likely to possess monopsony power in the short term rather in the long term. Longer periods of time permit persons to search for alternatives elsewhere. Moreover, there is greater assurance to prospective employees that observed differentials are not transitory and are likely to persist over a sufficiently long period of time to make a move financially attractive. The possibility that hospitals are monopsonists in the short term but not in the long term raises a legitimate question about the "run" one actually observes in a particular data base. It is quite possible that the inferences about monopsony power one makes from empirical analysis are quite sensitive to the nature of the data employed.

Third, the slope of the nurse supply curve facing a hospital depends on the responsiveness of nurse hours of work to wages *as well as* the responsiveness of geographic movements to earnings differentials. To the extent that nurses work hours are wage elastic, the slope of the supply curve will be more elastic, and the ability of hospitals to exercise monopsony power will be correspondingly less. Some studies suggest that nurse hours of work are highly wage elastic [such as Sloan and Richupan (1975)] while others suggest a rather small work-hours response [such as Bognanno, et al. (1974)].

There are essentially two ways to assess the existence of a monopsony when a wage rate is the dependent variable. First, product demand variables should demonstrate no impact on wages if the market is both competitive and in equilibrium. If the market contains monopsonistic elements and/or is basically competitive but in a temporary disequilibrium induced by an outward demand shift, variables hypothesized to have a positive impact on product demand should have a positive impact on wages. This type of empirical test can at best rule out a competitive equilibrium. In the present context, a temporary disequilibrium in a competitive market remains a possibility, even if such product demand variables as personal per capita income in fact have positive impacts on nurses' wages.

A second type of empirical test reflects the observation that monopsony is more likely the more highly concentrated a labor market is on the employers' side. When a single hospital is the dominant employer of nurses, a natural monopsony is a possibility. Where there is more than one such employer, collusion among employers is commonly thought to be more readily accomplished if there are only a few individual employers. Alternative measures appropriate for the second kind of test will be considered below as part of this review and in discussing our own work.

Four articles within the health services research field deal with the monopsony issue. Hurd (1973) estimated wage regressions for professional nurses using data from the U.S. Census and Bureau of Labor Statistics. His wage equation did not contain any product demand variables. Thus, he did not conduct the first test of monopsony power. He did, however, include a measure of employers' concentration, the percentage of non-Federal hospital employment accounted for by the eight largest hospitals in the Standard Metropolitan Statistical Area (SMSA). The coefficient of Hurd's concentration ratio variable was negative and statistically significant in all regressions presented. This evidence supports the argument that there are some noncompetitive elements in the market for professional nursing services.

Davis's (1973) evidence of monopsony power is more indirect. In contrast to Hurd's study, which dealt exclusively with professional nurses, Davis included all hospital personnel. One may thus have expected from the outset that Davis would have found no evidence of monopsony power, even if it had existed in some occupations. Certainly in view of the numerous potential employers of lower-skilled labor, even within a local market area, it would be surprising to find that hospitals possessed monopsony power as a general matter. Davis measured monopsony power by the number of hospitals per square mile in the state. Presumably if hospital labor markets are monopsonistic, wages will be lower in areas of lower hospital density. As Davis stated, her

> Evidence on the monopsony hypothesis is mixed. *Wages are insignificantly related to hospital density when the (hospital) facilities variables are included, but excluding specialized facilities leads to a significantly positive relationship.* [Our emphasis.] That is, wages are higher in areas with more hospitals, implying collusive agreements with hospitals either do not exist or break down when there are a large number of hospitals competing for labor. Because of the high correlation between facilities and hospital density, it is difficult to isolate the importance of each issue. Overall explanation is slightly higher when specialized facilities are included [p. 198].

Since the dependent variables, the average wage for the hospital (payroll divided by the total number of employees), encompasses the skill mix of the hospitals' work force as well as wage rates for each skill level, it is rather clear that any available and adequate measure of the hospital's case mix should have been included. Given that the facilities variables, proxies for case mix, should have been included as explanatory variables, and were in some variants, the Davis results imply on balance that, considering all types of personnel together, hospitals do not possess monopsony power.

The most recent, as well as the most comprehensive, published research on the monopsony issue as it relates to nurses is Landon and Link (1975) and Link and Landon (1976). Since both studies used the same data base and equation specification was similar in many respects, these studies should be assessed together. Landon and Link used data from their own survey of 520 hospitals which resulted in 317 usable responses.

Landon and Link gauged the extent of monopsony power in the market for nurses by including several alternative measures of hospital concentration as independent variables in their wage regressions. Landon and

Link's regressions included no hospital product demand variables. Thus, as with the other studies reviewed in this section, tests for monopsony power were exclusively of the second variety.

Landon and Link used three alternative measures of hospital concentration to test for a monopsony influence. The first was a four-firm concentration ratio, the percentage of total beds in the city accounted for by the four largest hospitals. Second, a Herfindahl Index was calculated by summing the squares of each firm's percentage share of the total market. When all beds in the city fall under the jurisdiction of a single hospital, such an index is one. When there are a large number of hospitals in a city, the index approaches zero. Third, an Entropy measure was calculated according to the formula $E = \sum_{i=1}^{n} S_i \ln S_i$ where E is the measure of concentration, S_i, hospital i's market share, and n, the number of hospitals in the city. In contrast to the other two measures, high values of E signify a high degree of competition.

In practice, Landon and Link found very little difference in the empirical results using the three measures, at least gauged in terms in statistical significance. Elasticities associated with the concentration measures are difficult to assess due to lack of pertinent information on variable means. Using means from our data base, we conclude that the elasticity relating nurses wages to the Herfindahl Index is about 0.05. Elasticities implied by the four hospital concentration ratio and the Entropy measure appear to be higher and lower, respectively. Caution is warranted as Landon and Link's parameter estimates are extremely sensitive to the wage equation's specification. Implied monopsony effects are much greater from regressions with few explanatory variables.

Quite a number of studies outside the health field deal with the monopsony issue. Tests for monopsony power generally have involved including various kinds of concentration measures. As a rule, evidence in favor of a monopsony has been found by investigators who have looked for it.[7] Important exceptions are Frey (1975) and Hall and Carroll (1973). These latter studies employed a test of (essentially) the first type and found that product demand variables have at best a small impact on teachers salaries.

Union Effects

The potential effects of unions in any context depends on their objectives and also on the constraints which limit unions' ranges of choices, including their relative power vis-à-vis employers. The question of union objectives has been debated for literally decades [Dunlop (1944), Ross (1948), Atherton (1973), for example] and is unlikely to be resolved by an single study. Considering a wide range of objectives and constraints, the following are possible consequences of collective bargaining on nurse employment and wages in hospital settings.

1. Offset in part or in full the hospital's monopsony (or oligopsony) power with a resultant increase in both professional nurse employment and wages.

2. Raise nurse wages, creating a temporary disequilibrium gap which is eventually closed by hiring freezes and the like, a process described by Reder (1959).

3. In bargaining for better working conditions for professional nurses and/or improvements in the quality of nursing service, affect the production function according to which the hospital operates with the result that professional nurse employment rises. Given an upward sloping nurse supply curve, wages would increase with increases in employment.

Both Davis and Landon and Link also tested for the impact of unionization on wages. The Davis study did not employ a direct measure of unionization at a particular hospital, but instead included variables that describe the impact of a threat of unionization. Citing Miller and Shortell (1969), Davis argued that hospitals located in geographic areas where they are legally required to bargain are more likely to have union contracts. Moreover, she recognized that hospitals located in geographic areas in which a high proportion of the labor force is unionized are more likely to be unionized. Presumably, such areas have a political climate favorable to unions, and persons with the expertise needed to organize workers are more readily available. Variables representing state labor laws, requiring private nonprofit hospitals to recognize a collective bargaining unit when a majority of employees of a unit request recognition, and the percentage of nonagricultural employees in a state to a union were included as explanatory variables. Neither demonstrated a statistically significant effect on average hospital wage rates.

Landon and Link (1975) included two union variables in their nurse wage regressions. The first was a dummy variable taking the value one if 75 percent or more of nurses in the hospital belong to a union and was zero otherwise.[8] A second was a union interaction variable, the product of the first variable and a binary variable which was one for states with 30 percent or more of the state's labor force unionized. Coefficients of the first variable proved to be statistically significant or nearly so in all regressions. Those for the second had lower associated t-ratios but nevertheless suggested an interaction effect. One may infer from Landon and Link's diploma salary regression that unionization raises nurses' salaries by about 5 percent.[9]

The effects of unionization on wages have been assessed in numerous studies covering many industries. Recently, there has been considerable interest in the impact of unions on wages in the public sector. As a rule, significant effects have been found, but the magnitude of effects has varied markedly from study to study.[10]

Ideally, it would be possible to gauge the impacts of unions experimentally. This type of approach is *far* more expensive than the nonexperimental methods typically employed by economists. However, as several economists have argued, most notably Ashenfelter and Johnson (1972), Schmidt and Strauss (1976), and Lee (mimeo.), there is good reason to believe that wages and unionization are jointly determined. If so, ordinary least square (OLS) estimates of the partial impact of unionization on wages are biased. It can be shown that if wages have a positive impact on the demand for union coverage, the OLS parameter estimate associated with the union variable in the wage regression will be upward-biased [Ashenfelter and Johnson (1972)].

The case for the positive impact of wages on union coverage is both theoretical and empirical. Conceptually, there is a strong argument for treating unionization as a normal good, in Pencavel (1971). Not only may unions secure higher wages, but they process workers' grievances and obtain and maintain a member's seniority rights. Empirically, the parameter estimate on the wage variable in regressions with union membership as the dependent variable has proved to be positive and significant in several studies, each using somewhat different econometric techniques and data bases.[11] Furthermore, when techniques that specifically take simultaneity into account have been employed, the estimated impact of collective bargaining on wages has tended to fall (as contrasted with the corresponding OLS estimate) rather substantially. Although simultaneous equation estimation has often been judged to be unsuccessful in cross-sectional analysis, previous research on the topic of union's effects suggests that these types of estimators should at least be attempted.[12]

"Philanthropic Wage Setting"

Feldstein (1971) has documented the substantial increase in occupation-specific wage rates within the hospital sector during the course of the 1950s and 1960s. By the late 1960s, hospital wage rates in certain occupations and cities slightly exceeded wage rates paid workers in the same occupations and cities who had nonhospital employers. Feldstein attributed some of hospital employees wage rate gains to increased demand for the hospital's product, the result of improvedth rd-party coverage and rising patient incomes. According to Feldstein, a portion of these hospital wage rate increases reflect real costs, that is, payments necessary to attract labor from other sectors. But he suggested that another portion represents pure transfer payments to hospital workers. By pursuing this "philanthropic wage policy," as Feldstein termed it, hospital administrators may be meeting one of their own objectives, namely, to improve the welfare of hospital staff as well as of patients.

In support of the philanthropic hypothesis, Feldstein first presented data showing that many hospitals in the late 1960s paid personnel in some clerical and housekeeping occupations higher wages than did employers in other sectors. Second, he argued that standard economic theory cannot explain why salaries for interns and residents at such hospitals as the Massachusetts General Hospital (MGH) have increased dramatically in recent years even though applications for intern and residency positions at these high prestige hospitals have exceeded available places by far. In situations where there is excess demand for places, salaries would normally be expected to fall, not rise.

The philanthropic wage hypothesis provides a possible and interesting explanation of recent hospital wage behavior. However, Feldstein's evidence is at best weakly suggestive. For one, narrowing wage differentials are inadequate by themselves because, even if we examine specific occupations, intra-occupational variations in personal attributes of employees are not held constant. Hospitals may have raised hiring standards *and* wage rates in response to the demand factors Feldstein mentioned. Higher-quality workers may yield benefits to the hospital in terms of reduced labor turnover, lower worker absenteeism rates, fewer difficulties in day-to-day management and the like. Only after adjusting for worker attributes is it possible at all to speak of a philanthropic wage effect as it has been defined. Even then, a few difficulties remain. For example, hospitals may have to grant unusually high wage increases if they desire to expand employment rapidly. What appears to be philanthropy may be an effort on the part of hospital employers to offset labor's transactions costs associated with changing jobs.

Certainly Feldstein did not mean to apply the concept to for-profit hospitals, but rather to not-for-profit hospitals. The test of Feldstein's hypothesis in our study relates to whether, holding a number of factors constant, not-for-profit hospitals pay higher wages. It should be emphasized that Feldstein's hypothesis is very difficult to formalize. Unless the supply of nurses schedule is completrate an ely inelastic, a highly restrictive and unrealistic assumption, paying hospital employees rents would generate an excess supply of prospective employees. The hospital would then have to use some nonmonetary method of rationing its scarce positions. The model used in our study relies entirely on the price mechanism.

III. CONCEPTUAL FRAMEWORK FOR OUR EMPIRICAL ANALYSIS

In general, research on wage-setting has not relied on an explicit theoretical framework. Although the comparative statics of a model even as simple as the one presented in this section are ambiguous, formulating an explicit framework is important for understanding the role of specific wage determinants.

The market for the hospital's services and the professional nurse factor market are assumed to be imperfectly competitive.[13] The hospital is assumed to be a factor price-taker in the markets for other, lower-skilled labor inputs and capital inputs.[14]

We assume that the hospital's decision makers possess a preference function (U). It includes the quantity of service (X), the quality of services (Y), and profits or cash flow (π) as arguments:

$$U = U(X,Y,\pi;E_1). \tag{1}$$

The exogenous variable E_1 permits variation in hospital preferences. If $\partial U/\partial X$ and $\partial U/\partial Y$ are zero and $\partial U/\partial \pi$ is constant, one has the traditional profit-maximizing case under certainty, a reasonable assumption for the proprietary hospital. The majority of hospitals are operated on a "not-for-profit" basis, which may well mean that they are willing to "purchase" additional units of quantity and/or quality at the cost of cash flow.

Profits are defined as:

$$\pi = R(X,Y;E_2) - W(L;E_3) \cdot L - r \cdot N \tag{2}$$

where:

R = current revenue from patient service (either directly from the patient or from insurance);
W = professional nurse compensation;
L = quantity of professional nurse labor;
r = exogenous factor price of "another" input;
N = quantity of the "other" input;
E_1 and E_2 = exogenous variables pertinent to each of the functions.

The R function includes the patient demand schedule for the hospital's services. The inclusion of quality (Y) in R (rather than in U alone) implies that one should observe interhospital variation in Y on grounds that persons in different market areas are willing to pay differing amounts for quality (e.g., due to income differentials). For purposes of empirical analysis of input choice decisions and/or wages, it does not matter how quality is defined. As an endogenous variable, quality does not appear explicitly in the reduced-form equations for these variables. The set of-variables represented by E_2 includes demographic variables and such variables as per capita income.

The function W is upward-sloping if hospitals possess a degree of monopsony power in the market for professional nurses' services. Exogenous factor supply variables (E_3) include (1) characteristics of the hospital's surrounding community, e.g., whether the hospital is located in inner city or rural area; (2) characteristics of the hospital itself, e.g., whether the hospital is affiliated with a nursing school, and (3) measures of the hospital's dominance in the local marekt for professional nurses. More will be said about this third kind of E_3 variable below.

Hospital technology is embodied in the hospital production function:

$$\theta(X,Y,L,N;E_4) = 0 \qquad\qquad (3)$$

Given that the production function incorporates quality, the notion of input "inferiority" in the production of quality, particularly with regard to lower-skilled labor categories, becomes a real possibility. For example, RNs may be far more productive in high-quality settings than are LPNs. The possibility of input inferiority is a source of ambiguity in comparative statistics analysis based on our model.[15]

The hospital selects optimal levels of X, Y, L, and N by maximizing ϕ:

$$\phi = U(X,Y,(R(X,Y;E_2) - W(L;E_3)\cdot L - r\cdot N);E_1) + \lambda\phi(X,Y,L,N;E_4). \quad (4)$$

Once values for these four endogenous variables have been obtained, values of R and W may be obtained by substitution. Given an upward sloping nurses' supply curve, exogenous factors that raise optimal nurse staffing levels also raise their wage. Comparative statics analysis may be used to deduce the direction of effect (positive or negative) specific exogenous variables have on endogenous variables. Unfortunately, even this simple model is too complex to allow us to deduce predicted effects of exogenous variables without making a number of additional assumptions, some of which may be somewhat arbitrary.[16] Therefore, it is best to use the above equations as a means of classifying exogenous variables, and, in broad terms, as a basis for evaluating our empirical results. Questions of direction and magnitude of effects must be settled empirically.

IV. DATA AND EMPIRICAL SPECIFICATION

Data Sources

The primary data source for this is the Survey of Hospital Directors of Nursing conducted by the authors and associates at the University of Florida during 1973. A total of 1,011 hospitals located in all parts of the

United States were sent questionnaires; 707 returned them. After various screens, slightly over 500 hospitals are available for the empirical analysis on nurse wage determination.

This survey offers several advantages for the conduct of this study. First, data are available on wages for nurses with specific kinds of nursing degrees and on-the-job experience. Wages are directly observable, not derived by dividing a wage bill by full-time equivalents. Second, a substantial amount of data on hospital fringe benefits, working conditions, and locational amenities are available. Third, since the hospital's address is known, we were able to merge additional information.[17] To characterize the neighborhood in which the hospital is located (variables belonging to the E_3 factors), we used ZIP code data if the hospital is located within an SMSA. Since hospitals generally draw patients from outside their immediate neighborhoods, the demand variables have been defined for the hospital's county.

Wages of non-RN personnel are estimated for each of the 147 county groups; the 1970 1/100 Public Use Sample of the U.S. Census provided 1969 wage estimates which were updated using the U.S. Bureau of Labor Statistics 1969 and 1972 hospital wage survey reports. Geographic real wage differentails in a competitive labor market largely reflect differences in community amenities. Ideally, the wage measure would correspond to a geographic area that is homogeneous in this regard. One may reasonably expect substantial variation in the size of such areas. The county groups are defined on the basis of economic activity and commuting patterns, and, for this reason, are appropriate for our purpose.

Finally, some explanatory variables correspond to the state. In some cases, it is desirable conceptually to use a state variable, such as state regulatory legislation or measures of the extent of professional nurse training in the state. In others, a variable corresponding to a smaller geographic area would be more appropriate if data were available at a more desegregated level. The latter type of variable has been excluded from regressions presented in the following sections.

All monetarily expressed variables have been deflated by an area price index. One [described in Steinwald and Sloan (1974)] is defined for the state (DFL1); the other permits variation within as well as among states (DFL2). While the latter measure would appear to be more sensitive, it appears to introduce undesirably large differences in cost-of-living between metropolitan peripheries and contiguous area classified as nonmetropolitan.

Dependent Variable (WAGE1)

The dependent variable is WAGE1, the starting monthly salary of nurses with a diploma and no on-the-job experience at the current hospital or elsewhere. This particular wage is highly correlated with wages for nurses in other degree and experience categories. The wage equation's explanatory variables fall into the exogenous variable categories described in the previous section. Some fall into more than one category, as we indicate. Since the focus of this study is on the performance of a few explanatory variables, the discussion of many variables will be brief. Sloan and Elnicki (1976) provide a more detailed variable specification, and also discuss the roles of explanatory variables excluded after preliminary empirical work.

Demand (E.)

As discussed earlier, if the nurses' market is imperfectly competitive or competitive but in short-run disequilibrium, wages will be higher in areas with high demand for the hospital's product.

Past empirical work indicates that real per capita disposable income (INC, defined for the hospital's county) has a positive impact on hospital patient days.[18] Unfortunately, evidence on the demand for aspects of hospital quality is lacking. Our patient health status measure is SICK, disability day per 1,000 persons aged 15 to 65. This variable is defined for the hospital's major city, if the hospital is outside such a city but within an SMSA, and for the rural areas of the state as a whole if the hospital is not located within an SMSA. A variable representing the percentage of the county's population aged 65 and over was included in initial regressions, but it was consistently insignificant.

The availability of physicians in the hospital's market may affect the demand for hospital services in several ways. A greater availability of physicians may cause a shift from hospital care toward ambulatory care, thus reducing the demand for the former. Although in-patient and ambulatory care are substitutes in this sense, hospital quantity (X) may also be seen as complementary in that patients are admitted to a hospital only on a physician's recommendation.[19] The latter positive effect may be more important in the case of specialist physicians who spend a larger portion of their practice time in operating or delivery rooms and on hospital rounds. The variables PHYSG and PHYSP measure, respectively, the number of nonhospital-based, patient-care, general practice and specialist physicians per 10,000 county population.[20] In some variants, PHYSG and PHYSP are combined into a single variable termed MD.

The rationale for including population density measures in hospital demand equations also relates to spatial factors. Patients in low-density areas must, holding other factors constant, travel longer distances for ambulatory care. When multiple patient visits for a given diagnosis are involved, it may be preferable to hospitalize. Since patients for whom ambulatory care is a technical alternative have less serious illnesses, a higher admission rate in low-density areas may be at least partly offset by shorter lengths of stay. Also, less complex cases generate less demand for "quality" (input-intensive) hospital services. For this study, we have selected the percentage of the county population living in urban areas (URB) to present this effect.

By the 1970s, virtually the entire U.S. population has coverage for hospital services. However, there are substantial geographic differences in the nature of such coverage. A variable measuring the percentage of the hospital's county population covered by cost-based insurance was included initially, but it was always highly insignificant and therefore has been omitted in the regressions presented below.

Factor Supply (E_3)

These variables describe the attractiveness of the hospital's environment to professional nurses. The Survey of Hospital Directors of Nursing asked hospital respondents to rate the hospital's parking facilities in terms of safety. The variable SAFE ($= 1$ if the facilities are only "moderately safe" or "unsafe") is in effect a proxy for the likelihood of crimes against persons and property in the hospital's immediate vicinity. The variable HDENS measures the percentage of families living in housing with 1.5 or more persons per room. Areas with this amount of space per person are likely to be very poor; HDENS is defined for the hospital's ZIP code area for hospitals in SMSAs and for the county for hospitals outside SMSAs.

Nurses may have different reservation wages for work in hospitals affiliated with educational institutions or programs. The variables MEDSC, MEDSA, and NURSC identify hospitals which, respectively, are part of a medical school complex, affiliated with a medical school but not part of a school complex, and those affiliated with a nursing school. All of these variables could also be construed to belong to the E_1 and E_4 variable sets, and for this reason their parameters cannot be fully attributed to nurse preferences.

The Survey of Hospital Directors of Nursing asked a large number of questions pertaining to working conditions and fringe benefits. In the interest of economy in terms of numbers of explanatory variables, hospital fringe benefits and work conditions are characterized by a set of "package" variables defined in Table 1. Each variable takes the value one if the hospital satisfies Table 1's criteria for a respective package. Ideally, one would specify these variables to be jointly determined with wages. However, in view of the paucity of information on exogenous determinants of fringe benefits and working conditions, we did not feel able to adequately specify equations for these variables at this time.

Our measure of the hospital's importance in the local market for professional nurses in MON—the hospital's beds as a percentage of all hospital

Table 1. Definitions of "Package" Variables

Variable	Definition	Proportion Satisfying Criteria
HOMEPG	Adequate or very adequate housing for RNs within walking distance of the hospital or subsidized housing is provided by the hospital.	0.33
LEAVEPG	RN vacation and sick leave days per year greater than the survey means (RN employed one year).	0.21
EDUCPG	In-service education is budgeted for by hospital and hospital offers its own refresher courses or the hospital subsidizes them (if taken elsewhere).	0.38
WORKPG	Secretaries or clerks at nursing stations; RNs frequently determine their own schedules; diploma graduates can fill supervisory positions; percent of RNs always working the same shift greater than survey mean; percent of supervisory positions filled internally greater than mean; and day notice given for a permanent shift change is greater than mean or not applicable.	0.13
INSURPG	Subsidized, convertible life insurance; subsidized convertible health insurance; all full-time RNs are eligible for a retirement plan after a waiting period; and hospitals' retirement contribution is not lost on termination after a waiting period or sickness and disability insurance is subsidized by hospital.	0.15
CHILDPG	Hospital fully or partly subsidizes day care or maternity leaves *are* covered by sick leave.	0.35

beds in the county. Given the high proportion of hospitals that are monopolists in their local product markets, the MON variable is probably highly correlated with concentration measures used in past research on monopsony (such as Landon and Link's (1975) research). However, there is an important conceptual difference. In our work, MON accounts for interhospital variations in the slope of the nurse labor supply function [W($\cdot$)]. As MON rises, this function's slope is hypothesized to become *less* elastic. Concentration measures in other studies generally refer to the ease of organizing and maintaining a cartel. Once the wage is set by the cartel, it is exogenous to individual hospitals. That is, W($\cdot$) is infinitely elastic except in cases in which the monopsony is natural rather than contrived. Natural monopsonies may occur when hospitals are monopolists in their product market areas.

We also considered concentration variables based on RN employment. But in counties where the hospital accounts for a large share of hospital employment, any error in the denominator of the monopsony variable would be common to the dependent variable as well. An error might arise, for example, if the hospital temporarily deviated from what it considers to be its optimal professional nurse employment level.

Effects of collective bargaining on wages are captured by the variable UNION (= 1 if the hospital has a collective bargaining agreement covering professional nurses). In the first set of regressions, UNION will be considered exogenous. In latter regressions, we will treat it as jointly determined with wages. The "UNION" equation will be specified in a later section.

The most relied-upon policy instrument for affecting the supply of professional nurses, both in the aggregate and in spatial terms, are public expenditures on nurse training. The rationale given at both Federal and state legislative levels is that nurses who receive their training in a given area are likely to remain there. This reasoning implicitly places an important weight on the transactions costs of moving (either for psychological reasons or the direct financial outlays themselves) and/or legal restrictions (such as licensure) that impede movement. Although references to retention probabilities (from nursing school to work) are often cited as evidence, they do not tell the whole story, since higher proportions of "home-grown" nurses may affectively discourage immigration of nurses from other areas. However, if, on the whole, the pool of potential migrants is comparatively small because nurses are immobile, a locality may successfully increase its pool of nurses by means of training. According to the American Nurses' Association (1974a), most states offer reciprocity to other states; licensure per se is probably not an important barrier to mobility. Our measure of nurse training is NSTU, the ratio of graduates of nursing schools in the state per 10,000 state population. We have selected a state training measure because nursing students are eligible for state-subsidized education throughout the state in which they claim residence.

Preference-Production Function (E_1 and E_4)

Empirically, preference and production function variables (and, in some cases, factor supply variables) are virtually inseparable. The hospital's case mix may vary systematically with hospital ownership. The variables PROPRI (= 1 for proprietary hospitals) and VOLUN (= 1 for voluntary hospitals) distinguish private from state-local government hospitals. Inclusion of the variable PROPRI permits us to evaluate the philanthropic wage hypothesis. As noted above, the education affiliation variables MEDSC, MEDSA, and NURSC may also be construed as belonging to this category.

In this and related work on professional nurse staffing in hospitals, we assume hospital beds (BEDS) to be exogenous. Unfortunately, no theory exists with which to predict the size of individual hospitals (without, of course, reference to the number of beds in a previous period).

Prices of Other Inputs (r)

Only Ehrenberg (1974) has dealt explicitly with the impact of non-RN wages on RN staffing. In that study, the dependent variable was the ratio of full-time RN equivalents employed by the hospital to full-time equivalent (FTE) LPNs employed by the hospital. One of the explanatory variables was the annual payroll cost per FTE RN divided by the annual payroll cost per FTE LPN. As can be easily shown (a point Ehrenberg recognized), this method for constructing the relative wage variable introduces error-in-variables, and the resulting bias may cause a negative wage coefficient, even if the true coefficient were zero. Since a major objective of Ehrenberg's study was to ascertain whether hospitals are in fact cost-minimizers, which is indicated if the relative wage coefficient is negative, this bias is very unfortunate. Little confidence can therefore be placed on the reported negative coefficient Ehrenberg reports.

In our study, wage data for non-RNs from the 1970 U.S. Census, updated to 1974 using Bureau of Labor Statistics hospital wage surveys have been merged with our survey of hospitals. Our measures are WAGE2, real hourly wages of hospital LPNs, aides and orderlies; and WAGE3, real hourly wages of other non-RN personnel, including hospital clerical, labor, and service employees. In terms of mean percentages of hospital's total wage bill, the latter is 2.2 times more important than the former labor category. We also included a measure of real wages of other hospital professional and managerial personnel in preliminary regressions. This variable, however, proved to be insignificant and highly collinear with the other wage variables.

It is reasonable to expect that some of the "amenity" variables listed above are also source of wage differentials for non-RNs. With both "amenity" and non-RN amenity effects not captured by non-RN wages. To the extent that RN and non-RN preferences differ, one would expect to observe independent amenity effects on RN staffing and real RN wages.

Regulation

The rapid rise in hospital costs has led to a plethora of controls in an effort to temper the rate of cost increase. Probably the two most potentially important regulatory mechanisms to arise in recent years are certificate-of-need laws (CN) and prospective reimbursement (PR).

Under CN, a local planning agency has the right to place legal restrictions on capital investments they deem unnecessary or to prevent the hospital from receiving capital and operating revenues relating to unapproved projects. Conceptually, CN controls the levels of specific hospital inputs. In the process of hospitals' remaximizing, it is not surprising to find compensatory responses to such restraints.

Salkever and Bice's (1976) analysis indicated that while CN has decreased bed construction, assets per bed have increased, presumably on types of equipment not subject to regulation and on regulated items during "grace" periods which such laws tend to provide. The hospital's use of labor inputs and hence wages rates are assumed to be likewise affected by CN. The variables CN1 and CN2 identify, respectively, states with CN prior to 1972 and those with laws implemented during 1972–1973.[21]

In principle, PR is a method for paying hospitals according to "fee schedules" fixed prior to the start of the year they apply. After a set period, the schedules may be revalued according to a formula, budget review, or negotiation [Dowling (1974)]. Aside from this feature, there is considerable variation in PR, in terms of the number of insurance programs covered, the methods for setting rates, and whether the hospital's participation in PR is compulsory or voluntary. As of 1973, only New Jersey and New York had mandatory PR programs for both Medicaid and Blue Cross. If PR has any impacts at all, it is likely to have them in these two states because of their programs' relatively broad coverage and mandatory nature. Hospitals in these states are identified in our analysis by the variable PR.[22]

Functional Form

For purposes of the regression analysis, all continuous variables are in log form, and all binary variables are linear. Expressed in this form, all continuous variable parameters have the constant elasticity property.

V. EMPIRICAL RESULTS: WAGE REGRESSIONS WITHOUT FRINGE BENEFITS–WORKING CONDITIONS VARIABLES

The discussion of empirical results consists of three sections. In the first, wage regressions *not* containing the package explanatory variables are discussed. These results are presented in Table 2.

Empirical evidence on the product demand variables relates to the first test of monopsony power. If wages tend to be high in high-product demand areas, there is empirical support for the monopsony hypothesis, or, alternatively, of a recent demand shift leading to a temporary disequilibrium in a market essentially competitive in the long run. In our research on professional nurse staffing in hospitals (not reported here), area per capita income (INC), the first product demand variable, had a positive impact on nurse staffing levels.[23] The INC variable also has a significantly

Table 2. Nurse Wage Regressions without Hospital Nonwage Offerings

Explanatory variable	Dependent variable — WAGE1				
	I	II	III	IV	V[a]
INC	0.118[b]	0.101[b]	0.118[b]	0.115[b]	0.036
	(0.033)	(0.034)	(0.033)	(0.034)	(0.035)
SICK	0.055[c]	0.059[c]	0.050	0.047	0.033
	(0.027)	(0.026)	(0.027)	(0.027)	(0.026)
PHYSG	-0.014	-0.010	-0.012	- -	- -
	(0.010)	(0.010)	(0.010)	(-)	(-)
MD	- -	- -	- -	0.012	0.011
	(-)	(-)	(-)	(0.012)	(0.012)
PHYSP	0.008[c]	0.004	0.008[c]	- -	- -
	(0.003)	(0.004)	(0.003)	(-)	(-)
URB	- -	- -	- -	- -	0.003
	(-)	(-)	(-)	(-)	(0.002)
SAFE	0.020	0.020	0.020	0.020	0.028[c]
	(0.012)	(0.012)	(0.012)	(0.012)	(0.012)
HDENS	0.030[b]	0.030[b]	0.028[b]	0.028[b]	0.023[b]
	(0.007)	(0.007)	(0.007)	(0.007)	(0.007)
MEDSC	0.036	- -	0.034	0.048	0.012
	(0.025)	(-)	(0.025)	(0.025)	(0.025)

Table 2. (Continued)

Explanatory variable	I	II	III	IV	V[a]
Dependent variable — WAGE1					
NURSC	– –	– –	– –	– –	0.017
	(-)	(-)	(-)	(-)	(0.013)
MEDSA	0.031	– –	0.034	0.037	0.029
	(0.020)	(-)	(0.025)	(0.020)	(0.020)
UNION	0.026	0.031	0.019	0.020	0.039c
	(0.018)	(0.018)	(0.018)	(0.018)	(0.018)
MON	-0.006	-0.010c	-0.009	-0.009	-0.010c
	(0.005)	(0.005)	(0.005)	(0.005)	(0.005)
NSTU	-0.052b	-0.052b	-0.062b	-0.072b	-0.082b
	(0.019)	(0.018)	(0.018)	(0.018)	(0.018)
VOLUN	-0.010	-0.013	-0.014	– –	-0.016
	(0.013)	(0.012)	(0.012)	(-)	(0.012)
PROPRI	0.017	0.016	– –	0.021	0.013
	(0.021)	(0.021)	(-)	(0.020)	(0.021)
BEDS	– –	0.020b	– –	– –	– –
	(-)	(0.007)	(-)	(-)	(-)
WAGE2	0.063	0.065	0.063	0.072	0.008
	(0.053)	(0.052)	(0.053)	(0.053)	(0.052)
WAGE3	0.240b	0.223b	0.247b	0.253b	0.240b
	(0.064)	(0.064)	(0.063)	(0.064)	(0.059)
CN1	– –	– –	0.063c	0.069c	0.071c
	(-)	(-)	(0.031)	(0.031)	(0.029)
CN2	(-)	(-)	(0.015)	(0.015)	(0.015)
	– –	– –	0.017	0.021	0.016
PR	– –	– –	-0.069c	-0.074c	-0.047
	(-)	(-)	(0.031)	(0.031)	(0.030)
CONSTANT	4.71	4.74	4.74	4.72	5.81
	(-)	(-)	(-)	(-)	(-)
	$R^2 = 0.31$	$R^2 = 0.32$	$R^2 = 0.31$	$R^2 = 0.31$	$R^2 = 0.28$
	$F(15,487) = 14.5^b$	$F(14,488) = 16.1^b$	$F(17,487) = 13.1^b$	$F(16,488) = 13.5^b$	$F(19,485) = 9.8^b$

[a]   Uses DFL2

[b]   Significant at the 1% level.

[c]   Significant at the 5% level.

Numbers in parentheses are standard errors.

positive effect on nurse wages in the first four regressions in Table 2. The fifth regression uses an alternative deflator that permits cost-of-living variations within states (DFL2). To the extent that the deflators contain measurement errors, it can be shown that the INC parameter estimate will be positively biased when WAGE1 is the dependent variable (since both dependent and explanatory variables use the same deflator). The fact that INC parameter estimates are higher in the first four regressions raises the possibility that the second deflator more accurately measures area cost-of-living. This inference, however, is not very convincing because parameter estimates of other explanatory variables, such as WAGE2 and WAGE3, which have also been deflated, are either higher in the fifth regression than in the other regressions or are unaffected by the choice of price deflator.

On balance, the INC coefficients in Table 2's regressions lend support to the view that the market for nursing services contains monopsonistic elements, or at least, is a temporary disequilibrium. Nurses wages also are shown to be higher in geographic areas containing relatively large proportions of unhealthy persons. However, although the positive coefficients on PHYSP are encouraging, the poor performances of PHYSG and the variable MD (the sum of the two physician variables) do not support the view that hospitals exercise monopsony in this market.

Our measure of the hospital's importance in the local market for professional nurses MON consistently shows a negative impact on nurse wage levels with associated t-values greater than one in every variant. However, the MON elasticities are in the 0.01 range, far too small to suggest that monopsony is an overpowering force on the average. Our estimates are somewhat smaller than Landon and Link's. However, Landon and Link included comparatively fewer explanatory variables and the coefficients of Landon and Link's monopsony measures tended to decline as explanatory variables were added.

The coefficients of the two locational amenity variables, SAFE and HDENS, have plausibly positive signs in all regressions. In both cases, the coefficients imply small compensating wage differentials. The positive coefficients of the three educational affiliation variables MEDSC, MEDSA, and NURSC are inconsistent with the view that nurses prefer to work in such settings. Our research on nurse staffing in hospitals indicates that hospitals with formal educational affiliations tend to have higher levels of nurse staffing per hospital bed. To secure more nurses, such hospitals have to pay higher wages.

Parameter estimates corresponding to our UNION variables consistently exceed their standard errors and are sometimes significant at the 5 percent level. However, these estimates imply small impacts on wages. The largest UNION coefficient suggests that unions raise professional nurses wages by four percent.

Our estimate of unionization's impact is very close to Landon and Link's (1975) estimate of unionization's direct effect. Their union variable took the value one if 75 percent or more of nurses were unionized, and was zero otherwise. In our research, UNION assumes the value one if "there is a collective bargaining agreement in your (the respondent's) hospital covering RNs.'' Landon and Link noted, based on experimentation with alternative measures, that their results on unionization effects were reasonably invariant with respect to the precise way the union variable was specified. Certainly the consistency between Table 2 and Landon and Link's research on union's wage impacts lend further support to their finding. As in Table 2, they considered collective bargaining at the level of the individual hospital to be exogenous. We shall relax this assumption in section VII.

Landon and Link also included an interaction term in their wage regressions to capture union "threat" effect on nurses' wages. When added to the direct union effect, the total union effect was about twice the size of the effect associated with the UNION variable in Table 2. We have also experimented with a "threat" effect variable in preliminary regressions, but not ones interacting with UNION. In our preliminary work, inclusion of a union threat variable contributed nothing to explaining interhospital variations in nurses' wages. Therefore, this variable has been excluded as an explanatory variable in Table 2.

One reason underlying differences in the performance of the union threat variable, as with our lowest marginal impact of hospital concentration, may relate to the number of explanatory variables included in Landon and Link's as compared with regressions. Landon and Link included far fewer explanatory variables.

The VOLUN and PROPRI coefficients are fully inconsistent with Feldstein's philanthropic wage hypothesis. In fact, the proprietaries appear to pay nurses about 2 to 4 percent more than other hospitals. To maintain this hypothesis in the face of Table 2's evidence would require an argument that owners of for-profit hospitals also grant wages to employees in excess of the minimum amount required to obtain a given quantity of nursing services. Although such hospitals may find it advisable to pay more than the minimum to reduce turnover or obtain more capable nurses, it is doubtful that for-profits would be motivated by charitable considerations per se.

The Table 2 regressions permit one to examine the effect of hospital ownership on nurses' wages, holding a large number of factors constant. Elnicki and Sloan (1975) presented a table reporting mean wages for nurses by type of nursing degree and nurse experience. Mean wages offered by proprietaries were consistently higher than corresponding wages for voluntary and government hospitals. The percentage differences among hospital ownership types, evident from the table of means, are about the same as those implied by Table 2's VOLUN and PROPRI parameter estimates.

The NSTU parameter estimates are uniformly negative and statistically significant at the 1 percent level. This result implies that increased nursing school output in a state tends to depress nurses' entry wages in hospitals located in the state. This result is consistent with our research on nurse staffing in hospitals [Sloan and Elnicki (1976)], where we found that professional nurse staffing levels in hospitals are higher in states where nurse training is extensive.

The regulation variables show professional nurses' wages (adjusted for area cost-of-living differences) to be higher by about 6 to 7 percent in states with certificate-of-need laws (CN) prior to 1972, and lower by about 5 to 7 percent in New Jersey and New York, the states (as of 1973) with the broadest mandatory prospective reimbursement (PR) coverage. These results are suggestive, but they should mainly be used to encourage further work on this topic. An important extension would be to gauge regulation's impact using a time series of cross sections (including observations on hospitals before and after the regulatory device was instituted) in order to verify that the regulation variables measure regulation as opposed to unspecified "state" effects.

VI. EMPIRICAL RESULTS:
WAGE REGRESSIONS WITH FRINGE
BENEFITS–WORKING CONDITIONS VARIABLES

In preliminary work, we developed a wage measure that included a monetary equivalent of various fringe benefits offered nurses by the hospital. The empirical results, however, differed only slightly from the results presented in Table 2. Furthermore, because of information on fringe benefits was not as well reported in our survey as was information on wages, the number of complete observations available for analysis was smaller.

In this section, we shall use another approach. Nonwage benefits are included as explanatory variables in regressions with the hospital's starting monthly salary for the diplomate (WAGE1) as the dependent variable. Wages represent only one, albeit important, form of nurse compensation. The hypothesis investigated in this section is that wages tend to be lower in hospitals offering comparably generous quantities of specific nonwage benefits. If so, one may make the inference that the "average" beginning diplomate values these benefits.

Table 3 gives simple correlations among wage, nonwage benefit, ownership, and union variables. These patterns are especially noteworthy. First, there are as many positive correlations between WAGE1 and individual nonwage benefit variables as there are anticipated negative correlations. If there are indeed compensating wage differentials for benefits

Table 3. Wage and Nonwage Offering Correlations

	WAGE1	HOMEPG	LEAVEPG	EDUCPG	WORKPG	INSURPG	CHLDPG	SAFE	VOLUN	PROPRI	UNION
WAGE1	1.00	0.11[b]	0.00	-0.00	0.00	0.13[b]	-0.03	0.13[b]	-0.02	0.09[b]	0.12[b]
HOMEPG		1.00	0.04	0.09[b]	0.03	0.11[b]	-0.12[b]	-0.02	0.17[b]	-0.02	0.00
LEAVEPG			1.00	-0.01	0.05[b]	-0.03	0.03	0.09[b]	-0.11[b]	-0.04	-0.03
EDUCPG				1.00	0.02	0.10[b]	0.06[b]	0.02	0.15[b]	-0.11[b]	0.07[b]
WORKPG					1.00	-0.02	-0.02	-0.00	0.01	0.00	0.00
INSURP						1.00	-0.02	0.04	0.19[b]	-0.04	0.06[b]
CHILDPG							1.00	0.06[b]	-0.11[b]	-0.03	0.03
SAFE								1.00	-0.02	0.02	0.03
VOLUN									1.00	[a]	-0.03
PROPRI										1.00	-0.04
UNION											1.00

[a] Correlation is meaningless.
[b] Significant at the 5% level.

241

valued by nurses, at least the partial (as opposed to the simple correlations shown in the table) must be negative. Second, simple correlations among the benefit variables themselves tend to be weak. There are negative as well as positive signs on these correlations. Third, while the correlation between the proprietary hospital dummy variable PROPRI and WAGE1 is positive and significant, the correlations between PROPRI and the benefit package variables tend to be negative. This may be due to the small mean size of for-profits, which may make hospital provision of certain types of benefits comparatively costly. Fourth, with the exception of the LEAVEPG, voluntary hospitals tend to be relatively generous in their benefit offerings. Judging from the negative simple correlations of VOLUN and PROPRI, it is apparent that government hospitals provide the highest levels of vacation and sick leave. This pattern is also seen in the table of mean values, based on data from the Survey of Hospital Directors of Nursing, presented in Elnicki and Sloan [1975]. Fifth, the positive simple correlation between WAGE1 and UNION is by far the highest among the correlations in the column of UNION correlations. It is doubtful that the UNION variable would have performed very well, had we estimated regressions with each of the package variables as the dependent variables.

Table 4 contains two nurses' wage regressions with the package variables included. All monetarily expressed variables are deflated by DFL1, our state price index. Variant I only contains the benefits variables. Variant II is based on precisely the same specification as Table 2's first regression. Variant II's R^2 is only slightly higher than its Table 2 counterpart, but this regression's F-statistic is lower because several of the benefit variables coefficients are statistically insignificant.

If hospitals with attractive offerings are able to hire nurses at lower wages, coefficients of variables HOMEPG through CHILDPG should have negative signs. In Variant I, negative signs are only observed in the cases of LEAVEPG, and EDUCPG, but neither of the two parameter estimates is statistically significant.

In Variant II, when a number of exogenous wage determinants are included, LEAVEPG, EDUCPG, and CHILDPG have anticipated negative signs, and the first two are statistically significant at the five percent level or nearly so. If a hospital provided all three, our results suggest that wages would be almost 6 percent lower than if none of the three were provided. But an equal number of variables HOMEPG, WORKPG, and INSURPG have unanticipated positive parameter estimates.

Link and Landon (1976) also included benefits variables in some variants of their nurse wage regressions. Link and Landon described their nonmonetary benefits variables as follows:

Table 4. Wage Regressions with Hospital Nonwage Offerings

Explanatory variables	I	II
HOMEPG	0.030^b	0.024^b
	(0.013)	(0.011)
LEAVEPG	-0.000	-0.026^b
	(0.015)	(0.013)
EDUCPG	-0.006	-0.021
	(0.012)	(0.011)
WORKPG	0.001	0.007
	(0.018)	(0.016)
INSURPG	0.042^a	0.023
	(0.017)	(0.015)
CHILDPG	-0.008	-0.010
	(0.012)	(0.011)
SAFE	0.042	-0.024^b
	(0.014)	(0.012)
INC	$--$	0.120^a
	(0.26)	(0.033)
SICK	$--$	0.050
	(0.10)	(0.026)
PHYSG	$--$	-0.016
	(-0.15)	(0.010)
PHYSP	$--$	0.007^b
	(0.27)	(0.003)
HDENS	$--$	0.030^a
	(0.20)	(0.007)
MEDSC	$--$	0.047
	(0.12)	(0.026)
MEDSA	$--$	0.029
	(0.12)	(0.020)
UNION	$--$	0.026
	(0.11)	(0.018)
MON	$--$	-0.008
	(-.30)	(0.005)
NSTU	$--$	-0.056^a
	(-0.22)	(0.018)
VOLUN	$--$	-0.018
	(-0.06)	(0.013)
PROPRI	$--$	0.006
	(0.10)	(0.021)
WAGE2	$--$	0.076
	(0.29)	(0.052)
WAGE3	$--$	0.213^a
	(0.32)	(0.063)
CONSTANT	6.48	4.694
	(-)	(-)
	$R^2 = 0.05$	$R^2 - 0.33$
	$F(7,501) = 3.9^a$	$F(21,487) = 11.5^a$

[a] Significant at the 1% level.
[b] Significant at the 5% level.
Numbers in parentheses are standard errors when there is a parameter estimate; otherwise, they are partial correlations.

In addition to starting salary, the surveyed hospitals (by L-L) were asked to list nonmonetary factors which they felt were significant in recruiting nurses. From these responses a series of dummy variables was created to indicate whether or not the hospital included in its list a particular class of benefits. The four classes of benefits found most frequently in the responses were included in this study. They were, one, educational benefits (teaching programs available, teaching hospital, paid tuition for advanced study, etc.); two, shift benefits (nurses can choose their own shift, freedom to work the same shift all the time, etc.); three, new hospital (new facility, excellent facilities, etc.); and four, parking-transportation (free, convenient parking, convenient to public transportation, etc.) [p. 153]

Although details in specification differ, Link and Landon's first variable roughly corresponds to EDUCPG, L-L's second very roughly to WORKPG, and L-L's fourth to SAFE. Our Survey of Hospital Directors of Nursing did not collect data on the age of the hospital's facilities. Link and Landon did not include variables analogous to HOMEPG, LEAVEPG, INSURPG, and CHILDPG. They found shift benefits to be associated with lower nurse wages, but their parking-transportation variable had an unanticipated positive impact while our SAFE parameter estimate makes sense (SAFE = 1 if hospital parking is "unsafe" or "moderately safe"). Although plausibly negative, their shift benefits parameter estimate was insignificant at conventional levels. The education benefits and new facilities variables performed very poorly.[24]

There are a number of nonmutually exclusive explanations for the presence of some positive benefit parameter estimates as well as some negative estimates below significance at conventional levels. First, it is possible that these benefits are simply not very important to professional nurses, and, as a result, the parameter estimates wander about. Second, nurses may be ignorant of the levels of hospital offerings and may consider the costs of obtaining such information to be quite high. These two points are related, since nurses would presumably be willing to incur the search costs if they valued the kinds of offerings represented by the above package variables highly. Third, the offerings may be important but poorly measured by Link and Landon's survey and by us. Although poor measurement cannot be ruled out, Sloan (1976b) found similar results using still another data base. Finally, the market could be out of equilibrium. Really all one can say currently is that the intrinsic value to professional nurses of the types of nonwage offerings we have analyzed remains to be demonstrated. As defined, such offerings as WORKPG and INSURPG may primarily be useful to the nurse who intends to stay with her employer for a substantial amount of time. The mean tenure of a nurse with any given hospital employer is quite short [Sloan (1975a)].

VII. EMPIRICAL RESULTS: WAGE REGRESSIONS WITH UNIONIZATION ENDOGENOUS

As discussed in our literature review, a rather convincing case can be made for gauging the impact of collective bargaining within a simultaneous equation framework in which both wages and collective bargaining activities are jointly determined. In this section, we specify collective bargaining equation. Then two-stage least squares estimates of the two equations are presented and evaluated.

Collective Bargaining Equation

As above, collective bargaining is measured by the variable UNION, which assumes the value one if the hospital has a collective bargaining agreement covering RNs. With UNION as the dependent variable, the following are the explanatory variables.

The nurse wage (WAGE1) is included for reasons explained in the literature review. If collective bargaining coverage is a normal good, higher wages will shift the demand for unionization function outward (with price in this function including such items as union dues). Organizing costs per potential member are plausibly lower in larger hospitals, in areas where there is extensive unionization in nonhospital sectors, and when the hospital is closely affiliated with other large employers, such as state or municipal governments. Hospital size is represented by BEDS; COLLB is the fraction of the state nonagricultural labor force represented by unions; the variables VOLUN and PROPRI account for differences by hospital ownership.

Organization is likely to be facilitated by state laws favorable to collective bargaining. Using data from U.S. Department of Labor (1975) and *Iowa Law Review* (1971–72), we developed a variable identifying states with favorable laws affecting collective bargaining in state-local government hospitals (STRG) and voluntary hospitals (STRP). The STRG dummy variable is based on separate series for state and municipal hospitals. The Department of Labor data source rated state laws on a scale from one to four, according to the extent to which they are favorable to collective bargaining in state and local government employment settings. In constructing STRG, values of four were recoded to one; all other values were recoded to zero. The variable STRP assumes the value one if the state includes private nonprofit hospitals within their labor statutes.[25]

Tables 5 and 6 present the results of our two equation models in which both unionization and nurses' wages are considered endogenous. The equations have been estimated by both ordinary least squares (OLS) and two-stage least squares (TSLS).

Table 5. Unionization Regressions

Explanatory variables	1. OLS	2. TSLS
WAGE1	0.344[a]	0.513[a]
	(0.107)	(0.229)
BEDS	−0.004	-0.010
	(0.014)	(0.016)
COLLB	0.140[a]	0.141[a]
	(0.003)	(0.034)
STRG	0.039	0.039
	(0.045)	(0.045)
STRP	0.054	0.050
	(0.041)	(0.041)
VOLUN	-0.050	-0.044
	(0.037)	(-0.037)
PROPRI	-0.065	-0.072
	(0.054)	(0.054)
CONSTANT	-2.54	-3.63
	(-)	(-)

$$R^2 = 0.07$$
$$F(5,507) = 5.70^a$$

[a] Significant at the 1% level.

Referring to Table 5, it is evident that WAGE1 has a positive impact on the probability that nurses have some form of collective bargaining representation using both OLS and TSLS. The implied effect is even greater when TSLS is used. Judging from the COLLB coefficients, the presence of substantial collective bargaining activity in the state's nonagricultural sector overall makes it more likely that hospital-based nurses organize. Once one has taken this factor into account, state laws are not an important independent influence. On the average, nurses employed in state and local hospitals are more likely to be covered by a collective bargaining agreement. Although Elnicki and Sloan's (1975) two-way tabulations indicated that a higher proportion of large hospitals have collective bargaining agreements covering nurses, BEDS exhibits no effect in Table 5's regressions.

Specifying unionization as an endogenous independent variable not only reduces the estimated impact of unions on wages, but, as seen in Table 6, results in a sign reversal. The coefficient associated with UNION

Table 6. Wage Regressions with Unionization Endogenous

Explanatory variables	1. OLS	2. TSLS
INC	0.114^a	0.057
	(0.033)	(0.037)
SICK	0.053^b	0.049
	(0.026)	(0.030)
PHYSG	-0.014	-0.005
	(0.010)	(0.011)
PHYSP	0.008^a	0.012^a
	(0.003)	(0.004)
SAFE	0.019	0.025
	(0.012)	(0.013)
HDENS	0.028^a	0.027^a
	(0.007)	(0.008)
MEDSC	0.030	0.015
	(0.024)	(0.027)
MEDSA	0.028	0.065^b
	(0.019)	(0.032)
UNION	0.025	-0.160
	(0.018)	(0.143)
MON	-0.008	-0.006
	(0.005)	(0.005)
NSTU	-0.055^a	-0.035
	(0.018)	(0.030)
VOLUN	-0.014	-0.036^b
	(0.012)	(0.016)
WAGE2	0.063	0.042
	(0.052)	(0.060)
WAGE3	0.236^a	0.304^a
	(0.063)	(0.086)
CONSTANT	4.77	5.32
	(-)	(-)

$$R^2 = 0.31$$
$$F(14,498) - 15.7^a$$

[a] Significant at the 1% level.
[b] Significant at the 5% level.

falls from 0.025 using OLS to -0.160 with TSLS.[26] Marked reductions in the size of estimated unionization coefficients are also reported in Ashenfelter and Johnson (1972) and Schmidt and Strauss (1976) when two stage methods rather than OLS was used. Some negative coefficients are reported in the former article. One should not make much of the negative UNION coefficient per se, but the reduction in this coefficient is probably meaningful. Ordinary least squares estimates of unions' effects on wages may well be upward-biased as a general matter.

VII. SUMMARY AND CONCLUSION

Four issues have been emphasized: the use of monopsony power by hospitals in the market for nursing services; the effects of unions on nurses' wages; relationships among wage and nonwage benefits; and the philanthropic wage hypothesis.

The possible existence of monopsony or monopsonistic elements in the market for professional nursing services is more than a scholarly issue. In recent years policy makers in the health-manpower field have been concerned about inequalities in the geographic distribution of health manpower, including professional nurses. If, for example, it could be demonstrated that hospitals located in one-hospital communities exercise monopsony power, policy makers would be likely to look at nurse staffing levels in rural areas quite differently. Low staffing would be the result of an optimizing hospital's deliberate choice rather than sheer inability to attract nurses, as such terms are used outside of economics.

As mentioned above, there are a number of ways to gauge the presence of monopsony power. In part, one's measure depends on whether one views monopsony as potential or contrived. Our tests suggest that monopsony effects are at most small, and our results are also to a degree consistent with a basically competitive market in a temporary disequilibrium. Evidence from other recent studies indicated somewhat larger impacts, but the effects were very sensitive to equation specification.

Inquiring into the monopsony issue has probably progressed as far as it can go with the types of methods employed by us and others. Certainly, it would be useful to ascertain the prevalence of employer cartels and to develop more explicit models to predict the circumstances under which they are likely to be formed and to be effectively maintained.

Ordinary least squares parameter estimates in wage regressions presented in this paper imply that collective bargaining agreements raise wages by approximately 2 to 4 percent. These estimates only apply to nurses working in hospitals with collective bargaining agreements. Our preliminary tests for union "threat" effects yielded nothing. Although we have estimated no regressions with specific nonwage benefits as dependent variables, it appears very unlikely, judging from patterns among simple correlations, that collective bargaining would demonstrate a significant effect on the provision of nonwage benefits.

Treating unionization as endogenous eliminated even the two to four percent effect. Given the tremendous growth in collective bargaining in the hospital sector, this is clearly a result worth verifying with other data bases. If union coverage is indeed a normal good, it must yield returns to covered members. Further research on the multifaceted payoffs from such coverage is also warranted.

A hedonic approach has been used to assess the desirability of specific nonwage benefits to professional nurses. Although there has been a substantial amount of research on the monopsony issue and on collective bargaining, using single equation methods, research on the supply of and demand for nonwage benefits is still in its infancy. Our results suggest nurses are willing to sacrifice small amounts of money at best for selected nonwage benefits. Possible explanations of our findings were given in section VI.

We have conducted a test of the philanthropic wage hypothesis. Valid questions about the hypothesis can be raised on a theoretical level. Given results contained in this paper, it would appear very doubtful that the hypothesis has an empirical basis either.

There is an unmistakable link between the extensiveness of nurse training in a state and entry wages of nurses in the state. This evidence is consistent with the finding reported in Sloan and Elnicki (1976) that the ratio of graduates from nursing schools in the state to state population exerts a positive impact on professional nurse staffing in hospitals. If policy makers desire to raise employed nurse-to-population ratios in a particular area, they may accomplish this by expanding the area's nursing school enrollments.

Our rather preliminary assessments of the effects of forms of regulation, certificate-of-need (CN) and prospective reimbursement (PR) suggest (1) that CN has raised the levels of both RN staffing [as reported in Sloan and Elnicki (1976)] and wages, and (2) that PR has had a negative impact on wage rates. Our CN results, which run counter to conventional wisdom, are broadly consistent with prior research on certificate-of-need [Salkever and Bice (1976)] which showed assets per bed to increase under CN while the number of beds tend to decrease. However, our results on these regulatory instruments, which are based on a single cross section, should be replicated with a time series of observations on individual hospitals before firm policy statements are made.

FOOTNOTES

*This research was supported in part by Contract #N01-NU-24264 between the Division of Nursing, U.S. Department of Health, Education, and Welfare (USDHEW) and the University of Florida and Grant #7-R01-H502590 awarded to Vanderbilt University by the National Center for Health Services Research, USDHEW. The authors wish to thank Roger Feldman, Lawrence Kenny, and G. S. Maddala for comments on earlier drafts. They are in no way responsible for what remains. A much earlier version of this paper was presented at the Atlantic Economic Association Meetings, Washington, D.C., October 1976.

1. U.S. Department of Health, Education, and Welfare (1974).

2. Letter from Mr. Wayne Emerson, American Nurses' Assocaition to Frank Sloan. According to the most recent Inventory of Registered Nurses, there were 1.1 million employed RNs in 1972. See American Nurses' Association (1974b).

3. See Seidman (1971) and Walther and LeGros (1976).

4. The hedonic approach is described in Griliches (1971).

5. According to Yett (1970), "In a survey of the thirty-one largest metropolitan hospital-associations, all but one association of the fifteen replying reported having established successful 'wage-standardization programs. (The association that did not already have such a program asked for information' on how to establish one.)'' (p. 378.) Unfortunately, this quote does not reveal the prevalence of such organizations, the coverage of such contracts (whether it only includes a wage ceiling which is only rarely binding), nor the provisions for compelling individual hospitals to comply with association decisions. To the extent that such arrangements effectively constrain a number of hospitals' ability to set professional nurse wages, empirical analysis of professional nurse wage-setting by individual hospitals becomes untenable.

6. Data on geographic movements of professional nurses are presented in Sloan (1975b, 1976a).

7. See, for example, Landon and Baird (1971), Schemenner (1973), and Ehrenberg and Goldstein (1975).

8. According to Landon and Link, "In preliminary regressions not included in this paper, other measures of unionization were tested, including percent unionized, a dummy equal to one if there was any union membership and zero otherwise. Unionization was always significant, and its coefficient had the predicted sign'' [Landon and Link (1975)], p. 654.

9. Unlike our study which is based on starting salaries of diploma graduates, Landon and Link presented regressions with starting salaries of baccalaureate and diploma graduates. The results for the two groups were quite similar. We collected baccalaureate, associate degree, and diploma salaries; the correlations among the salary variables are quite high.

10. See, for example, Ashenfelter (1971), Baird and Landon (1972), Ehrenberg (1972, 1973a, 1973b), Ehrenberg and Goldstein (1975), Frey (1975), Getz and Vahaly (1976, mimeo.), Hall and Carroll (1973), Kasper (1970), Schmenner (1973), and Thorton (1971).

11. Ashenfelter and Johnson (1972), Schmidt and Strauss (1976), and Lee (1978).

12. Frequently, it is difficult to find good instruments in cross-sectional analysis, and the resulting parameter estimates tend to be very imprecise.

13. As justification for the hospital product market assumption, variations in hospitals quality, ownership, and so on probably serve to differentiate the hospital's product. Transportation factors, pertaining to both patient and the referring physician, tend to limit the product market to a localized geographic area. Finally, given that the vast majority of hospital expenditures are covered in full or part by insurance, the payoff from searching for a lower price may be minimal.

14. In contrast to professional nurses, less specialized labor has viable employment opportunities both in and outside the local health sector. The market for hospital capital inputs is, for all practice purposes, national.

15. See Hadar (1971) for a discussion of input inferiority.

16. Comparative statics solutions depend on the signs of cross-partials (a) between pairs of endogenous variables and (b) between endogenous and exogenous variables. Unfortunately, there exists no set of restrictions on the type (a) cross-partials that by itself satisfies the second-order condition—unless, of course, one assumes that some of the cross-partials are zero; however, such restrictions generally come at high cost in terms of reality—for example, $\frac{\partial^2 \phi}{\partial Y \partial N}$ might be considered zero, but not if one wants to incorporate the possibility of inferior inputs. The comparative statics analysis also requires that one sign cross-partials of type (b). Although past research provides some evidence on some of the parameters of the underlying structural equations, there is generally insufficient detail. For instance, it seems reasonable to assume that quality is far more patient income elastic than is quantity. But this is only a maintained hypothesis, and, given the large number of plausible explanatory variables, one would have to make many such assumptions. Ambiguity in comparative statics is by no means unique to this study. See Archibald (1965).

17. Additional details are presented in Schaeffer and Sloan (1975). The Survey instrument has been reproduced in Elnicki and Sloan (1975).

18. See Davis and Reynolds (1976), Feldstein (1971), and Newhouse and Phelps (1976). Patient days are the product of the number of admissions and the length-of-stay per admission. Income elasticities associated with admissions have always been lower than those for length-of-stay. In fact, in two studies—Davis and Russell (1972) and Rosenthal (1964)—income has a negative impact on admissions. However, as Davis and Russell noted, the negative sign on income may reflect the absence of adequate health status measures in these equations.

19. Evidence from previous studies on the effect of physician availability on hospital use is mixed. Both positive and negative signs have been reported in hospital demand studies. See Davis and Reynolds (1976), Feldstein (1971), and Newhouse and Phelps (1976).

20. At first glance, it would appear preferable to include cross-price terms for ambulatory services rather than physician-population ratios. But such price data are unavailable at a level below the state, and the general practitioner-specialist distinction is not made in any published series on state physician prices.

21. We thank David Salkever for providing the data on CN.

22. The New Jersey and New York programs are described in detail in Bauer and Clark (1974a, 1974b).

23. See Sloan and Elnicki (1976).

24. Link and Landon (1976) obtained a more precise new hospital facilities parameter estimate when they omitted an area cost-of-living variable. We do not put much emphasis on this regression because omission of a price index is a potentially serious source of specification bias.

25. Our source is *Iowa Law Journal* (1971–1972). The list of states differs from a list given in Miller and Shortell (1969) and subsequently used for regression analysis by Davis (1973). After checking, we determined that the Iowa list is the accurate one.

26. The PROPRI variable has been eliminated from the Table 6 regressions because the Vanderbilt version of TSLS does not have sufficient core space to permit us to estimate an equation with 15 explanatory variables and a constant term. Based on our OLS regression results, it is reasonable to assume that dropping PROPRI has essentially discernible effect on the estimated coefficients of the other variables.

REFERENCES

American Nurses' Association (1974a), *Facts About Nursing,* Kansas City: American Nurses' Association.

――― (1974b), *The Nation's Nurses! 1972 Inventory of Registered Nurses,* Kansas City: American Nurses' Association.

Archibald, G. C. (February 1965), "The Qualitative Content of Maximizing Models," *Journal of Political Economy* LXXIII, No. 1: 36.

Ashenfelter, O. (January 1971), "The Effect of Unionization on Wages on the Public Sector: The Case of Firemen," *Industrial and Labor Relations Review* 24, No. 2: 191–203.

――― and Johnson, George E. (October 1972), "Unionism, Relative Wages, and Labor Duality in U.S. Manufacturing Industries," *International Economic Review* 13, No. 3: 488–508.

Atherton, W. N. (1973), *Theory of Union Bargaining Goals,* Princeton, N.J.: Princeton University Press.

Baird, W. M. (1969), "Barriers to Collective Bargaining in Registered Nursing," *Labor Law Journal* 20: 42–46.

――― and Landon, J. (April 1972), "The Effects of Collective Bargaining on Public School Teachers' Salaries: Comment," *Industrial and Labor Relations Review* 25, No. 3, 410–417.

Bauer, K. G. and Clark, A. R. (1974a), *The New Jersey Budget Review Program,* Boston: Harvard Center for Community Health and Medical Care.

――― and ――― (1974b), *New York: The Formula Approach to Prospective Reimbursement;* Boston: Harvard Center for Community Health and Medical Care.

Bognanno, M. F., Hixson, J. S., and Jeffers, J. R. (Winter 1974), "The Short-Run Supply of Nurse's Time," *The Journal of Human Resources* IX, No. 1: 80–94.

Davis, K. (Spring 1973), "Theories of Hospital Inflation: Some Empirical Evidence," *The Journal of Human Resources* 8, No. 2: 181–201.

――― and Reynolds, R. (1976), "The Impact of Medicare and Medicaid on Access to Medical Care," in R. Rosett, ed., *The Role of Health Insurance in the Health Services Sector,* New York: National Bureau of Economic Research, pp. 391–425.

――― and Russell, L. (May 1972), "The Substitution of Hospital Outpatient Care in Inpatient Care," *Review of Economics and Statistics* 54, No. 2: 109–120.

Dowling, W. L. (September 1974), "Prospective Reimbursement of Hospitals," *Inquiry* XI, No. 3: 163–180.

Dunlop, J. T. (1944), *Wage Determination under Trade Unions,* New York: Macmillan.

Ehrenberg, R. (1972), *The Demand for State and Local Employees,* Lexington, Mass.: D. C. Heath.

――― (December 1973a), "Heterogeneous Labor, Minimum Hiring Standards and Job Vacancies in Public Employment," *Journal of Political Economy* 81, No. 4: 1442–1452.

―――, "Municipal Government Structure, Unionization, and the Wages of Fire Fighters," *Industrial and Labor Relations Review* 27, No. 1: 36–48.

――― (Winter 1974), "Organizational Control and the Economic Efficiency of Hospitals," *The Journal of Human Resources* 9, No. 1: 21–32.

――― and Goldstein, G. S. (July 1975), "A Model of Public Sector Wage Determination," *Journal of Urban Economics,* Vol. 2, No. 3, July, 1975, pp. 223–245.

Elnicki, R. A. and Sloan, F. (1975), "Normative Measures of Nurse Distribution: Evidence from the Survey of Directors of Nursing," in F. A. Sloan, *The Geographic Distribution of Nurses and Public Policy,* Washington, D.C.: Division of Nursing, U.S. Department of Health, Education, and Welfare.

Feldstein, M. S. (1971), *The Rising Cost of Hospital Care*, Washington, D.C.: Information Resources Press.

Frey, D. E. (1975), "Wage Determination in Public Schools and the Effects of Unionization," in D. Hamermesh, ed., *Labor in the Public and Nonprofit Sectors*, Princeton, N.J.: Princeton University Press, pp. 183–219.

Getz, M. and Vahaly, J. (1976) "Determinants of Fire Fighter Compensation," mimeo.

Griliches, Zvi (1971), *Price Indexes and Quality Change*, Cambridge, Mass.: Harvard University Press.

Hadar, J. (1971), *Mathematical Theory of Economic Behavior*, Reading, Mass.: Addison-Wesley.

Hall, W. and Carroll, N. (January 1973), "The Effects of Teachers' Organization on Salaries and Class Size," *Industrial and Labor Relations Review* 26, No. 2: 834–841.

Hurd, R. W., (May 1973) "Equilibrium Vacancies in a Labor Market Dominated by Non-Profit Firms: The 'Shortage' of Nurses," *The Review of Economics and Statistics* 55, No. 2: 234–240.

Iowa Law Review (1971–1972), "Exemption of Nonprofit Hospital Employees from the National Labor Relations Act: A Violation of Equal Protection," 73: 412–450.

Kasper, H. (October 1970), "The Impact of Collective Bargaining on Public School Teachers' Salaries," *Industrial and Labor Relations Review* 24, No. 1: 57–72.

Landon, J. and Baird, R. (December 1971), "Monopsony in the Market for Public School Teachers," *Americna Economic Review* 61, No. 5: 966–971.

——— and Link, C. R. (1975), "Monopsony and Union Power in the Market for Nurses," *Southern Economic Journal* 41, No. 4: 649–659.

Lee, Lung-Fei (June 1978) "Unionism and Wage Rates: A Simultaneous Equations Model with Qualitative and Limited Dependent Variables," *International Economic Review* 19, No. 2: 415–433.

Link, C. R. and Landon, J. H. (Winter 1976), "Market Structure, Nonpecuniary Factors, and Professional Salaries: Registered Nurses," *Journal of Ecomomics and Business* 28, No. 2: 151–155.

Miller, J. D. and Shortell, S. M. (August 1969), "Hospital Unionization: A Study of the Trends," *Hospitals* 43: 67–73.

Newhouse, J. P. and Phelps, C. E. (1976), "New Estimates of Price and Income Elasticities of Medical Care Services," in R. Rosett, ed., *The Role of Health Insurance in the Health Services Sector*, New York: National Bureau of Economic Research, 261–312.

Pencavel, John H. (January 1971), "The Demand for Union Services: An Exercise," *Industrial and Labor Relations Review* 24, No. 2: 180–190.

Reder, M. W. (1959), "The Theory of Occupational Wage Differentials," *American Economic Review* 44: 833–852.

Rosenthal, G. (1974), *The Demand for General Hospital Facilities*, Chicago: American Hospital Association.

Ross, A. M. (1948 and 1956) *Trade Union Wage Policy*, Berkeley and Los Angeles: University of California Press.

Salkever, D. S. and Bice, T. W. (Spring 1976), "The Impact of Certificate-of-Need Controls on Hospital Investment," *The Milbank Memorial Fund Quarterly, Health and Society* 54, No. 2: 185–214.

Schaeffer, R. and Sloan, F. (1975), "Purposes and Design of the Two Surveys," in F. Sloan, *The Geographic Distribution of Nurses and Public Policy*, Washington, D.C.: Division of Nursing, United States Public Health Service, pp. 65–79.

Schmenner, R. (February 1973), "The Determination of Municipal Employee Wages," *Review of Economics and Statistics* 36, No. 1: 83–90.

Schmidt, Peter and Straus, Robert (February 1976), "The Effect of Unions on Earnings and Earnings on Unions: A Mixed Logit Approach," *International Economic Review* No. 1: 204–212.

Seidman, Joel (January 1971), "State Legislation on Collective Bargaining by Public Employees," *Labor Law Journal* 22, No. 1: 13–22.

Sloan, Frank A., "Determinants of Nurse Retention in Current Employment and Nurse Hours of Work," in F. A. Sloan, *The Geographic Distribution of Nurses and Public Policy,* Washington, D.C.: Division of Nursing, U.S. Department of Health, Education, and Welfare, pp. 185–212.

—— (1976a), "Interstate Migration of Professional Nurses and their Families," in F. A. Sloan, *Equalizing Access to Nursing Services: The Geographic Dimension,* Final Report on Contract #N01-NU-24264 between the Divison of Nursing, U.S. Department of Health, Education, and Welfare, and the University of Florida, pp. 109–144.

—— "Nurse Mobility Patterns," in F. A. Sloan, *The Geographic Distribution of Nurses and Public Policy.* Washington, D.C.: Division of Nursing, U.S. Department of Health, Education, and Welfare, pp. 141–162.

—— (1976b) "Nurse Retention in Current Employment," in F. A. Sloan, *Equalizing Access to Nursing Services: The Geographic Dimension,* Final Report on Contract #NO1-NU-24264 between the Division of Nursing, U.S. Department of Health, Education, and Welfare, and the University of Florida, pp. 177–210.

—— and Elnicki, Richard A. (1976), "Professional Nurse Staffing in Hospitals," in F. A. Sloan, *Equalizing Access to Nursing Services: The Geographic Dimension,* Final Report on Contract #N01-NU-24264 between Division of Nursing, U.S. Department of Health, Education, and Welfare, and the University of Florida, pp. 23–71.

——, and Richupan, Somchai (1975) "Short-Run Supply Responses of Professional Nurses: A Microanalysis," *The Journal of Human Resources* X, No. 2: 241–257.

Steinwald, Bruce, and Sloan, Frank (October 1974), "Determinants of Physicians' Fees, *Journal of Business* 47: 493–511.

Thorton, R. (1971), "The Effect of Collective Teacher Negotiations on Relative Teacher's Salaries," *Quarterly Review of Economics and Business* 11: 37–46.

U.S. Department of Health, Education, and Welfare, (1974) *Nursing Personnel in Hospitals: 1972 Survey of Hospitals Registered with the American Hospital Association.* Washington, D.C.: Division of Nursing, United States Public Health Service.

U.S. Department of Labor (1975), *Public Sector Labor Relations Information Exchange; Summary of State Policy Regulations in Public Sector Labor Relations,* Washington, D.C.: Government Printing Office.

Walther, Peter D. and LeGros, Robert R. (1976), "The Health Care Industry under the 1974 Amendments to the National Labor Relations Act," *Labor Law Developments,* pp. 83–108.

Yett, D. E. (1970) "The Chronic 'Shortage' of Nurses: A Public Policy Dilemma," in H. Klarman, ed., *Empirical Studies in Health Economics,* Baltimore: The Johns Hopkins University Press, pp. 357–389.

NURSE MARKET POLICY SIMULATIONS USING AN ECONOMETRIC MODEL*

Robert T. Deane

Donald E. Yett**

I. INTRODUCTION

The market for professional nurses is a fascinating and important topic for economic analysis. It's participants on the supply side constitute the largest health manpower occupation requiring formal training and licensing. Over 95 percent of them are female, which makes nursing the largest almost exclusively female occupation other than domestic self-employment. They produce a service which is often described as a "necessity" rather than a "want," and which many public health authorities believe was in short supply from the start of World War II until quite recently.[1]

Research in Health Economics, Vol. 1, pp 255–300.

Considering the sense of urgency attached to the "shortage" of nurses, it is not surprising that Congress initiated a massive nurse training subsidy program in 1964.[2] A short while later, in a totally unrelated move, Congress enacted the Medicare and Medicaid programs (titles XVIII and XIX of the Social Security Act). Although the purpose of these programs was to provide adequate health care to the elderly and indigent, they also had the effect of further increasing the demand for nurses.

Given the size and scope of Federal intervention on both the supply and demand sides of the nurse market, it is surprising that no attempt was made to forecast in advance the likely net impacts of these subsidy programs. Perhaps it was because the traditional health planning tools of trend projections and ratio maintenance techniques are not capable of making such forecasts. This task requires a model which explicitly treats both nurse demand and supply and their interactions. The purpose of this paper is to describe the development of such a model.[3]

Section II describes the salient characteristics of the nurse market and the key relationships reflected in the model. The structure of the model is summarized in section III. Simulation results are presented in section IV, and section V contains conclusions and a description of further work ongoing.

II. THE NURSE MARKET[4]

Most nurses are either secondary wage earners or plan to be in the near future. As a result, they exhibit very low levels of wage-induced geographic mobility. This fact, combined with the site-specific nature of the service produced, means that local area nurse markets have a high degree of autonomy (i.e., conditions in other areas have little effect on the behavior of either nurses or employers of nurses in a given locality).

Hospitals account for approximately 70 percent of total nurse employment and, thus, constitute the dominant employers in virtually all local nurse markets. Indeed, their influence is so pervasive that most nurse markets can best be characterized in terms of the degree of employer competition in their hospital sectors. Hospitals in rural areas are often monopsonistic nurse employers. Those in other areas are oligopsonists.[5] In communities with a small number of hospitals, oligopsonistic wage policies require no formal coordination. And large urban areas almost universally have hospital associations which operate "wage standardization" programs [Yett (1965), p. 100]. The existence of these programs confirms that the members believe if they acted individually each could have a noticeable effect on nurse wages. Because of this belief they voluntarily join together to avoid costly "wage wars" which would have little overall effect on nurse employment or job vacancies.[6]

The fact that urban hospitals adhere to association wage recommendations (in the absence of effective enforcement mechanisms) strongly suggests that each believes it faces a rather steep nurse supply curve. Numerous independent estimates of nurse supply elasticity support this belief.[7] Further support is provided by a Los Angeles area hospital nurse mobility study [Payne (1970), Payne and Yett (1971)].[8] Less than 2 percent of the job changes observed involved a "wage-induced" move into or out of the area. Moreover, all of the wage-induced mobility flows *within* the area were extremely small—including: shifts between hospital and non-nursing employment (nil), wage-induced re-entry into the nurse labor force (0.5 percent), intra-area hospital moves (3 percent), and shifts between hospitals and other types of nurse employment (2.3 percent).

Faced with supply curves which exhibit significant positive slopes, oligopsonistic and monopsonistic hospital employers report that they want to hire more nurses than they can at existing wage levels. Unfilled positions of this sort are called "equilibrium job vacancies." They are quite different from unfilled positions arising as a result of dynamic increases in demand relative to supply. The latter—which can be filled given sufficient time for the necessary market adjustments—are called "effective vacancies."[9] They exist in all fields of nursing, whereas the former are found only in the hospital fields.

Approximately 15 percent of all active nurses are employed as private duty or office nurses. In both fields wages are directly tied to those paid by hospitals rather than their own market conditions. Virtually all private duty employment is arranged through nurse registries, which, as a matter of policy, set their basic rates in conformity with hospital staff nurse wages. As a result, complaints of large numbers of unfilled private duty requests have been common. By contrast, the amenities associated with office nurse employment are such that physicians find it easy to recruit at the same wages paid by the hospitals in which they also practice. Job vacancy rates are low, and complaints of nurse shortages were never widespread in this field.

In general, the highest-paid nurses are those who work in industries where they constitute only a small percentage of the total work force. In such industries nurse salaries are administratively set on the basis of wages paid to the majority of workers. Thus, for example, industrial nurse wages closely correspond to the wages of production workers. Public health nurses are commonly covered by civil service pay scales. Boards of education pay school teachers approximately the same salaries as primary and secondary school nurses; and nurse educator salaries are comparable to those of other college instructors.

Since their wage-setting practices result in paying "above scale" relative to hospitals, these nurse employers face what they perceive to be horizontal supply curves at the wages they offer. They could pay lower salaries without encountering serious "shortages." The fact that they do not do so means that the benefits of low vacancies (indeed "waiting lists" are common), low turnover, and long tenure outweigh the small additional payroll cost. As long as this continues to be true, employment practices in these fields will have little or no effect on the general level of nurse salaries.

III. THE MODEL

Model Overview

The model treats the nurse market as being made up of ten separate fields:[10] hospital directors of nursing service, nurse supervisors, head nurses, and general duty nurses, nurse educators, office, private duty, public health, school, and industrial nurses. For each of these fields, the model explains actual employment, desired employment, vacancies, vacancy rates, job quits, retirements, and annual hires. In addition, it estimates all wages except those for nurse educators, public health, school, and industrial nurses, which are exogenous to the model. Since the model explicitly incorporates monopsonistic/oligopsonistic elements into the four hospital nurse fields, the number of "equilibrium" vacancies and "equilibrium" vacancy rates are also estimated for each of these fields. In addition, it generates estimates of total nurse employment, the nurse labor force, the total stock of nurses, participation rates, unemployment, and other pertinent variables. In total the model explains 131 variables; and yet it requires the manipulation of only 24 exogenous variables for forecasting purposes.

In order to embody the market theory of section II, the model should be local in character. On the other hand, the data available apply to the total industry. The result is a model which, instead of representing any *single* local market, represents an average[11] or *typical* local market but, because industry-wide data are used, forecasts aggregate quantities. Therefore, the model presented below retains explicitly its microeconomic theoretical basis, yet deals with aggregate quantities; and, with minor modification, is capable, given sufficient data, of handling conditional predictions of individual markets.

The mathematical formulation chosen is similar to that reported by

Charles C. Holt and Martin H. David in Holt (1970) and Holt and David (1966). Holt and David view the labor market

> as a complex stochastic process that involves interaction among many participants. Their actions are governed by fairly complex relationships arising from the objectives and constraints of firms and families. Thus, the labor market is not considered in terms of such relatively simple constructs as supply and demand schedules (p. 74).

To be sure, equations appear in the model of the nurse market that represents schedules of demand and supply, but the solution process is much more complex than simply finding the intersection of these schedules. As Holt describes it:

> The general approach considers the worker, both in his skills and preferences, to be complex and unique. Jobs similarly are considered to have unique and complex sets of requirements and rewards. The successful pricing of a worker and a job that leads to employment requires the mutual satisfaction of worker and employer and depends on many characteristics of job and worker. To obtain the large amounts of information necessary for making choices, substantial resources and time are consumed by employer and employee in search. . . . [It] follows that knowledge will be costly and highly imperfect, so that blind random search necessarily will play an important role [Holt (1970), pp. 54–55].

Two of the stocks in the model, the number of unemployed nurses and the number of job vacancies, interact to represent "a random search process through which a nonstandard worker and a nonstandard job are somewhat matched to satisfy certain wage and skill criteria established by firm and worker" [Holt and David (1966), p. 74.] The net result of this interaction is a flow of new hires which reduces both the stock of unemployed workers and the stock of job vacancies and increases the stock of employed workers.

This random search process provides the theoretical basis for the hiring procedure contained in the model. However, the equations of the model are used to generate estimates of proportions (probabilities of being hired) which are then applied to the stock of available positions or vacancies to determine the number of these positions which get filled by new hires. This procedure is used in lieu of a random sampling of probability density functions (as in Monte Carlo experiments) in order to determine the flow of new hires during the simulation year.

There are ten separate fields of nursing inlcuded in the model, each of which maintains a stock of vacancies. Employers in these ten nursing fields are continually trying to find suitable nurses to fill these positions. In their search for these nurses, the employers are restricted to the pool of unemployed nurses. Employers in all ten nursing fields compete for prospective employees out of the *same* pool of unemployed nurses.

Since the data interval chosen is one year, the filling of vacancies from the pool of unemployed occurs annually. Immediately before the hiring process takes place, the pool of potential nurse employees is calculated by adding the net change in the nursing labor force from last period to this period and the number of nurses who quit during the year and are seeking other nursing positions to the stock of unemployed nurses remaining after *last* year's hiring round (last period's stock of unemployed). By the same token, the number of nursing positions in each nursing field for which personnel are sought just prior to the hiring process is calculated by adding the net change in the number of positions vacated during the year in each field to the stock of effective vacancies remaining unfilled from last year's hiring round (last period's stock of effective vacancies in each nursing field).

Thus, from one period to the next, the number of vacant positions which are potentially fillable is allowed to accumulate in each nursing field and, at the same time, the common pool of unemployed nurses who are seeking to fill these positions is likewise accumulating. Finally, at the end of the year (or the beginning of the next year), the model initiates the hiring process in which nurse employers in each of the ten nurse fields hire nurses from the pool of unemployed to fill vacancies in their fields. Each hire, of course, simultaneously reduces the common pool of unemployed by one and vacancies in one of the ten nurse fields by one.

The model explicitly provides that at the end of the hiring process a stock of unemployed nurses will remain along with some unfilled vacancies in each of the ten nurse fields. In other words, in no field is the probability of filling all the accumulated effective vacancies equal to one. While the estimated probabilities or proportions vary substantially among the ten nurse fields, each is determined in large part by the same factor—the size of the pool of potential employees (normalized for the size of the labor force). The larger the pool of unemployed nurses relative to the size of the labor force, the larger the proportion of each field's vacancies that will be filled.

The growth of the pool of unemployed nurses during the year, as well as the growth of the number of fillable vacancies in each nurse field during the year are, in large part, dependent on key behavioral relationships in the model. A large portion of the accumulation of the pool of unemployed during the year is due to changes in the nurse labor force. Such changes are calculated by applying age-specific participation rates to age cohorts of the stock of living nurses. The stock of living nurses between the ages of 20 and 79, inclusive, is found by survivor weighting the number of graduates from nursing schools for the previous 60 years (including the current year). The participation rates, however, are functions of nurse wages, price levels, past participation rates, and other selected variables, and, therefore, are highly sensitive to current nurse market conditions.

The growth in the number of effective vacancies in each field of nursing is determined in large part by the number of new positions created during the year which are fillable. These new positions are calculated by comparing the *change* in the desired employment of nurses from last period to this period in each field of nursing.[12] The desired employment of nurses in each nurse field is a function of the money wage, the product price, the desired employment last period, the equilibrium vacancy rate (hospital fields only), and other field-specific variables. As with nurse participation, the desired employment of nurses in each nurse field is, therefore, highly sensitive to nurse market conditions.

Basic Stock-Flow Relationships

The complete model is presented, along with all variable definitions, in the Appendix. In order to reduce the complexity of the presentation, a simplified version of the model will be presented here. Figure 1 presents the key stocks and flows of the model and their interrelationships in an abbreviated schematic. In this schematic, stocks are represented by boxes and flows by lines.

The stock of trained nurses *not* in the labor force, the labor force reserve (RSRV), is increased by new graduations of trained nurses (GRAD)[13] and decreased by total deaths from the stock of trained nurses (DIES) and the annual change in the nurse labor force (CHNG). The stock of unemployed nurses in the labor force (UNEM) is increased by the annual change in the nurse labor force (CHNG), annual quits (QUIT), and annual retirements (including deaths of those employed) (RETR), while being decreased by total hires (HIRE). The total stock of effective vacancies which firms are seeking to fill (TVSE) is incremented by the flow of total vacancies created during the year (TVFE) and decreased by total hires (HIRE) which fill vacancies. The stock of employed nurses (EMPL) is decreased by the flow of quits (QUIT) and retirements (RETR) and is increased by the flow of total hires (HIRE).

The relationships between these stocks and flows as presented in Figure 1 can also be expressed as accounting identities with negative subscripts indicating a time lag:[14]

Figure 1:   Basic Nurse Market Stocks and Flows

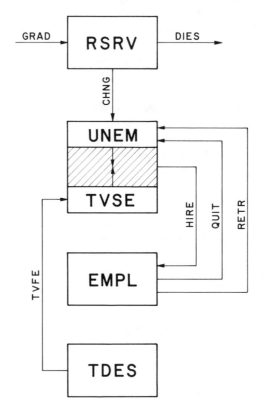

$$RSRV \ - RSRV_{-1} \equiv GRAD - DIES \ - CHNG \tag{1}$$

$$UNEM - UNEM_{-1} \equiv RETR + QUIT + CHNG - HIRE \tag{2}$$

$$TVSE \ - TVSE_{-1} \equiv TVFE - HIRE \tag{3}$$

$$EMPL \ - EMPL_{1} \ \equiv HIRE \ - QUIT - RETR \tag{4}$$

Several points of clarification concerning these relationships should be added. Implicit in Figure 1 is that all hires are to be from the pool of unemployed. This is why all additions to the labor force (CHNG) and all quits (QUIT) are shown as increments to UNEM. This does not explain why retirements (RETR) (which includes the flow of deaths from the stock of employed) are shown as an increment to the stock of unemployed nurses instead of an increment to the nurse labor force reserve (RSRV).

The answer lies in the nature of the flow, CHNG. The annual change in the nurse labor force is, conceptually at least, the algebraic sum of two flows, one of which is positive (all entrants to the labor force) and the other negative (all withdrawals from the labor force). Since CHNG is the net sum of these two flows, its inclusion in equation (2) would understate the change in the stock of unemployed by the amount of RETR (all withdrawals from the *employed* labor force) if RETR were not added back in the equation.[15]

While the net changes in the labor force (CHNG) are conceptually the algebraic sum of all entrants into the labor force and all withdrawals from the labor force, its determination is best achieved through its definition. Equation (5) therefore defines CHNG as:

$$CHNG = LBFS - LBFS_{-1} \qquad (5)$$

From Figure 1 and equation (3) it is evident that the total flow of effective vacancies (TVFE)[16] is a *gross flow* rather than a flow of net vacancies. TVFE is seen as the *only* flow which increases the total stock of effective vacancies (TVSE). Therefore, since it is obvious that every time a quit or a retirement occurs a position is vacated, TVFE must include those vacancies created by QUIT and RETR. This being the case, *net* effective vacancies are equivalent to the change in the desired level of employment (TDES):

$$TDES - TDES_{-1} \equiv TVFE - QUIT - RETR \qquad (6)$$

While it is quite possible that net effective vacancies may be negative (desired employment decreases), it is highly improbably that the flow of gross effective vacancies (TVFE) will be negative. For this to occur, desired employment would have to decrease by an amount greater than the annual quits (QUIT) and retirements (RETR). Such an event is highly unlikely given the average turnover in the nurse market. Note also that in Figure 1 the direction of the flow of TVFE is from the box labeled TDES and yet equation (6) shows TVFE as increasing TDES. This unusual treatment occurs because the flow of vacancies is determined, in part, by the change in desired employment rather than vice versa. Rearranging equation (6), we have:

$$TVFE \equiv TDES - TDES_{-1} + QUIT + RETR \qquad (7)$$

In this case, we have a flow determined by a change in a stock rather than the usual situation of a change in a stock being brought about by a flow.

Figure 1 also shows the flow DIES regulating the nurse labor force reserve (RSRV), and therefore, the stock of living nurses (STOK). The number of annual deaths of trained nurses (DIES) is a reduction in the stock of living nurses (STOK). But, instead of being calculated directly via survivor rates, the flow DIES is calculated from the past and present stocks of living nurses (STOK) and new nursing student graduations (GRAD):

$$DIES \equiv STOK_{-1} - STOK + GRAD \qquad (8)$$

There are a few other relationships among the stocks referred to in Figure 1 that are not explicitly represented by the schematic. The total nurse labor force (LBFS) minus the stock of employed nurses (EMPL) equals the stock of unemployed nurses (UNEM). The total stock of trained nurses (STOK) minus the stock of nurses in the labor force (LBFS) is equal to the stock of nurses *not* in the labor force (RSRV); and the total stock of effective nurse vacancies (TVSE) is the difference between the desired level of nurse employment (TDES) and the stock of employed nurses (EMPL). These definitions are expressed as accounting identities as follows:

$$UNEM \equiv LBFS - EMPL \text{ (if EMPL} > LBFS, UNEM = 0) \qquad (9)$$

$$RSRV \equiv STOK - LBFS \qquad (10)$$

$$TVSE \equiv TDES - EMPL \qquad (11)$$

Equation (9) also contains a constraint such that, if EMPL is greater than LBFS, UNEM is set equal to zero. Conceptually, within the context of the model, a negative value for UNEM is absurd. As a practical matter, UNEM can be expected to engage the constraint occasionally. LBFS and EMPL are both large numbers of about the same size. Therefore, small percentage errors in either LBFS, EMPL, or both can produce extremely large percentage errors in UNEM. The net result is that predicted UNEM can be expected to have a large variance and occasionally be negative during simulation.

Other key stocks which did not appear explicitly in Figure 1, but which appeared quite often in the equations above, are the total nurse labor force (LBFS) and the total stock of living nurses (STOK). The stock of living nurses (STOK) is found by applying the survivor weights (SRWT) to annual nursing school graduations (GRAD) as in equation (12). The negative subscripts indicate a time lag. The total nurse labor force (LBFS) is found by applying a participation rate (PART) to the stock of living nurses (STOK) as shown in equation (13).

$$STOK \equiv \sum_{0}^{59}(GRAD_{-i} \cdot SRWT_{-i}) \qquad (12)$$

$$LBFS \equiv STOK \cdot PART \qquad (13)$$

Basic Behavioral Relationships

Up to this point, Figure 1 and equations (1) to (13) have attempted to explain only the accounting relationships between the stocks and flows in a simplified representation of the final model. None of the equations accompanying Figure 1 contain any behavior relationships. This section will complete the abbreviated model by introducing behavioral functions which are representative of those present in the full model. Expected signs of coefficients are shown below each term in the function.

Three of the flows and one of the stocks in Figure 1 are behaviorally determined. That is, the mathematical expressions used to calculate these quantities are classified as behavioral equations rather than identities. The flow of quits (QUIT) is a function of the last period's level of employment as shown in equation (14).

$$QUIT = f(\underset{+}{EMPL_{-1}}) \qquad (14)$$

The functional relationship is positive and most likely proportional, so that the larger the level of employment last period, the larger the number of quits during the year. Equation (15) explains the determination of the annual flow of nurse retirements (RETR).

$$RETR = f(\underset{+}{DIES \cdot PART_{-1}}, \underset{+}{EMPL_{-1}/LBFS_{-1}}) \qquad (15)$$

The annual flow of retirements of those employed (RETR), which includes deaths of those employed, is a positive function of both the total number of deaths and retirements from the nurse labor force (DIES $\cdot$ PART$_{-1}$) during the year, and the proportion of the nurse labor force employed last (EMPL$_{-1}$/LBFS$_{-1}$). The last term is included because DIES $\cdot$ PART$_{-1}$ measures deaths and retirements from the nurse labor force from year t-1 to year t and RETR is to measure only those deaths and retirements from nursing of those *employed* in year t-1.

The average wage of nurses (WAGE) is determined endogenously, and is explained by the following functional representation:

$$WAGE = f(\underset{+}{EMPL + TVSE}, \underset{-}{LBFS}, \underset{+}{PRIC}) \qquad (16)$$

Thus, the wage of nurses (WAGE) depends positively on the total number of positions that *can be filled* at that wage (EMPL + TVSE) and the general price level (PRIC), and negatively on the size of the nurse labor force (LBFS). The general price level (PRIC) is determined exogenously to the model.[17]

While equation (16) may be thought of as a supply equation, the function which explains the total desired employment of nurses may be thought of as a demand equation. While there are ten fields of nursing in the complete model, each with a different set of independent variables, the independent variables shown in equation (17) are those for the hospital nurse fields only. The independent variables are the average daily patient census in short term, nonfederal, general hospitals (CENS) and the product wage which is the average wage of nurses (WAGE) divided by the index of average daily hospital charges (PRA1).

$$\text{TDES} = f(\underset{+}{\text{CENS}}, \underset{-}{\text{WAGE/PRA1}}) \qquad (17)$$

The desired employment of nurses (TDES) appears on Figure 1 as a stock. This leaves the flow of annual hires (HIRE) as the last variable in Figure 1 to be explained. The flow of hires in each annual period is a result of the interaction of the accumulated stock of unemployed nurses and the accumulated stock of nurse vacancies. Figure 1 shows the interaction between these two stocks as the shaded area from which the flow of hires (HIRE) originates.

The shaded area in Figure 1 is the random job search process discussed earlier. In the model, however, an equation is used to generate a single point estimate of the proportion of total vacancies that will be filled during the search process. This proportion (or probability of vacancies being filled) is a positive function of the number of nurses seeking to fill the vacant positions normalized for the size of the labor force.

That is, the larger the accumulated stock of those unemployed relative to the total nurse labor force, the greater the proportion of accumulated vacancies that will be filled. The accumulation of unemployed nurses just prior to the initiation of the hiring process can be deduced from equation (2) above as: $\text{UNEM}_{-1} + \text{QUIT} + \text{RETR} + \text{CHNG}$. Normalizing for the size of the labor market, we then have

$$Z = (\text{UNEM}_{-1} + \text{QUIT} + \text{RETR} + \text{CHNG}) / \text{LBFS} \qquad (18)$$

By the same token, the accumulation of the stock of effective vacancies just prior to the initiation of the hiring process can be deduced from equation (3) above as: $\text{TVSE}_{-1} + \text{TVFE}$. Therefore, the proportion of these accumulated vacancies filled in the hiring process is a positive function of the accumulated stock of unemployed nurses relative to the nursing labor force (Z),

$$\text{HIRE} / (\text{TVSE}_{-1} + \text{TVFE}) = \underset{+}{g(Z)} \qquad (19)$$

or the number of hires is represented by

$$HIRE = [TVSE_{-1} + TVFE] \cdot g(Z). \tag{20}$$

But, since from equation (3) we have

$$TVSE_{-1} + TVFE + TVSE + HIRE \tag{21}$$

then equation (20) can be rewritten as

$$HIRE = TVSE \cdot f(Z), \text{ where } f(Z) = g(Z) / (1 - g(Z)). \tag{22}$$

The expression $f(Z)$ in equation (22) represents a mapping of $g(Z)$ from zero to infinity into a space of zero to one, and vice versa. Therefore, no matter what the estimate of $f(Z)$, as long as it is positive, a value between zero and one is assured for the proportion of vacancies being filled, $g(Z)$.

The last endogenous variable to be explained does not appear in Figure 1, but it is important in determining the proportion of the stock of living nurses (STOK) that participates in the labor force (LBFS). This proportion is shown in equation (13) as PART. The participation rate (part) is a positive function of the average nurse wage (WAGE) and last period's participation rate ($PART_{-1}$), and a negative function of the average wages of all female workers (AVF1) and the general price level (PRIC). Both of the later quantities are exogenous to the model.

$$PART = f(WAGE, PART_{-1}, AVF1, PRIC) \tag{23}$$
$$\quad\quad\quad + \quad\quad + \quad\quad - \quad\quad -$$

Equation (23) completes the presentation of the simple model portrayed in Figure 1. The final model is much more complex, but contains the same basic elements as the simple model. Before presenting the simulation results of the final model, one added feature should be incorporated into the simple model. This is the existence of "equilibrium" vacancies.

Introducing Equilibrium Vacancies

The introduction of market imperfections, such as monopsony and oligopsony, into the nurse market alters the relationship between annual changes in the desired level of employment and the flow of net effective vacancies, equation (6). It also affects the relationship between the desired level of employment and the actual level of employment, equation (11). As discussed earlier, these types of market imperfections imply the existence of vacancies that will remain unfilled even when the market is in static equilibrium.[18] The employer would like to fill these vacancies *at the prevailing wage* but cannot. On the other hand, some of these vacancies *could* be filled at higher wages, but to do so is inconsistent with profit maximizing (or loss minimizing) behavior. These vacancies are called "equilibrium" vacancies, which are to be distinguished from "effective" or "disequilibrium" vacancies.[19]

Thus, it is apparent that the difference between the desired level of employment (TDES) and the actual level of employment (EMPL) is not only due to the existence of a stock of effective vacancies (TVSE), but also to the existence of a stock of equilibrium vacancies. If TVRT is equal to the equilibrium vacancy rate, then the stock of equilibrium vacancies is equal to TVRT • TDES[20] and equation (11) becomes:

$$TVSE \equiv TDES - TVRT \cdot TDES - EMPL \qquad (24)$$

By the same token, the presence of equilibrium vacancies makes the change in the desired level of employment equal to the net flow of *total* vacancies rather than the net flow of *effective* vacancies. To determine the latter quantity, all equilibrium vacancies must be excluded,[21] so that equation (6) then becomes:

$$EMPL + TVSE - EMPL_{-1} - TVSE_{-1} \equiv TVFE - QUIT - RET \equiv R \qquad (25)$$

If monopsony or oligopsony is not present in the market (TVRT=0), then equation (24) reduces to equation (11) and equation (25) reduces to equation (6).

Detailed Stock-Flow Relationships

Figure 2 presents a detailed schematic of the stocks and flows of the final model. Time will not be taken here to describe the remaining identities and behavioral relationships, but the reader is referred to the in-depth discussion in Deane and Yett (1979), Chapter II, for such details. At this point, the description of the basic model should have provided enough general knowledge of the sectors of the model and how it works to facilitate the interpretation of the simulation results presented below.

IV. SIMULATION RESULTS[22]

The estimated model was tested by evaluating its ability to track the 1947–1966 historical period, after which it was used to conduct policy sensitivity experiments and to make "forecasts" to 1973. Since the model predicts values for such a large number of variables, it is not possible to describe, in each case, the effects on all of them.[23] Instead, only the

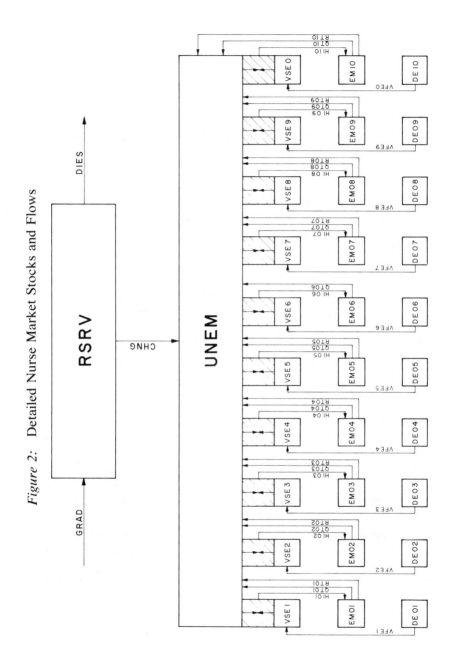

Figure 2: Detailed Nurse Market Stocks and Flows

269

effects on the most aggregative variables are reported (except when special effects on other variables are notable).

Historical Tracking

The model was used to simulate the period 1947–1966, and the results were compared with actual historical values as a test of its tracking ability. Since the same data were used in this test as were used to estimate the model, this might not appear to be a very severe test. However, just because the individual equations of the model displayed a good fit to the data over the historical period (i.e., the R^2s were high) does not guarantee that their solutions together (either joint or recursive) will produce estimates which closely approximate the historical data. When equations which were originally estimated on an equation-by-equation basis are solved simultaneously, the values for a particular period may contain an accumulation of errors, resulting in significant deviations from the target values. Indeed, the individual equations may fit well over the entire simulation period, their joint solution may produce reasonable predictions for one or two periods, and yet by the *end* of simulation interval the solution values obtained over a number of periods may vary considerably from historical data. This is because solution values of previous periods are used in the simulation as lagged values of endogenous variables for the current period. Consequentty, errors are cumulative, and each succeeding period of the simulation run is subject to greater error. If no such accumulation of errors is observed, then the model has met an extremely severe test.

Two summary statistics were calculated to show how close the solution values from simulation are to the historical or target values. The first, the Mean Percentage Error (MPE), is the average of the errors (expressed as a percentage of the historical or target value) of all endogenous variables for each time period. The second, the Root Mean Squared Error (RMSE), is the square root of the average of the squared errors (expressed as percentages of the historical values) of all endogenous variables for each time period. The MPE was less than five percent in absolute value for all 20 years in the period. In all but four of the years it was below three percent. While these gross error statistics are very small, care must be exercised in their interpretation. Just as large values of MPE can result from large errors on only one or two variables, small values of MPE can be the result of large but compensating errors on individual variables for the same period. The RMSE values for eight of the years (1947, 1951, 1952, 1957, 1963–1966) were below 10 percent. For six years (1953, 1956, 1959–1962) they were between 10 and 15 percent. Although the RMSE

Table 1. Policy Sensitivity and Historical Tracking Results for Selected Variables and Years

Variable	Year	Historical	Historical Tracking	Demand Subsidy	Training Subsidy	Demand Training and Subsidies
Average Nurse Wage ($ per month)	1948	202.8	199.7	199.7	199.7	199.7
	1952	246.7	249.7	249.7	249.7	249.7
	1956	287.6	289.5	308.6	289.5	308.6
	1961	357.0	349.2	372.3	340.4	360.5
	1966	453.1	450.9	496.2	411.8	445.8
Total Employment	1948	325,600	325,300	325,300	325,300	325,300
	1952	376,300	385,200	385,200	385,200	385,200
	1956	433,100	441,900	450,800	441,900	450,900
	1961	511,800	516,100	526,800	521,100	533,100
	1966	579,900	582,200	624,200	600,600	620,600
Total Labor Force	1948	330,800	327,500	327,500	327,500	327,500
	1952	382,400	389,500	389,500	389,500	389,500
	1956	440,200	443,800	451,500	443,800	451,500
	1961	520,100	516,600	521,700	522,700	529,400
	1966	589,300	595,200	610,300	618,700	640,000
Total Unemployment	1948	5,250	2,276	2,276	2,276	2,276
	1952	6,100	4,282	4,282	4,282	4,282
	1956	7,050	1,897	673	1,858	634
	1961	8,300	452	0	1,623	0
	1966	9,400	13,060	0	18,030	19,440
Total Effective Vacancies	1948	46,200	41,650	41,650	41,650	41,650
	1952	59,870	55,520	55,520	55,520	55,520
	1956	85,780	77,230	85,550	77,250	85,570
	1961	112,600	106,700	113,000	110,500	116,500
	1966	126,600	127,300	105,200	131,800	138,900

values for the remaining years were over 15 percent, only the value for 1949 exceeded 20 percent (21.39). Taken together, these results indicate that: (i) the model's tracking performance is poorest for 1949 and 1950 (as indicated by the MPE); (ii) rather large errors for 1948, 1954, and 1955 had opposite signs, and these tended to cancel each other when calculating the MPE; and (iii) the model's tracking performance is better during the latter part of the period, suggesting that no serious problem of error accumulation exists.

Examination of the predictions of selected variables (shown in Table 1) also indicates that the model tracks fairly accurately. In fact, all trackings were highly accurate, except in the case of unemployment. Such a result is not surprising, however, since unemployment is calculated as a small residual between two very large quantities—the labor force and total employment. Consequently, even quite small errors in these quantities can produce large errors in predicted unemployment.

Policy Sensitivity

In order to explore the sensitivity of the solution values of the model to changes in selected equation parameters and/or exogenous variables, three different policy experiments were conducted and the results were compared to the solution set obtained for the historical period. The experiments chosen were: (1) the introduction of a demand subsidy, (2) a nurse training subsidy, and (3) both of these simultaneously.

(1) *The Demand Subsidy*—The first policy sensitivity test was the introduction of a demand subsidy similar to Medicare and Medicaid. For this experiment five of the 24 exogenous variables subject to manipulation were changed. These variables were: the annual mean income of phtsicians, the index of daily hospital service charges, the subsidy dummy variable appearing in the hospital nurse desired employment equations, and the average daily patient census in all hospitals and in non-Federal, short-term general hospitals.

The demand subsidy was specified to cause a 20 percent increase in the utilization of hospital services by elderly persons [Wilkin (1968), pp. 999–1004], which, in turn, implied an increase is approximately five percent in overall hospital utilization. Accordingly, the values of the average daily patient census in all hospitals and in non-federal, short-term general hospitals were increased each year from 1953[24] to 1966 by five percent above the historical experience. Also, the demand subsidy was specified to increase physicians' income by 10 percent above the historical values for each year [*Medical Economics* (July 24, 1967), pp. 102–131]. Finally, the index of average daily hospital charges was assumed to be 10 percent higher than the historical value for each year. The Medicare dummy variable (DUMZ) appearing in the hospital nursing desired employment equations was also activated (set equal to one) in each year.

Table 1 shows that the specified demand subsidy produced a sizable increase in the simulated number of nurses employed by 1966 relative to the historical tracking figures. At the same time, the total stock of effective nurse vacancies declined (mainly in the general duty and private duty fields); and the average nurse wage increased (due to wage increases in all fields where the wage is endogenous). These changes were the net result of a shift in the demand for nurses and a simultaneous movement upward along the demand curve. The increase in wages also produced a larger labor force through increased participation rates. Note that the levels of unemployment in 1961 and 1966 have been set at zero. This is because the demand subsidy increased employment to such an extent that it caught and passed the also-increased labor force.[25]

Although the demand subsidy experiment clearly put pressure on various sectors of the nurse market, none of the economic results were undesirable. Both the labor force and employment increased. Wages increased in what had previously been regarded as a depressed-wage industry. Vacancies and unemployment both decreased showing that many positions were either filled because of increased hiring activity induced by rising wages, or done away with because of the higher wage cost that would have to be incurred in filling them. And finally, nurse graduates were projected to face a market in which they would have little difficulty securing positions at relatively high wages.

(2) *Nurse Training Subsidy*—The second sensitivity test was the introduction of a nurse training subsidy. This experiment was patterned after the 1963 recommendations of the Surgeon General's Consultant Group on Nursing [(1963), p. 22], whose recommended goal was to increase annual nursing school graduations from approximately 30,000 to 53,000 over a nine-year period. In setting up this experiment it was assumed that the number of graduates would meet the recommended goals by type of program in 1965; with Associate Degree programs going from 252 in 1956 to 5,000, Diploma programs from 25,905 in 1957 to 40,000, and Baccalaureate degree programs from 3,652 in 1958 to 8,000.[26]

Table 1 shows the results of the training subsidy experiment on selected key variables. As a result of declining wages (relative to the historical experience) more nursing services were demanded and nurse employment increased. Total effective job vacancies also increased somewhat relative to the historical tracking. However, this increase was due almost entirely to the effect of the depressed wage on the flow of *private duty* nurse desired employment. Nevertheless, the nurse labor force increased dramatically, owing to the large number of young recent graduates who are the least sensitive to wage influences. This combination of forces, of course, produced some nurse unemployment, which by 1966 approached a rate of three percent (vs. 2.2 percent without the training subsidy).

The economic results of this experiment then were, on balance, undesirable. Even though total nurse employment grew, total job vacancies also increased, wages were depressed below levels already considered low, and unemployment increased. This policy resulted in large numbers of new graduates being produced while, at the same time, job prospects and wage levels deteriorated.

(3) *Demand and Nurse Training Subsidies*—The third policy sensitivity test was the introduction of both the demand subsidy of experiment one and the nurse training subsidy of experiment two simultaneously. The same variables and parameters were changed by the same amounts as described above for each program separately. The object of this test was to see in what manner, and to what degree, the two programs either reinforced or counterbalanced each other. For example, given the implied market situation from the demand subsidy experiment, one might be tempted to advocate a simultaneous subsidy of nurse training in order to alleviate the "tightness" of the market.

Table 1 shows the values of key variables for selected years after initiating both subsidies. Initially the results paralleled those of implementing the demand subsidy alone because, while it was initiated immediately, the training subsidy program was phased in over a number of years. Once the training subsidy program was fully implemented, however, its effects tended to dominate those of the demand study. For example, the level of unemployment and total effective job vacancies by 1966 were higher than in the historical tracking, and higher than in the case of the training subsidy alone. Moreover, there was an increase in job vacancies in virtually all fields of nursing.[27] At the same time, nurse wage levels were depressed below those of the historical tracking—although they remained above those produced by the training subsidy program alone. The net effect of both policies operating simultaneously is that wages remained depressed while effective job vacancies and unemployment were larger than ever.

The nurse labor force grew substantially as a result of both the high levels of nursing school graduations (due to the training subsidy) and the rise in nurse wage levels (due to the demand subsidy). Consequently, the two policies acted to reinforce each other with respect to unemployment, although separately they produced opposite effects. Likewise, the two policies acting in concert resulted in larger numbers of job vacancies. The demand subsidy produced an upward shift in the demand for nurses, while, at the same time, the training subsidy depressed nurse wages and caused a movement down the demand curve. Both effects increased the amount demanded. However, owing to the depressed wage levels, hiring activity could not keep pace and the number of job vacancies increased.

To summarize, the net results of the simultaneous implementation of both subsidies were depressed wages with increased levels of job vacancies and nurse unemployment. Thus, instead of counteracting each other as anticipated, the effects of the two policies tended to be mutually reinforcing with respect to the size of the nurse labor force, unemployment, and job vacancies.

V. CONCLUSIONS

It is interesting to note that adding the number of nurses in fields not covered by the model (approximately 40,000) and the 72.4 percent of the 1967 and 1968 basic nurse program graduates who are expected to be employed to the number of nurses employed in the endogenous fields in 1966 yields a figure for total nurse employment of approximately 680,500. This is slightly more than the *1970 goal* advocated by the Surgeon General's Consultant Group on Nursing [(1963), p. 54], which, in turn, was the basic justification for the Nurse Training Act (NTA) of 1964. It is also the level of employment actually achieved in 1969. However, the actual number of nursing school graduations in 1968/1969–42,196–was considerably below the 53,000 figure the Surgeon General's Consultant Group on Nursing [(1963), p. 54], said would be necessary to meet its 1970 employment goal. The fact is that the NTA subsidy program contributed little to the attainment of the goal set by the Surgeon General's Consultant Group on Nursing. The growth in nurse employment was mainly due to increased labor force participation in response to the wage effects of Medicare and Medicaid, and to the movement of members of the large World War II graduating classes into the age cohorts with higher labor force participation rates.

If the NTA of 1964 had been as effective in increasing nursing school entrants as intended, there would have been a dramatic increase in the ratio of nursing school enrollments to the number of female high school graduates, which did not occur. Such an increase, along with the intended reduction in the nurse school dropout rate, would have caused at least double the observed increase in graduations. As indicated by the results of our policy simulations, the impacts on nurse job vacancies, unemployment, and wages would also have been quite large. Moreover, since Medicare and Medicaid were enacted shortly after the NTA went into effect, the marginal impacts on vacancies and unemployment would have been amplified. Indeed, given that the large World War II graduating classes were moving into age cohorts associated with high labor force participation rates, the resulting unemployment would have been substantial. The fact that no such market conditions were observed further supports the conclusion that the initial economic impacts of the NTA were nil.

However, since the original NTA in 1964, there has been a steady flow of legislation increasing the amounts and types of nurse training subsidies. This legislation includes the 1966 amendments to the Nurse Training Act of 1964, the Health Manpower Act of 1968, the Nurse Training Act of 1971, and the Nurse Training Act of 1975. But unless Congress and the President are convinced soon that nurse training subsidies are not the correct solution for diminishing the nurse "shortage" complaints, it is likely that growing unemployment will become the nurse market issue of greatest concern in the next decade.

It is our hope that the refinements now being made to the preliminary model described here will result in a final version capable of accurately forecasting the likely consequences of future policies to alleviate the anticipated future nurse market problems.[28] It is, of course, entirely possible that the massive training subsidies of the past twelve years will—in a sense—be justified by the enactment of National Health Insurance. The final version of our model should help to determine the extent to which that may occur, and what, if any, remedial measures such action would be required.

APPENDIX

VARIABLES AND EQUATIONS

This Appendix is divided into two closely related sections. Section I contains an alphabetical listing of the variables endogenous to the model and an alphabetical listing of the variables exogenous to the model. Section II consists of a listing of the equations of the model, separated into identities and behavioral equations.

I. Variables

This section contains an alphabetical listing of the 131 endogenous variables of the model in Part A and an alphabetical listing of the 87 exogenous variables in Part B. In addition to the variable name (the four character names used in the computer algorithm are utilized) and the variable description, each variable is assigned a number and a form code. The assigned number will facilitate cross-referencing the other section of this Appendix, and the form code should aid in the understanding of the nature of each variable.

Since the model is a stock-flow model, some of the endogenous variables have flow dimension and others have stock dimension. The flow variables are labeled with an "F" and the stock variables with an "S." Those endogenous variables not representing stocks or flows of nurses or nurse positions are labeled with an "O."

A.   Endogenous

Number	Name	Form	Description
1	CHNG	F	annual change in the labor force
2	DE01	S	desired employment of general duty nurses
3	DE02	S	desired employment of directors of nursing service
4	DE03	S	desired employment of nursing supervisors
5	DE04	S	desired employment of head nurses
6	DE05	S	desired employment of office nurses
7	DE06	S	desired employment of private duty nurses
8	DE07	S	desired employment of public health nurses
9	DE08	S	desired employment of school nurses
10	DE09	S	desired employment of nurse educators
11	DE10	S	desired employment of industrial nurses
12	DIES	F	number leaving the stock of trained nurses annually via death and retirement
13	EM01	S	number of general duty nurses employed
14	EM02	S	number of directors of nursing service employed
15	EM03	S	number of nursing supervisors employed
16	EM04	S	number of head nurses employed
17	EM05	S	number of office nurses employed
18	EM06	S	number of private duty nurses employed
19	EM07	S	number of public health nurses employed
20	EM08	S	number of school nurses employed
21	EM09	S	number of nurse educators employed
22	EM10	S	number of industrial nurses employed
23	EM00	S	number of nurses employed by hospitals
24	EMPL	S	total number of nurses employed
25	GRAD	F	annual graduates from nursing schools
26	HI01	F	number of general duty nurses hired
27	HI02	F	number of directors of nursing service hired
28	HI03	F	number of nursing supervisors hired
29	HI04	F	number of head nurses hired
30	HI05	F	number of office nurses hired
31	HI06	F	number of private duty nurses hired
32	HI07	F	number of public health nurses hired
33	HI08	F	number of school nurses hired
34	HI09	F	number of nurse educators hired
35	HI10	F	number of industrial nurses hired
36	LBFS	S	number of nurses in the labor force

Number	Name	Form	Description
37	PT01	O	participation rate of nurses, ages 20-24
38	PT02	O	participation rate of nurses, ages 25-34
39	PT03	O	participation rate of nurses, ages 35-44
40	PT04	O	participation rate of nurses, ages 45-54
41	PT05	O	participation rate of nurses, ages 55-64
42	PT06	O	participation rate of nurses, ages 65-79
43	QT01	F	number quitting general duty nurse positions
44	QT02	F	number quitting director of nursing service positions
45	QT03	F	number quitting nurse supervisor positions
46	QT04	F	number quitting head nurse positions
47	QT05	F	number quitting office nurse positions
48	QT06	F	number quitting private duty nurse positions
49	QT07	F	number quitting public health nurse positions
50	QT08	F	number quitting school nurse positions
51	QT09	F	number quitting nurse educator positions
52	QT10	F	number quitting industrial nurse positions
53	QUIT	F	total quitting all nurse positions
54	RETR	F	total deaths and retirements from nurse employment
55	RSRV	S	number of trained nurses not in the labor force
56	RT01	F	deaths and retirements of general duty nurses
57	RT02	F	deaths and retirements of directors of nursing service
58	RT03	F	deaths and retirements of nursing supervisors
59	RT04	F	deaths and retirements of head nurses
60	RT05	F	deaths and retirements of office nurses
61	RT07	F	deaths and retirements of public health nurses
62	RT08	F	deaths and retirements of school nurses
63	RT09	F	deaths and retirements of nurse educators
64	RT10	F	deaths and retirements of industrial nurses
65	SK01	S	number of trained nurses, ages 20-24
66	SK02	S	number of trained nurses, ages 25-34
67	SK03	S	number of trained nurses, ages 35-44
68	SK04	S	number of trained nurses, ages 45-54
69	SK05	S	number of trained nurses, ages 55-64
70	SK06	S	number of trained nurses, ages 65-79
71	ST01	S	number of trained nurses, ages 21-25
72	ST02	S	number of trained nurses, ages 26-35

Number	Name	Form	Description
73	ST03	S	number of trained nurses, ages 36-45
74	ST04	S	number of trained nurses, ages 46-55
75	ST05	S	number of trained nurses, ages 56-65
76	ST06	S	number of trained nurses, ages 66-79
77	STOK	S	total number of trained nurses
78	TDES	S	total desired employment of nurses
79	TVSA	S	total number of actual vacancies
80	TVSE	S	total number of effective vacancies
81	TVSR	S	total number of reported vacancies
82	UNEM	S	number of unemployed nurses
83	VFE1	F	general duty nurse vacancies created during year
84	VFE2	F	director of nursing service vacancies created during year
85	VFE3	F	nurses supervisor vacancies created during year
86	VFE4	F	head nurse vacancies created during year
87	VFE5	F	office nurse vacancies created during year
88	VFE6	F	private duty nurse vacancies created during year
89	VFE7	F	public health nurse vacancies created during year
90	VFE8	F	school nurse vacancies created during year
91	VFE9	F	nurse educator vacancies created during year
92	VFE0	F	industrial nurse vacancies created during year
93	VRT1	O	equilibrium vacancy rate for general duty nurses
94	VRT2	O	equilibrium vacancy rate for directors of nursing service
95	VRT3	O	equilibrium vacancy rate for nurse supervisors
96	VRT4	O	equilibrium vacancy rate for head nurses
97	VSA1	S	total vacancies for general duty nurses
98	VSA2	S	total vacancies for directors of nursing service
99	VSA3	S	total vacancies for nurse supervisors
100	VSA4	S	total vacancies for head nurses

Number	Name	Form	Description
101	VSE1	S	effective vacancies for general nursing service
102	VSE2	S	effective vacancies for directors of nursing service
103	VSE3	S	effective vacancies for nurse supervisors
104	VSE4	S	effective vacancies for head nurses
105	VSE5	S	effective (total, reported) vacancies for office nurses
106	VSE6	S	effective (total, reported) vacancies for private duty nurses
107	VSE7	S	effective (total, reported) vacancies for public health nurses
108	VSE8	S	effective (total, reported) vacancies for school nurses
109	VSE9	S	effective (total, reported) vacancies for nurse educators
110	VSE0	S	effective (total, reported) vacancies for industrial nurses
111	VSR1	S	reported vacancies for general duty nurses
112	VSR2	S	reported vacancies for directors of nursing service
113	VSR3	S	reported vacancies for nurse supervisors
114	VSR4	S	reported vacancies for head nurses
115	VTR1	O	reported vacancy rate for general duty nurses
116	VTR2	O	reported vacancy rate for directors of nursing service
117	VRT3	O	reported vacancy rate for nurse supervisors
118	VTR4	O	reported vacancy rate for head nurses
119	VTR5	O	reported (total, effective) vacancy rate for private duty nurses
120	VTR6	O	reported (total, effective) vacancy rate for office nurses
121	VTR7	O	reported (total, effective) vacancy rate for public health nurses
122	VTR8	O	reported (total, effective) vacancy rate for school nurses
123	VTR9	O	reported (total, effective) vacancy rate for nurse educators
124	VTR0	O	reported (total, effective) vacancy rate for industrial nurses

125	WAGE	O	mean monthly wage of all nurses in current dollars
126	WG01	O	median monthly wage of general duty nurses in current dollars
127	WG02	O	median monthly wage of directors of nursing service in current dollars
128	WG03	O	median monthly wage of nurse supervisors in current dollars
129	WG04	O	median monthly wage of head nurses in current dollars
130	WG05	O	mean monthly wage of office nurses in current dollars
131	WG06	O	mean monthly wage of private duty nurses in current dollars

B.   Exogenous

Number	Name	Description
1	AVF1	median monthly wage of all females in current dollars
2	CENS	average daily patient census in nonfederal short-term general hospitals in the United States, in thousands
3	DUMX	residual adjustment dummy variable, 1947 = 1
4	DUMY	Korean war dummy variable, 1950 and 1951 = 1
5	DUMZ	medicare dummy variable, 1966 = 1
6	ENRL	total nursing school enrollment
7	ENRB	enrollments in four-year programs
8	GRDA	graduates of 2-year programs
9	GRDD	graduates of 3-year programs
10	GRDB	graduates of 4-year programs
11	MDIN	annual mean income of physicians, in thousands of current dollars
12	MDPP	number of nonfederal physicians in private practice
13	POPT	population of the U.S., in thousands
14	PRA1	index of daily hospital service charges, 1966 = 1.0
15	PRIC	Consumer Price Index, 1966 = 1.0
16	PUPE	number of elementary school pupils, in thousands
17	PUPS	number of secondary school pupils, in thousands
18	SLP1	slope of the general duty nurse supply curve
19	SLP2	slope of the directors of nursing service supply curve
20	SLP3	slope of the nurse supervisors supply curve

Number	Name	Description
21	SLP4	slope of the head nurses supply curve
22	SR01	survivor rate — age 21
23	SR02	survivor rate — age 22
24	SR03	survivor rate — age 23
25	SR04	survivor rate — age 24
26	SR05	survivor rate — age 25
27	SR06	survivor rate — age 26
28	SR07	survivor rate — age 27
29	SR08	survivor rate — age 28
30	SR09	survivor rate — age 29
31	SR10	survivor rate — age 30
32	SR11	survivor rate — age 31
33	SR12	survivor rate — age 32
34	SR13	survivor rate — age 33
35	SR14	survivor rate — age 34
36	SR15	survivor rate — age 35
37	SR16	survivor rate — age 36
38	SR17	survivor rate — age 37
39	SR18	survivor rate — age 38
40	SR19	survivor rate — age 39
41	SR20	survivor rate — age 40
42	SR21	survivor rate — age 41
43	SR22	survivor rate — age 42
44	SR23	survivor rate — age 43
45	SR24	survivor rate — age 44
46	SR25	survivor rate — age 45
47	SR26	survivor rate — age 46
48	SR27	survivor rate — age 47
49	SR28	survivor rate — age 48
50	SR29	survivor rate — age 49
51	SR30	survivor rate — age 50
52	SR31	survivor rate — age 51
53	SR32	survivor rate — age 52
54	SR33	survivor rate — age 53
55	SR34	survivor rate — age 54
56	SR35	survivor rate — age 55
57	SR36	survivor rate — age 56
58	SR37	survivor rate — age 57
59	SR38	survivor rate — age 58
60	SR39	survivor rate — age 59

Number	Name	Description
61	SR40	survivor rate — age 60
62	SR41	survivor rate — age 61
63	SR42	survivor rate — age 62
64	SR43	survivor rate — age 63
65	SR44	survivor rate — age 64
66	SR45	survivor rate — age 65
67	SR46	survivor rate — age 66
68	SR47	survivor rate — age 67
69	SR48	survivor rate — age 68
70	SR49	survivor rate — age 69
71	SR50	survivor rate — age 70
72	SR51	survivor rate — age 71
73	SR52	survivor rate — age 72
74	SR53	survivor rate — age 73
75	SR54	survivor rate — age 74
76	SR55	survivor rate — age 75
77	SR56	survivor rate — age 76
78	SR57	survivor rate — age 77
79	SR58	survivor rate — age 78
80	SR59	survivor rate — age 79
81	TCEN	average daily patient census in all hospitals, in thousands
82	VALU	value added of manufacturing in U.S., in millions of current dollars
83	WG07	median monthly wage of public health nurses in current dollars
84	WG08	median monthly wage of school nurses in current dollars
85	WG09	median monthly wage of nurse educators in current dollars
86	WG10	mean monthly wage of industrial nurses in current dollars
87	WHOL	wholesale price index, 1966 = 1.0

II. Equations

The model contains a total of 131 equations. Each is classified as either an identity or a behavioral equation. Part A contains the identities and Part B contains the behavioral equations. Each equation has a unique endogenous variable as a dependent variable. Therefore, equations in both Parts A and B are presented alphabetically according to their dependent variables. Each equation in each part is assigned a number to facilitate cross-referencing. In addition, the number appearing in parentheses in column I.A. is the number previously assigned to the dependent variable when it was defined in section I, Part A.

Many of the equations in Part B may appear at first glance to be identities rather than behavioral equations. However, these equations are true by assumption and are empirically refutable whereas identities are true by definition and are not empirically refutable. Parameters in these equations were assigned a priori.

Parameters in many other equations were also found through some analytical procedure or from a priori knowledge. The remaining parameters were determined via regression analysis. The latter are easily recognizable because their standard errors appear in parentheses below each coefficient. These coefficients (and standard errors) are shown rounded to the nearest four significant digits because this limitation was required by the algorithm when conducting simulation calculations. The coefficient of determination is reported for equations containing these parameters and the standard error of the estimate is reported in parentheses below the dependent variable. Unless otherwise indicated, all regressions were run on data for the period 1948 to 1966 using ordinary least squares. The data used for the regressions are presented in Deane and Yett (1979), Appendix B.

Finally, the equations presented below often employ summations for the sake of brevity. Since so many summations are used, the indices used in the summations have been standardized. The use of the index "i" is restricted to indicating the number of years lagged and ages, and can assume values of 01 to 59. For example, if $i = 10$, then $SRi = SR10$, which is the current survivor rate for those of age thirty ($i + 20$). By the same token, $GRAD_{-i} = GRAD_{-10}$, which is the graduating class ten years ago, the survivors of which are now of age 30 (assuming all graduates were age 20 at graduation). Therefore, when $i = 10$, $GRAD_{-i} \cdot SRi = GRAD_{-10} \cdot SR10 =$ the number of nurses graduating ten years ago who are currently living.

The index "j" is used to denote a particular field of nursing and may assume values of 01 to 10 or alternatively 0 to 9. For example when $j = 08$, $EMj = EM08 =$ employment in field 8 (school nursing). The last index, "k," is used to indicate the age cohort and may assume values from 01 to 06. For example, when $k = 03$, $PTk = PT03 =$ participation rate of nurses ages 35–44.

A. Identities

Number	I.A.	Equation		
1	(1)	CHNG	$\equiv$	$\mathrm{LBFS} - \mathrm{LBFS}_1$
2	(12)	DIES	$\equiv$	$\mathrm{STOK}_1 - \mathrm{STOK} + \mathrm{GRAD}$
3	(13)	EM01	$\equiv$	$\mathrm{DE01} - \mathrm{DE01} \cdot \mathrm{VRT1} - \mathrm{VSE1}$
4	(14)	EM02	$\equiv$	$\mathrm{DE02} - \mathrm{DE02} \cdot \mathrm{VRT2} - \mathrm{VSE2}$
5	(15)	EM03	$\equiv$	$\mathrm{DE03} - \mathrm{DE03} \cdot \mathrm{VRT3} - \mathrm{VSE3}$
6	(16)	EM04	$\equiv$	$\mathrm{DE04} - \mathrm{DE04} \cdot \mathrm{VRT4} - \mathrm{VSE4}$
7	(17)	EM05	$\equiv$	$\mathrm{DE05} - \mathrm{VSE5}$
8	(18)	EM06	$\equiv$	$\mathrm{DE06} - \mathrm{VSE6}$
9	(19)	EM07	$\equiv$	$\mathrm{DE07} - \mathrm{VSE7}$
10	(20)	EM08	$\equiv$	$\mathrm{DE08} - \mathrm{VSE8}$
11	(21)	EM09	$\equiv$	$\mathrm{DE09} - \mathrm{VSE9}$
12	(22)	EM10	$\equiv$	$\mathrm{DE10} - \mathrm{VSE0}$
13	(23)	EM00	$\equiv$	$\sum_{01}^{04} (\mathrm{EMj})$
14	(24)	EMPL	$\equiv$	$\sum_{01}^{10} (\mathrm{EMj})$
15	(36)	LBFS	$\equiv$	$\sum_{01}^{06} (\mathrm{PTk} \cdot \mathrm{SKk})$
16	(53)	QUIT	$\equiv$	$\sum_{01}^{10} (\mathrm{QTj})$
17[29]	(54)	RETR	$\equiv$	$\sum_{01}^{05} (\mathrm{RTj}) + \sum_{07}^{10} (\mathrm{RTj})$
18	(55)	RSRV	$\equiv$	$\mathrm{STOK} - \mathrm{LBFS}$
19	(65)	SK01	$\equiv$	$\sum_{01}^{10} (\mathrm{GRAD}_{-i} \cdot \mathrm{SRi}) + \mathrm{GRAD}$
20	(66)	SK02	$\equiv$	$\sum_{05}^{14} (\mathrm{GRAD}_{-i} \cdot \mathrm{SRi})$
21	(67)	SK03	$\equiv$	$\sum_{15}^{24} (\mathrm{GRAD}_{-i} \cdot \mathrm{SRi})$
22	(68)	SK04	$\equiv$	$\sum_{25}^{34} (\mathrm{GRAD}_{-i} \cdot \mathrm{SRi})$

44

Number	I.A.	Equation

23   (69) $SK05 \equiv \sum\limits_{35}^{59} (GRAD_i \cdot SRi)$

24   (70) $SK06 \equiv \sum\limits_{45}^{59} (GRAD_i \cdot SRi)$

25   (71) $ST01 \equiv \sum\limits_{01}^{05} (GRAD_i \cdot SRi)$

26   (72) $ST02 \equiv \sum\limits_{06}^{15} (GRAD_i \cdot SRi)$

27   (73) $ST03 \equiv \sum\limits_{16}^{25} (GRAD_i \cdot SRi)$

28   (74) $ST04 \equiv \sum\limits_{26}^{35} (GRAD_i \cdot SRi)$

29   (75) $ST05 \equiv \sum\limits_{36}^{45} (GRAD_i \cdot SRi)$

30   (76) $ST06 \equiv \sum\limits_{46}^{59} (GRAD_i \cdot SRi)$

31   (77) $ST01 \equiv \sum\limits_{01}^{06} (SKk)$

32   (78) $TDES \equiv \sum\limits_{01}^{10} (DEj)$

33   (79) $TVSA \equiv \sum\limits_{1}^{4} (VSAj) + \sum\limits_{5}^{9} (VSEj) + VSE0$

34   (80) $TVSE \equiv \sum\limits_{0}^{9} (VSEj)$

35   (81) $TVSR \equiv TVSE_1 + TVSA - TVSA_1$

36 [30]   (82) $UNEM \equiv LBSF - EMPL$ if $LBFS > EMPL$,

                                          0 Otherwise

37   (83) $VFE1 \equiv VSE1 + EM01 - VSE1_1 - EM01_1$
                      $+ QT01 + RT01$

38   (84) $VFE2 \equiv VSE2 + EM02 - VSE2_1 - EM02_1$
                      $+ QT02 + RT02$

39   (85) $VFE3 \equiv VSE3 + EM03 - VSE3_1 -$
                      $+ QT03 + RT03$

Number	I.A.	Equation	
40	(86)	VFE4 $\equiv$	VSE4 + EM04 $-$ VSE4$_1$ $-$ EM04$_1$ + QT04 + RT04
41	(87)	VFE5 $\equiv$	VSE5 + EM05 $-$ VSE5$_1$ $-$ EM05$_1$ + QT05 + RT05
42[3][1]	(88)	VFE6 $\equiv$	VSE6 + EM06 · VSE6$_1$
43	(89)	VFE7 $\equiv$	VSE7 + EM07 · VSE7$_1$ $-$ EM07$_1$ + QT07 + RT07
44	(90)	VFE8 $\equiv$	VSE8 + EM08 · VSE8$_1$ $-$ EM08$_1$ + QT08 + RT08
45	(91)	VFE9 $\equiv$	VSE9 + EM09 · VSE9$_1$ $-$ EM09$_1$ + QT09 + RT09
46	(92)	VFE0 $\equiv$	VSE0 + EM10 · VSE0$_1$ $-$ EM10$_1$ + QT10 + RT10
47	(97)	VSA1 $\equiv$	DE01 $-$ EM01
48	(98)	VSA2 $\equiv$	DE02 $-$ EM02
49	(99)	VSA3 $\equiv$	DE03 $-$ EM03
50	(100)	VSA4 $\equiv$	DE04 $-$ EM04
51	(101)	VSE1 $\equiv$	VSE1$_1$ + VFE1 $-$ HI01
52	(102)	VSE2 $\equiv$	VSE2$_1$ + VFE2 $-$ HI02
53	(103)	VSE3 $\equiv$	VSE3$_1$ + VFE3 $-$ HI03
54	(104)	VSE4 $\equiv$	VSE4$_1$ + VFE4 $-$ HI04
55	(105)	VSE5 $\equiv$	VSE5$_1$ + VFE5 $-$ HI05
56	(106)	VSE6 $\equiv$	VSE6$_1$ + VFE6 $-$ HI06
57	(107)	VSE7 $\equiv$	VSE7$_1$ + VFE7 $-$ HI07
58	(108)	VSE8 $\equiv$	VSE8$_1$ + VFE8 $-$ HI08
59	(109)	VSE9 $\equiv$	VSE9$_1$ + VFE9 $-$ HI09
60	(110)	VSE0 $\equiv$	VSE0$_1$ + VFE0 $-$ HI10
61	(115)	VTR1 $\equiv$	VSR1/(EM01 + VSR1)
62	(116)	VTR2 $\equiv$	VSR2/(EM02 + VSR2)
63	(117)	VTR3 $\equiv$	VSR3/(EM03 + VSR3)
64	(118)	VTR4 $\equiv$	VSR4/(EM04 + VSR4)
65	(119)	VTR5 $\equiv$	VSE5/(EM05 + VSE5)
66	(120)	VTR6 $\equiv$	VSE6/(EM06 + VSE6)
67	(121)	VTR7 $\equiv$	VSE7/(EM07 + VSE7)
68	(122)	VTR8 $\equiv$	VSE8/(EM08 + VSE8)
69	(123)	VTR9 $\equiv$	VSE9/(EM09 + VSE9)
70	(124)	VTR0 $\equiv$	VSE0/(EM10 + VSE0)
71	(125)	WAGE $\equiv$	$\sum_{01}^{10}$ (EMj · WGj)/EMPL

B. Behavioral Equations

Number	I.A.	Equation		
1^{32}	(2)	DE01 (5659)	$=$	$208700 - 33.62\,(WG01/PRA1) + 471.3\,CENS$ $(44210) \qquad\qquad\qquad\qquad (63.57)$ $- 620500\,VRT1 - 11950\,DUMZ$ $(85290) \qquad\qquad (7085)$	$R^2 = .9936$
2^{32}	(3)	DE02 (215.3)	$=$	$14520 - .9862\,(WG02/PRA1) + 21.96\,CENS$ $(2105) \qquad\qquad\qquad\qquad\ (2.739)$ $- 55760\,VRT2$ (6966)	$R^2 = .9959$
3^{32}	(4)	DE03 (810.4)	$=$	$64700 - 3.9\,(WG03/PRA1) + 12.56\,CENS$ $(6733) \qquad\qquad\qquad\qquad (8.978)$ $- 154500\,VRT3 - 1267\,DUMZ$ $(15510) \qquad\qquad (1034)$	$R^2 = .9885$
4^{32}	(5)	DE04 (1091)	$=$	$65970 - 8.251\,(WG04/PRA1) + 84.74\,CENS$ $(8487) \qquad\qquad\qquad\qquad (11.91)$ $- 151000\,VRT4 - 3584\,DUMZ$ $(15810) \qquad\qquad (1370)$	$R^2 = .9946$
5	(6)	DE05 (1720)	$=$	$24730 - 2166\,(WG05/MDIN) + .2929\,MDPP$ $(16076)\ (496.5) \qquad\qquad (.05645)$	$R^2 = .9460$
6	(7)	DE06 (2283)	$=$	$59701 - 276.9\,(WG06/PRIC) + 224.0\,CENS$ $(23058)\ (106.5) \qquad\qquad\ (76.13)$ $+ 104.4\,(TCEN\text{-}CENS) - 120600\,(VFE1/DE01)$ $(19.44) \qquad\qquad\qquad (39062)$	$R^2 = .6885$

Number	I.A.	Equation	
7	(8)	$DE07 = -5189 - 7.511\,(WG07/PRIC) + .0398\,POPT$ $(412.5)\ \ (2915)\ \ (8.845)\ \ (.03556)$ $+ 1.102\ DE07_{-1}$ $(.09535)$	$R^2 = .9870$
8	(9)	$DE08 = 202.6 - .0686\,(WG08 - WG08_{-1})$ $(213.7)\ \ (269.1)\ \ (10.47)$ $+ 1.023\ DE08_{-1} + .1254\,(PUPE - PUPE_{-1})$ $(.021) (.192)$ $+ .1164\,(PUPS - PUPS_{-1})$ $(.2514)$	$R^2 = .9964$
9	(10)	$DE09 = [.0161 + .9519\,(DE09_{-1}/ENRL)$ $(.0066)\ \ (.1075)$ $- .00011\ WG09 + .2506\,(ENRB/ENRL)]\cdot ENRL$ $(.00005) (.0987)$	$R^2 = .9808$
10	(11)	$DE10 = 2778 - 7.567\,(WG10/WHOL - WG10_{-1}/WHOL_{-1})$ $(958.8)\ (12.03)$ $+ .8541\ DE10_{-1}$ $(.05781)$ $+ 13.35\,(VALU/WHOL - VALU_{-1}/WHOL_{-1})$ (12.00)	$R^2 = .9433$
11	(25)	$GRAD = GRDA + GRDB + GRDD$	

For equations 12 through 21 the variable Z is [33]

$$Z = (.5\ UNEM_{-2} + .5\ UNEM_{-1} + QUIT + CHNG + RETR)/LBFS$$

Number	I.A.	Equation

12^{34} (26)

$$HI01 = 212.4 - 868.3\,(Z \cdot WG01/WAGE)$$
$$(.4881) \qquad (64.46)\ \ (248.7)$$
$$+\ 915.0\,(Z \cdot WG01/WAGE)^2 - 3.635\,(VFE1/VFE1_{-1})$$
$$(241.4) \hspace{5cm} (1.446)$$
$$+\ 2.236\ DUMY \cdot VSE1$$
$$(.4041)$$

$$R^2 = .9562$$

13^{34} (27)

$$HI02 = [167.3 - 635.4\ Z + 608.5\ Z^2$$
$$(.4867) \quad (74.66)\ \ (270.3)$$
$$+\ 1.177\,(VFE2/VFE2_{-1}) + 1.674\ DUMY] \cdot VSE2$$
$$(.5131) \hspace{4cm} (.3863)$$

$$R^2 = .8846$$

14^{34} (28)

$$HI03 = [147.7 - 564.7\ Z + 544.7\ Z^2$$
$$(.5529) \quad (80.95)\ \ (293.2) \qquad (265.2)$$
$$+\ .8004\,(VFE3/VFE3_{-1}) + 1.92\ DUMY] \cdot VSE3$$
$$(.3792) \hspace{4cm} (.4399)$$

$$R^2 = .8592$$

15^{34} (29)

$$HI04 = [158.7 - 601.2\ Z + 580\ Z^2$$
$$(.2904) \quad (43.28)\ \ (143.28) \quad (141.8)$$
$$-\ 1.16\,(VFE4/VFE4_{-1}) + 1.834\ DUMY] \cdot VSE4$$
$$(.4204) \hspace{4cm} (.2312)$$

$$R^2 = .9483$$

16^{34} (30)

$$HI05 = 556.4 - 2102\ Z + 2006\ Z^2$$
$$(1.124) \quad (162.4)\ \ (588.5) \qquad (522.9)$$
$$+\ 2.158\,(VFE5/VFE5_{-1})] \cdot VSE5$$
$$(1.591)$$

$$R^2 = .8647$$

Number	I.A.	Equation		

$17^{34,35}$ (31) $HI06 = [- 10.54 + 16.36\ Z + 3.111\ (WG06/WAGE)$
            $(.1876)$ $(5.936)\ (3.137)$ (6.616)
                       $+ 7082\ (VFE6/VFE6_{-1})]\ \cdot\ VSE6$
                         $(.5302)$ $R^2 = .7869$

18^{34} (32) $HI07 = [251.2 - 921.0\ (Z\ \cdot\ VFE7/VFE7_{-1})$
         (2.415) $(182.5)\ (643.4)$
                    $+ 863.0\ (Z\ \cdot\ VFE7/VFE7_{-1})^2\ \cdot\ VSE7$
                    (565.8) $R^2 = .4510$

$19^{34,36}$ (33) $HI08 = [- 997.9 + 3547\ Z - 3.31\ Z^2$
           (2.191) (692.4) (2548) (2345)
                    $+ 5.974\ (VFE8/VFE8_{-1})]\ \cdot\ VSE8$
                    (3.31) $R^2 = .6260$

20^{34} (34) $HI09 = [- 32.48 + 64.16\ Z]\ \cdot\ VSE9$
         $(.7697)$ (4.82) (8.776) $R^2 = .7587$

21^{34} (35) $HI10 = [131.6 - 555.0\ Z + 583.8\ . \ Z^2$
         (1.913) $(276.1)\ (1001)$ (906.0)
                    $+ .003145\ VFE0]\ \cdot\ VSE0$
                    $(.00107)$ $R^2 = .6226$

22 (37) $PT01 = - .1592 + .6391\ (WAGE/AVF1)$
       $(.01210)$ $(.08360)(.08073)$
                    $+ 2.122\ (SK01_{-1}\ \cdot\ PT01_{-1}/LBFS_{-1})$
                    $(.4415)$
                    $- 3.206\ (SK01/STOK)$
                    $(.2628)$ $R^2 = .9843$

291

Number	I.A.	Equation
23	(38)	$PT02 = .3984 + .0002816\ WAGE - .1151\ PT02_{-1}$ $(.00719)\quad (.1106)\ (.0001598)\qquad (.1798)$ $+ 1.742\ (SK02_{-2} \cdot PT02_{-1}/LBFS_1)$ $(.5551)$ $- 1.667\ (SK02/STOK)$ $(.2507)$ $R^2 = .9439$
24	(39)	$PT03 = .2635 + .0001042\ WAGE + .2796\ PT03_{-1}$ $(.008254)\quad (.1789)\ (.00006471)\qquad (.1468)$ $+ 1.642\ (SK03_{-1} \cdot PT03_{-1}/LBFS_1)$ $(.7438)$ $- 1.482\ (SK03/STOK)$ $(.336)$ $R^2 = .9723$
25	(40)	$PT04 = .4410 + .0003677\ WAGE - .1389\ PT04_{-1}$ $(.005007)\quad (.04884)\ (.00008171)\qquad (.1176)$ $+ 2.234\ (SK04_{-1} \cdot PT04_{-1}/LBFS_1)$ $(.2771)$ $- 2.249\ (SK04/STOK)$ $(.2417)$ $R^2 = .9931$
26	(41)	$PT05 = .2756 + .0005284\ (WAGE/PRIC - WAGE_{-1}PRIC_{-1})$ $(.007107)\quad (.1264)\ (.0002900)$ $+ .3989\ PT05_{-1} + 2.219\ (SK05_{-1} \cdot PT05_{-1}/LBFS_1)$ $(.2914)\qquad\quad (1.088)$ $- 2.167\ (SK05/STOK)$ $(.8533)$ $R^2 = .9489$

Number	I.A.	Equation
27	(42)	$PT06 = .4594 + .001166 \ (WAGE/PRIC - WAGE_{-1}/PRIC_{-1})$ $\quad\quad\quad (.003178) \quad (.0118) \quad (.0005382)$ $\quad\quad\quad - 3.293 \ (SK06/STOK)$ $\quad\quad\quad\quad (.2299)$ $R^2 = .9309$
28	(43)	$QT01 = .669 \ EM01_{-1}$
29	(44)	$QT02 = .215 \ EM02_{-1}$
30	(45)	$QT03 = .215 \ EM03_{-1}$
31	(46)	$QT04 = .215 \ EM04_{-1}$
32	(47)	$QT05 = .116 \ EM05_{-1}$
33	(48)	$QT06 = EM06_{-1}$
34	(49)	$QT07 = .263 \ EM07_{-1}$
35	(50)	$QT08 = .0564 \ EM08_{-1}$
36	(51)	$QT09 = .1015 \ EM09_{-1}$
37	(52)	$QT10 = .1246 \ EM10_{-1}$
38	(56)	$RT01 = \left[\sum_{01}^{06} (PTk_{-1} \cdot (SKk_{-1} - STk)) \right] \cdot EM01_{-1}/LBFS_{-1}$
39	(57)	$RT02 = \left[\sum_{01}^{06} (PTk_{-1} \cdot (SKk_{-1} - STk)) \right] \cdot EM02_{-1}/LBFS_{-1}$
40	(58)	$RT03 = \left[\sum_{01}^{06} (PTk_{-1} \cdot (SKk_{-1} - STk)) \right] \cdot EM03_{-1}/LBFS_{-1}$

Number	I.A.	Equation		
41	(59)	RT04	=	$[\sum_{01}^{06} (PTk_{-1} \cdot (SKk_{-1} - STk))] \cdot EM04_{-1}/LBFS_{-1}$
42	(60)	RT05	=	$[\sum_{01}^{06} (PTk_{-1} \cdot (SKk_{-1} - STk))] \cdot EM05_{-1}/LBFS_{-1}$
43	(61)	RT07	=	$[\sum_{01}^{06} (PTk_{-1} \cdot (SKk_{-1} - STk))] \cdot EM07_{-1}/LBFS_{-1}$
44	(62)	RT08	=	$[\sum_{01}^{06} (PTk_{-1} \cdot (SKk_{-1} - STk))] \cdot EM08_{-1}/LBFS_{-1}$
45	(63)	RT09	=	$[\sum_{01}^{06} (PTk_{-1} \cdot (SKk_{-1} - STk))] \cdot EM09_{-1}/LBFS_{-1}$
46	(64)	RT10	=	$[\sum_{01}^{06} (PTK_{-1} \cdot (SKk_{-1} - STk))] \cdot EM10_{-1}/LBFS_{-1}$
47	(93)	VRT1	=	$(SLP1 \cdot PRIC)/(.02974 \cdot PRA1 + SLP1 \cdot PRIC)$
48	(94)	VRT2	=	$(SLP2 \cdot PRIC)/(1.014 \cdot PRA1 + SLP2 \cdot PRIC)$
49	(95)	VRT3	=	$(SLP3 \cdot PRIC)/(.2564 \cdot PRAI + SLP3 \cdot PRIC)$
50	(96)	VRT4	=	$(SLP4 \cdot PRIC)/(.1212 \cdot PRA1 + SLP4 \cdot PRIC)$
51	(111)	VSR1	=	$VSE_{-1} + VSA1 - VSA1_{-1}$
52	(112)	VSR2	=	$VSE2_{-1} + VSA2 - VSA2_{-1}$
53	(113)	VSR3	=	$VSE3_{-1} + VSA3 - VSA3_{-1}$
54	(114)	VSR4	=	$VSE4_{-1} + VSA4 - VSA4_{-1}$

Number	I.A.	Equation		
55	(126)	WG01	=	$[360.5 + SLP1\,(EM01 + VSE1) - .002277\ LBFS] \cdot PRIC$
56	(127)	WG02	=	$[427.2 + SLP2\,(EM02 + VSE2) - .002902\ LBFS] \cdot PRIC$
57	(128)	WG03	=	$[356.9 + SLP3\,(EM03 + VSE3) - .002492\ LBFS] \cdot PRIC$
58	(129)	WG04	=	$[325.6 + SLP4\,(EM04 + VSE4) - .002267\ LBFS] \cdot PRIC$

$$WG05 = 274.6 + .6993 \sum_{01}^{04} (EMj \cdot WGj/EM00)$$

(7.868) (49.6) (.0412)

$$- 37180\ SLP1$$

(8642)

$$R^2 = .9873$$

$$WG06 = 60.96 + .9715\ WG01 - 10460\ SLP1$$

(4.20) (26.31) (.0233) (4580)

$$R^2 = .9971$$

FOOTNOTES

*This report summarizes results obtained using a preliminary version of our model. The final version is now in preparation and will be contained in our forthcoming book, *An Econometric Model of the Market for Nurses,* which will provide a detailed description of the development of the final model and its uses.

**The authors are, respectively, Vice President and Acting Director of the Division of Economic Analysis, Applied Management Sciences, Inc., Washington, D.C; and Director of the Human Resources Research Center and Professor of Economics, University of Southern California. The research described in this paper was supported in part by U.S. Public Health Service Grant NU000274 from the Division of Nursing of the Bureau of Health Manpower, U.S. Department of Health, Education, and Welfare. The authors wish to express their appreciation to Michael D. Intriligator, who reviewed an earlier version of the manuscript, and John S. Greenless, whose many contributions were critical to the completion of the project. The assistance of Brian McGaven, Leslie Michaels, and Thomas Nagle is also gratefully acknowledged.

1. For a detailed discussion of these complaints see Yett (1975) and for a brief summary see Yett (1970).

2. For summary and analysis of Federal nurse training subsidy programs, see Yett (1975), Chapters 1 and 5.

3. One of the few other econometric models of the nurse market capable of being simulated is Benham's three-equation model [Benham (1971)]. It has not yet been used for forecasting, but if it were, only total nurses, average participation (and therefore employed nurses), and median nurse income could be estimated by state. For a brief review of four of the most recent nurse models, see Deane and Ro (1978).

4. This section is condensed from more detailed presentations in Deane and Yett (1979), Yett (1970, 1975).

5. For evidence in support of the contention that hospitals tend to be monopsonistic or oligopsonistic nurse employees see Yett (1970), p. 100, Hurd (1973), pp. 237–39, and Link and Landon (1975), pp. 654–658. Recent reports [(Davis (1973), Ehrenberg (1974), Feldstein (1971), and Sloan and Richupan (1975)] indicate that earlier hospital monopsony and oligopsony wage policies may have been curtailed in the post-Medicare/Medicaid period. As Sloan explains, ". . . if RN wage costs are fully reimbursed (to take an extreme position) the change in the RN wage bill to the hospital per unit of labor hired would be zero . . . [eliminating incentives for monopsonistic employment practices]. Of course, RN wages are not fully reimbursed, but the incentive for monopsonistic behavior has become less nevertheless. . . . Judging from recent data on RN vacancies and employment. . . , hospital RN vacancy rates have been declining at the same time that hospital employment of RNs is rapidly expanding. These trends are consistent with a decrease in the importance of 'equilibrium vacancies' over time . . ." [Sloan (1975), p. 51].

6. Given the existence of "wage standardization" programs, a case could be made for collusive oligopsony in which all members of the association would act as *one monopsonistic buyer.* Under such an arrangement, however, wag changes would be *small* and rather *frequent,* whereas in an oligopsonistic market the wage changes are *large* and *infrequent.* Historically, nurse wage changes tend to support the latter interpretation.

7. See Altman (1971), p. 132, Benham (1971), p. 249, Bognanno (1969), p. 96, Hixson (1969), p. 34, and Yett (1965), p. 99. Other studies of interest are: Bognanno et al. (1974) which indicates, as does Yett (1965) that the nurse supply function is only inelastic but may be backwardbending at some point; and Bishop (1973), which reports, as does Altman (1971) that the elasticity of supply is higher—but still inelastic—for married as contrasted with single nurses; and Sloan and Richupan (1975), which contains some (possibly biased) regres-

sion estimates of high married, and low single, nurse elasticities (as well as weak support for the eventual backward bending segment of the curve).

8. Also see Sloan (1975) for data on nurse lifetime mobility patterns and future intentions.

9. The nurse job vacancies that are reported for hospitals are probably not the sum of equilibrium and effective vacancies. Most likely reported hospital vacancies are the sum of effective vacancies and the *change* in equilibrium vacancies. If a budgeted position continues to remain unfilled, the hospital administrator will probably eliminate it when preparing the *next* year's budget because he is likely to lose any funds he continues to allocate for positions he cannot fill. See Kehrer (1970) for supporting evidence to this effect.

10. It excludes nurses in the armed forces, nurse anesthetists, research nurses in hospitals, and nurse instructors in practical nursing programs. These fields represent less than 5 percent of all employed nurses.

11. The model represents an ''average'' local market in that the elasticity of the industry demand (and supply) curve is the weighted average of those in the local markets [Stigler (1966), p. 42], and the ratio of the slope of supply to that of the value of the marginal product (the inverse of the ratio of the elasticities at the point of intersection) is directly related to the degree of monopsony or oligopsony present in the market.

12. In the case of the hospital nurse fields, not only the change in the desired employment must be taken into consideration, but also the change in the equilibrium vacancy rate. This is to insure that only the change in *effective* vacancies is counted.

13. Total annual nursing school graduates (GRAD) is not behaviorally determined. It is the algebraic sum of exogenous graduations from the three types of basic training programs—Associate Degree (GRDA), Diploma (GRDD), and Baccalaureate (GRDB).

14. It is not necessarily the case that all the relationships expressed here as equations nor all of the variables in these equations appear in the final model.

15. Equation (1), which also contains CHNG, presents a somewhat similar problem in that DIES, all deaths from the total stock of living nurses, is subtracted from the stock of those *not* in the labor force (RSRV).

16. TVFE does not appear as a variable in the final model. It is equivalent, however, to:

$$\sum_{0}^{9} \text{VFEj}.$$

17. In the description of the model in the Appendix, the wages for certain fields of nursing are also exogenous.

18. Static equilibrium is the type of equilibrium contemplated in classical economic theory where the stock of effective vacancies is equal to zero. A concept of equilibrium more appropriate for the model being discussed is that of stochastic equilibrium in which the stock of effective vacancies and unemployment are constant, and the flows of hires is equal to the flow of total effective vacancies which, in turn, is equal to the sum of the flows of retirements, quits, and the change in the labor force. HIRE = TVFE = QUIT + RETR + CHNG.

19. Equilibrium vacancies can be further broken down into ''reported'' and ''not reported'' vacancies.

20. Since the equilibrium vacancy rate (TVRT) is defined as TVRT = TVSM/TDES where TVSM is the total stock of equilibrium vacancies, then TVSM = TVRT./TDES.

21. Since TDES = EMPL + TVSE + TVSM (see quation [24]) then TDES − TVSM = EMPL + TVSE.

22. Since the simultaneous block of equations was non-linear and large, solution of the block required the use of iterative convergence routines. Convergence was achieved by employing an extensively modified version of Program SIMULATE supplied by the Social Systems Research Institute (SSRI) of the University of Wisconsin. For a description of the original version see Holt (1965) pp. 637–59

23. For more detailed descriptions, see Deane and Yett (1979) Chapters 3 and 4.

24. This year was chosen for the following reasons: (1) it avoided the unique conditions existing during the immediate post-World War II and the Korean War years, and (2) since some of the policy actions to be introduced take up to ten years to fully implement, as long a period as possible was desired to allow the model to develop fully the implications of the policies. Like the historical tracking, the policy experiments were simulated to 1966.

25. Since unemployment is calculated as a residual between two relatively large numbers (i.e. nurse labor force and employment) it was expected that some negative values for unemployment would result.

26. The 1966 graduate figures employed to generate the 1966 simulation figure of Table 1 were obtained via a linear extrapolation for each program goal for 1965.

27. The exceptions were for nurse educators, school nurses and public health nurses which represent only about 2,000 vacancies out of the total.

28. Forecasts made using the preliminary version of the model for the historical period 1966–1969 were, for the most part, quite accurate. Further modifications are aimed primarily at achieving the same level of performance when the model is used to make longer range forecasts.

29. RETR does not include "retirements" from field 6, private duty nursing.

30. Since UNEM is calculated as the difference between two large numbers of approximately the same magnitude, small errors in either or both of these numbers can create sizable fluctuations in UNEM, and may even result in a negative number. Whenever the latter situation arose, UNEM was set to zero rather than allowing it to remain negative.

31. The equation of nursing field 6, private duty nursing, is different from the others because $QT06 = EM06_{-1}$, and RT06 is not calculated separately ("retirements" for field 6 are included in the estimate of QT06).

32. The regression was run on the variable $(DEj + aj + \frac{WGj}{PRAI})$ rather than DEj alone because the coefficient "aj" had been found previously by analytical methods; hence no standard error is shown under aj. (j = 1, 2, 3, 4.)

33. Since UNEM is a small number that is estimated as the difference between two large numbers (LBFS and EMPL), the estimate of UNEM is subject to large errors. In order to prevent such errors from creating explosive oscillatory behavior in the model, the mean of two successive estimates on UNEM is used.

34. The regression was run on the variable $\frac{HIj}{VSEj}$ rather than HIj as shown. (j = 1, 2, 3, . . . 9, 10 or 0.)

35. Observations for the years 1948 and 1954 were excluded from the regression.

36. Observations for the years 1948 to 1953 were excluded from the regression.

37. Observations for the year 1947 wre included in the regression.

REFERENCES

Altman, Stuart H. (November 1971), *Present and Future Supply of Nurses*, DHEW Publication Number (NIH), 72–134 Bethesda, Md.: Division of Nursing, Department of Health, Education, and Welfare.

Benham, Lee (August 1971), "The Labor Market for Registered Nurses: A Three-Equation Model," *Review of Economics and Statistics* LIII: 246–252.

Bishop, Christine E. (February 1973), "Manpower Policy and the Supply of Nurses," *Industrial Relations* XII: 86–94.

Bognanno, Mario F. (1969), "An Economic Study of the Hours of Labor Offered by the Registered Nurse," unpublished Ph.D. disseration, University of Iowa.

———, Hixson, J. S., and Jeffers, J. R. (Winter 1974), "The Short-run Supply of Nurse's Time," *Journal of Human Resources* IX: 80–94.

Davis, Karen (Spring 1973), "Theories of Hospital Inflation: Some Empirical Evidence," *Journal of Human Resources* VIII: 181–201.

Deane, Robert T. and Yett, Donald E. (1979), *An Econometric Model of the Market for Nurses,* forthcoming.

———, and Ro, Kong-Kyun (1978), *Comparative Analysis of Four Manpower Requirements Models Developed by the Division of Nursing.* Final Report on Contract No. 231-77-0062 for the Division of Nursing, Bureau of Health Manpower.

Ehrenberg, Ronald G. (Winter 1974), "Organizational Control and the Economic Efficiency of Hospitals: The Production of Nursing Services," *Journal of Human Resources,* IX; 21–32.

Feldstein, Martin S. (1971), *The Rising Cost of Hospital Care.* Washington, D.C.: Information Resources Press.

Hixson, Jessie S. (1969), "The Demand and Supply of Professional Hospital Nurses: Intra-Hospital Resource Allocation," unpublished Ph.D. dissertation, Michigan State University.

Holt, Charles C. (1970), "Job Search, Phillips' Wage Relation, and Union Influence: Theory and Evidence," *Microeconomic Foundations of Employment and Inflation Theory,* Edmund S. Phelps (ed.), New York: W. W. Norton.

———, Charles C. (1965), "Validation and Application of Macroeconomic Models Using Computer Simulation," in *The Brookings Quarterly Economic Model of the United States,* James S. Duesenberry, Gary Fromm, Laurence R. Klein, and Edwin Huh, (eds.), Chicago: Rand McNally.

———, and David, Martin H. (1966), "The Concept of Job Vacancies in a Dynamic Theory of the Labor Market," in *The Measurement and Interpretation of Job Vacancies,* Robert Ferber (ed.). New York: National Bureau of Economic Research.

Hurd, Richard W. (May 1973), "Equilibrium Vacancies in a Labor Market Dominated by Non-Profit Firms: The 'Shortage' of Nurses," *Review of Economics and Statistics,* LV: 234–240.

Kehrer, Barbara F. (1970), "The Nursing Shortage and Public Policy: an Economic Analysis of the Demand for Hospital Nurses in Connecticut," unpublished Ph.D. dissertation, Yale University.

Link, Charles R., and Landon, John H. (April 1975), "Monopsony and Union Power in the Market for Nurses," *Southern Economic Journal* XLI: 649–659.

"Medicare's Economic Impact on Doctors" (July 24, 1967), (a symposium), *Medical Economics* XLIV: 102–131.

Payne, Richard D. (1970), "An Economic Analysis of Nurse Mobility Patterns," unpublished Ph.D. dissertation, University of Southern California.

——— and Yett, Donald E. (1971), "A Pilot Study of Nurse Mobility Patterns," final report on U.S. Public Health Service Grant NU 00328, Los Angeles: Human Resources Research Center, University of Southern California (processed).

Sloan, Frank A. (May 1975), *The Geographic Distribution of Nurses and Public Policy,* DHEW Publication No. (HRA) 75-53, Bethesda, Md.: Division of Nursing, Health Resources Administration, Department of Health, Education and Welfare.

———, and Richupan, Somchai (Spring 1975), "Short-Run Supply Responses of Professional Nurses: A Microanalysis," *Journal of Human Resources* X: 241–257.

Stigler, George J. (1966), *The Theory of Price,* 3rd. ed., New York: Macmillan.

Surgeon Generals' Consultant Group on Nursing (1963), *Toward Quality in Nursing: Needs and Goals,* Public Health Service Publication No. 992, Washington, D.C.: Government Printing Office.

Witkin, Erwin (September 1968), "Medicare and the Future of Health Services," *Journal of the American Geriatrics Society* XVI: 999–1004.

Yett, Donald E. (1975), *An Economic Analysis of the Nurse Shortage*, Lexington, Mass.: D. C. Heath.

———— (March 1970), "Causes and Consequences of Salary Differentials in Nursing," *Inquiry* VII 76– 101.

———— (1970), "The Chronic 'Shortage' of Nurses: A Public Policy Dilemma." *Empirical Studies in Health Economics*, Herbert Klarman (ed.). Baltimore: Johns Hopkins Press, 1970.

———— (February 1965), "The Supply of Nurses: An Economist's View," *Hospital Progress* XLVI 88– 102.

HEALTH STATUS MAXIMIZATION AND MANPOWER ALLOCATION*

Joseph Lipscomb, DUKE UNIVERSITY

Lawrence E. Berg, Virginia L. London, Paul A.

Nutting, INDIAN HEALTH SERVICE, TUCSON, ARIZONA

ABSTRACT

A production function for health services is introduced in which output—defined as expected improvement in population health status—is related explicitly to alternative allocations of real resources among competing disease programs. The production function is in the form of a mathematical program. whose objective function, technology matrix, and right-hand-side resource constraint parameters may be viewed, respectively, as the *outcome, process,* and *structural* elements of health-care delivery. Operationally, the model determines that allocation of labor inputs which results in the greatest aggregate (population-wide) expected improvement in health status; the latter

Research in Health Economics, Vol. 1, pp 301–401.
Copyright © 1979 by JAI Press, Inc.
All rights of reproduction in any form reserved.
ISBN 0-89232-042-7.

concept is defined in the sense of Bush (1975), except that here the disease process is modeled in a semi-Markovian framework. The authors have implemented the model on an experimental basis for two infant diseases, gastroenteritis and respiratory infections, that are highly prevalent among Indians in Arizona.

I INTRODUCTION

Consider the plight of a developing nation or territory where disease prevalence is high but the market for modern medical care is virtually nonexistent. If a ruling government, vested with the authority to designate and provide merit (public) goods, determines that the status quo is unacceptable, it must face some major normative and practical questions:

How much should be budgeted for health care overall?

What are the short-run and long-run supply characteristics of key inputs, particularly providers such as physicians and nurses?

Given expenditure and supply constraints, how can resources be allocated most efficiently, in two senses:

(1) choosing that mix and distribution of medical care goods and services which will lead to maximum social welfare, defined in some fashion; and

(2) for each good or service, using the cost-minimizing combination of inputs which meets minimum technical process standards of quality?

The purpose of this paper is to examine this third major issue, efficiency, by focusing on health-care resource allocation on an American Indian Reservation. The empirical results will consist of prescriptions for how certain health manpower should be employed to maximize expected improvement in population health status, the operational welfare criterion defined for the analysis. These findings are derived from a production function for health status, structured as a mathematical program whose allocation decisions reflect:

(a) the population's stated preferences for alternative levels of physical, social, and emotional functioning, i.e., for "states" of health;

(b) the expected efficacy of alternative disease treatment programs;

(c) the relative efficiency of alternative input combinations for producing each medical good or service; and

(d) ceilings on the absolute supply of certain inputs.

This paper does not deal with the important issues of determining the size of the health portion of a given public goods budget [see, for example, Musgrave (1959)]. Nor does it treat the more immediate problem of manpower supply planning in a (labor) market or nonmarket context [see, for example, Reinhardt (1975), and P. Feldstein (1973)]. We do inject these issues, if only briefly, to put the following analysis in perspective; in particular, we will proceed within a short-run framework where the size of the health budget (implicitly) and the supplies of key inputs (explicitly) are treated as fixed over an arbitrary period t.

These two global matters aside, much remains for analysis, as indicated in items (a)–(d) above. The major practical tasks involve determining the technical relationships among inputs and outputs and the impact on health status of various preventive and curative interventions. Perhaps the major conceptual challenge is securing a medical care product mix that is in accordance with population preferences, which, by assumption, cannot (at this point, at least) be registered in a marketplace or other naturally emerging public forum. The related issues here are numerous, and we note for now two crucial ones:

(1) Preferences for what? If medical care is regarded as an input into the production of the commodity health (1972), then the states of health rather than the services rendered become the final objects of choice. This view is somewhat analogous to Lancaster's (1976) notion that the attributes of a good, rather than the good per se, are the relevant choice variables in a model of utility maximization. But Lancaster's theory is positivistic and focuses on the individual, while our concern is one of public choice.

(2) How shall these preferences be brought to bear in the allocation decision process? In the classic spirit of representative democracy, the government's legislative or executive branches could be authorized to make specific allocation decisions. Or consumer planning councils could be imbued by law with the partial or sole authority for decision making. But the treatment of *individual* preferences is intentionally left unspecified in these traditional procedures, which amount to allocation by representation. Are there alternative mechanisms for supplying planners with information on preferences so that decisions can be based on an *explicit* aggregation of these? Then, in principle, one could test the sensitivity of "optimal" allocation both to assumed shifts in individual preferences and to the method of aggregation itself.

The theoretical framework for our analysis of these efficiency issues has its foundation in Fanshel and Bush (1970), Chen et al. (1975), Bush et al. (1972, 1973), and to some extent Torrance et al. (1973, 1976). Health status is defined in terms of expected population movement through non-disease-specific "function levels," which are assigned relative value weights on the basis of sampled population preferences, aggregated in some explicit fashion. Each disease is decomposed into clinical stages. Each stage is associated with a corresponding function level and is assigned the preference weight given that level by the population. The effectiveness of a particular health program is then gauged by its likely impact on the expected health state occupancy pattern of the target population, relative to a status quo pattern assumed to result were the program not instituted. In this paper the objective function will be given a new, semi-Markovian interpretation, which establishes a direct and natural correspondence between estimable model parameters and the traditional epidemiologic components of disease prevalence. Also, the constraint set here is structured for the allocation of physical resources rather than a budget. The result is that the specificity of resource allocation recommendations is increased, but at the expense of requiring much data linking medical care process to outcome.

The empirical work reported here is based on a Department of Health, Education, and Welfare study initiated jointly by the National Center for Health Services Research (NCHSR) and the Indian Health Service (IHS) in 1974. The first, and perhaps most important, purpose of that 15-month interagency effort was to establish an evaluation mechanism for assisting tribal health leaders and the IHS in determining how available health-care resources—particularly professional and para-professional providers—can be utilized to minimize the morbidity and mortality impacts of major acute and chronic problems. Most of this paper is devoted to developing some practical answers to that very practical question. Assisting the IHS's Office of Research and Development (ORD) in this effort was the Papago Indian tribe of Arizona.

The narrow the issues, we focus on two particular acute diseases in the Papago population, infant gastroenteritis and infant respiratory infections. Further, while our resource allocation models will deal explicitly with several categories of providers, the focus will be on the tribal outreach worker. These Community Health Representatives (CHR's) and Nutrition Aides (NA's) are vital components in the Papago health system. Consequently, it is important to examine the relationship between alternative assignments for these providers and population health status. In general, the kinds of data required for this analysis have not been available for large population groups. Health program impact information has usually been obtained either through adaptation of certain epidemiologic models from the clinical medicine literature [Torrance (1976)] or by the aggregation of expert medical opinion [Bush and Palreck (1973)]; expert judgment was employed where necessary in this study, as well.

In the next section the resource allocation model is introduced formally. For clarity in presentation, the parameters of the model are given in their most basic form. However, to make the best use of the epidemiologic and resource costs data available on the Papago tribe, it was necessary to refine, and sometimes complicate, these parameter specifications. Section III summarizes these refinements, which are described in more detail in Appendices A–D. The results of the analysis are in section (IV). Some extensions of the methodology are considered in the concluding section.

II SPECIFICATION OF A RESOURCE ALLOCATION MODEL[1]

(a) Desirable Properties

We believe that the health status-oriented allocation models of Bush et al. (1972, 1973), Chen et al. (1975) and Torrance *et al* (1973, 1976) represent significant advancements in the methodology of health program evaluation. In particular, they are designed to take explicit account of consumer preferences in allocating a given budget across programs to maximize health status improvement. Setting the allocation problem in an optimization context is important, for it forces budgetary decisions to be goal-directed.[2] Since our specific focus will be on the allocation of physical resources among disease programs, the model here must be structured to accomodate certain accompanying empirical complexities which have been naturally of lesser concern to these writers:

As noted earlier, the model must incorporate information on the processes of medical care. These processes must be linked simultaneously with the structure of care (the distribution of available inputs) and the outcome of care as summarized by a health status measure.

Information will be required on the types of resources potentially able to meet the health needs of a target population; the effective availability of each resource; alternative intervention strategies at each clinically-defined stage of each disease at which programs might be directed; the amount of each resource required to undertake each alternative intervention strategy; and the expected impact of each strategy on the health status of each sub-population (module) in the target population.

Like Chen et al. (1975) and Bush et al. (1973), we seek a delineation of the target population into modules, such that each is relatively homogeneous with respect to transitions among disease stages and durations of stay in stages. One might ideally define a module as a subpopulation whose members are at approximately the same *risk* to a particular disease. Individuals would be assigned to risk levels on the basis of certain predisposing characteristics (e.g., weight, age, sex) which have been linked with disease prevalence.

The resource-drain from non-intervention should be explicitly accounted for. Thus, for a given module one might have choices among interventions A, B, C—or not intervening at all. But the latter decision, to consign the module to the status quo, represents an intervention in one important sense: these module members will be consuming health care resources over time, perhaps eventually at a faster rate than would have been the case with early intervention. This, in time, would have the effect of shrinking the size and shape of the resource pool which supports the "active" interventions A, B, and C.

It may be particularly true with acute diseases, such as infant gastroenteritis and respiratory infections, that prevalence patterns are seasonal.
Since changes in expected prevalence within a module directly influence
the optimal set of intervention strategies and their associated resource
requirements, the model should acknowledge cyclical variations in those
epidemiologic parameters likely to be affected.

(b)   A New Discrete-Time Semi-Markov Resource Allocation Model

Unlike the formulation of Torrance et al. (1973, 1976), the resource
allocation model introduced below will have an explicit stochastic structure; and departing from the models of Bush et al. (1973), this structure
will be semi-Markovian rather than pure Markovian in thrust. The motiva-
tion for this departure is that a pattern of disease prevalence typically
involves not only transitions among states, but stays of *variable duration*
in each state. Because (in contrast to a pure Markovian model) a semi-
Markovian model treats these durations as random variables, it is a
natural framework for epidemiological analysis. However, there have
been comparatively few applications of semi-Markovian concepts to
health services delivery problems [for an excellent exception, see Kao
(1972)].

As a prelude to the resource allocation framework, a discrete-time
semi-Markovian model of disease prevalence will be developed. It will be
shown that, in the limit, the expected value of prevalence so defined is
equal to the product of the means of two random variables corresponding,
respectively, to incidence and duration-of-episode.

Let p_{ij} be the probability that a semi-Markov process which entered
state i on its last transition will enter j on its next transition; $p_{ij} \geq 0$ and
$\sum_{j=1}^{N} p_{ij} = 1$, for i, j = 1, . . . , N, where N is the number of states in the
model. These transition probabilities are, in fact, those of the Markov
process that is "imbedded" in the more general semi-Markovian formulation; see Howard (1971). One way to conceptualize a semi-Markov process
to imagine that after the process enters state i, it determines its next state
j according to the p_{ij}. Then, conditional on the choice of j, the process
holds in i for a time τ_{ij}. These holdings times are positive, integer-valued
random variables with densities $h_{ij}(s) = P(\tau_{ij} = s)$, for s = 1, 2, . . . , and for
all i and j. It is assumed that all holding time means, $\bar{\tau}_{ij} = \sum_{s=1}^{N} s\, h_{ij}(s)$, are
finite and that each holding time is at least one time unit in length so that
$h_{ij}(0) = 0$. In applications one can assign this fundamental time unit any
desired value. In his presentation, Howard also makes a distinction between *real* transitions (from state i to another state j) and *virtual* transi-

tions (from i to itself). However, there will be no advantage in maintaining this distinction here, and the exposition is simplified considerably by regarding all transitions as real. Thus, define

$$p_{ii} = \begin{cases} 0, \text{ if i is transient} \\ 1, \text{ if i is trapping (absorbing).} \end{cases}$$

To develop an expression for the prevalence of a health state over some finite period t, define

$$x_{ij}(n) = \begin{cases} 1, \text{ if the individual is in state j at time n, given that} \\ \quad \text{he entered i at time zero} \\ 0, \text{ otherwise.} \end{cases}$$

Then, following Howard (1971), the individual's total time in j over t, given an entry to i at time zero, is

$$pp_{ij}(t) = \sum_{n=0}^{t} x_{ij}(n),$$

where the pp notation indicates period prevalence for the individual. The expected value of this random variable is $\overline{pp}_{ij}(t) = \sum_{n=0}^{t} x_{ij}(n)$. But since $x_{ij}(n)$ is either zero or unity, $\overline{x}_{ij}(n) = \phi_{ij}(n)$, the so-called "interval transition probability" of *being in* state j at time n, given an entry into i at time zero. Thus, $pp_{ij}(t) = \sum_{n=0}^{t} \phi_{ij}(n)$. This definition of period prevalence corresponds to what Kao (1972) termed "time in recovery state" in his semi-Markovian model for predicting the recovery progress of coronary patients. From Kao, it is clear that the variance of $pp_{ij}(t)$ is $pp_{ij}(t) = \overline{pp}_{ij}(t)$ $(2\,\overline{pp}_{ij}(t) - 1 - \overline{pp}_{ij}(t))$.

Now each $\phi_{ij}(n)$ is a function of all the transition probabilities and holding time distributions, so that knowledge (or estimates) or these permits one to calculate (or estimate) pp_{ij} (t). For purposes here, the most useful expression for this interval transition probability is

$$\phi_{ij}(n) = \sum_{m=0}^{n} e_{ij}(m)\,{}^{>}w_{ij}(n-m),$$

where $e_{ij}(m)$ is the probability that an individual will enter state j at time m, given that he entered state i at time zero; and

$$^{>}w_j(n-m) = \sum_{r=n-m+1}^{\infty} \sum_{k=1}^{N} p_{jk} h_{jk}(r) = P(\tau_j > n - m),$$

the probability that the "waiting" time in j before the next transition is greater than $(n - m)$ time units. The semi-Markovian "entrance" probabilities [25] above can be determined from the recursive equation,

$$e_{ij}(m) = \delta_{ij}\, \delta(m) + \sum_{s=1}^{N} \sum_{q=0}^{m} p_{ih}\, h_{is}(q)\, e_{sj}(m - q), \text{ where } \delta_{ij} = \begin{cases} 1, \text{ if } i = j \\ 0, \text{ otherwise} \end{cases}$$

$$\delta(m) = \begin{cases} \text{and } 1, \text{ if } m = 0 \\ 0, \text{ otherwise.} \end{cases}$$

Then, by substitution, the expression for expected prevalence becomes

$$\overline{pp}_{ij}(t) = \sum_{n=0}^{t} \sum_{m=0}^{n} e_{ij}(m) \, {}^{>}w_j\, (n - m).$$

If i, the state of entry at period zero, is known with certainty, the above expression represents simply the expected prevalence of j over period t. Otherwise, the expected prevalence of j must reflect the fact that each i attains with only some probability at time zero. Kao (1972) handled this problem by employing data in which the probability of *being in* each coronary recovery state at the moment of hospital admission was assumed known. In essence, the patient's recovery progress was regarded as being governed by a semi-Markov process that went into effect, so to speak, only after his entry into the hospital.

In a more general view of disease prevalence, however, an individual's disease state occupancy pattern would be assumed to be governed continuously by a semi-Markov process. However, this poses a fundamental difficulty in calculating expected prevalence starting from some arbitrarily (randomly) chosen point in time. As Howard (1971) notes, the probability that the individual will be in i at this randomly chosen moment is ϕ_i, the limiting interval transition probability for state i. However, if the individual is found to be i, it is not likely, of course, that he has just entered i; rather, we must allow for the overwhelming likelihood that we have observed the individual in the midst of a holding time. (It should be noted though that since a discrete time process is assumed, the time remaining in the randomly entered state will be integer.) Consequently, both the probability that the next transition will be to j and the *remaining* holding time before that next transition will not be governed by the p_{ij} and $h_{ij}(m)$ defined earlier. Rather, they will be described by elements of the form (to use Howard's notation) $_rp_{ij}$ and $_rh_{ij}(m)$, which acknowledge the random manner in which the period of length t is initiated. Fortunately, as Howard shows, these latter quantities can be derived from the basic set of transition probabilities and holding time distributions:

$_r p_{ij} = p_{ij} \bar{\tau}_{ij} / \bar{\tau}_i =$ the probability that an individual observed in state i at a random moment will make his next transition to j,

$_r h_{ij}(m) = \sum\limits_{s=m}^{\infty} h_{ij}(s) / \bar{\tau}_{ij} = {}^> h_{ij}(m-1) / \bar{\tau}_{ij} =$ the probability that an individual observed in state i at a random moment will remain there m more time units, given that his next transition is to j.

Consequently, we can introduce the following expression for the expected prevalence of state j over a period of length t whose starting point is randomly selected:

$$_r p p_j(t) = \sum_{i=1}^{N} \phi_i \sum_{k=1}^{N} \sum_{m=0}^{t} {}_r p_{ik} \; {}_r h_{ik}(m) \left[\delta_{ij}.m + \sum_{n=0}^{t-m} \sum_{s=0}^{n} e_{kj}(s) \; {}^> w_j(n-s) \right],$$

where $\delta_{ij} = \begin{cases} 1, \text{ if } i = j \\ 0, \text{ otherwise.} \end{cases}$

This formulation acknowledges that (1) without further information, the state occupied at the randomly selected starting moment will be i with probability ϕ_i; (2) the probability that the next transition will be made m time units later to state k is $_r p_{ik} \cdot {}_r h_{ik}(m)$; (3) if $i = j$, the time before the first observable transition is included in the prevalence of j over t (thus the role of $\delta_{ij}.m$); and (4) after the first transition, the portion of the interval t remaining for analysis is $t - m$.

Alternatively, if one is interested in the expected prevalence of j over a period t which begins with the first transition after the random entry, one can write:

$$\overline{p p}_j(t) = \sum_{i=1}^{N} \phi_i \sum_{k=1}^{N} \sum_{m=0}^{\infty} {}_r p_{ik} \; {}_r h_{ik}(m) \left[\sum_{n=0}^{t} \sum_{s=0}^{n} e_{kj}(s) \; {}^> w_j(n-s) \right],$$

$$= \sum_{i=1}^{N} \phi_i \sum_{k=1}^{N} {}_r p_{ik} \left[\sum_{n=0}^{t} \sum_{s=0}^{n} e_{kj}(s) \; {}^> w_j(n-s) \right],$$

$$\text{since } \sum_{m=0}^{\infty} {}_r h_{ik}(m) = \sum_{m=0}^{\infty} {}^> h_{ij}(m-1) / \bar{\tau}_{ij} = \bar{\tau}_{ij} / \bar{\tau}_{ij} = 1,$$

by virtue of a well-known property of integral-valued random variables (see, for example, Feller (1968), pp. 264–266). This expression for period prevalence assumes that the interval of length t is initiated upon the first exit from the initial entry state i. As will be seen now, it permits one to derive a compact and intuitively appealing reformulation of the expected prevalence of state j over t as the product of the expected incidence of j over t and the expected duration-of-stay in j per entry.

$$\text{Let } y_{ij}(n) = \begin{cases} 1, \text{ if the individual enters state j at time n, given that he} \\ \quad \text{entered i at time zero} \\ 0, \text{ otherwise.} \end{cases}$$

Define $v_{ij}(t) = \sum_{m=0}^{t} y_{ij}(m)$, the number entries by the individual into j over t, given that he entered i at time zero. Then the mean of this random variable is $\bar{v}_{ij}(t) = \sum_{m=0}^{t} \bar{y}_{ij}(m) = \sum_{m=0}^{t} e_{ij}(m)$, where $e_{ij}(m)$ is the individual's probability of entering j at time m, given that he entered i at time zero. Next, rewrite $\overline{pp}_j(t)$ successively as:

$$\overline{pp}_j(t) = \sum_{i=1}^{N} \phi_i \sum_{k=1}^{N} {}_r p_{ik} \left[\sum_{s=0}^{t} e_{kj}(s) \sum_{n=s}^{t} {}^> w_j(n - s) \right]$$

$$= \sum_{i=1}^{N} \phi_i \sum_{k=1}^{N} {}_r p_{ik} \left[\sum_{s=0}^{T} e_{kj}(s) \sum_{n=0}^{t-s} {}^> w_j(n) \right].$$

Now if $t = \infty$, the expression becomes:

$$\overline{pp}_j(\infty) = \sum_{i=1}^{N} \phi_i \sum_{k=1}^{N} {}_r p_{ik} \; \bar{v}_{kj}(\infty) . \bar{\tau}_j,$$

since $\sum_{\substack{n=0 \\ (t \to \infty)}}^{t-s} {}^> w_j(n)$ converges to the mean of the random variable τ_j (Feller, (1968). For compactness, write $\bar{v}_j(t) = \sum_{i=1}^{N} \phi_i \sum_{k=1}^{N} {}_r p_{ik} \; \bar{v}_{kj}(t)$, the expected number of entries by an individual into state j over a period of length t which begins with the first transition following a randomly chosen moment. Then

$$\overline{pp}_j(\infty) = \bar{v}_j(\infty) \cdot \bar{\tau}_j.$$

This implies that the expected prevalence of state j over an unbounded horizon is equal to the product of the expected number of entries into j (the "incidence" of j) and the mean holding time in j (the "duration-of-stay" in j).[3] For finite t, the expression for expected prevalence becomes,

$$\overline{pp}_j(t) \doteq \bar{v}_j(t) \cdot \bar{\tau}_j,$$

since $\sum_{n=0}^{t-s} {}^> w_j(n) \doteq \bar{\tau}_j.$

Assuming that the disease process is, in fact, semi-Markovian, the results above imply:

For any t, one can forecast period prevalence (as defined by $\overline{pp}_j(t)$) by first obtaining estimates of all transition probabilities and holding time distributions and then employing the general formula above for $\overline{pp}_j(t)$.

If one is able to obtain (say, by experimental means) distinct, consistent estimates of the expected incidence of j and the expected duration-of-episode of j, one is justified in asymptotically treating the product of these two estimates as a consistent estimate of the expected prevalence of j. For large t, the product of these consistent estimates will approximate the expected prevalence of j over t (as defined by $\overline{pp}_j(t)$).

Note that this latter result does not merely imply that prevalence is equal to the product of incidence and duration—this identity must prevail *ex post* regardless of the assumed stochastic structure of prevalence. Rather, it specifies conditions under which one may forecast prevalence *(ex ante)* on the basis of available empirical evidence.

We turn finally to the resource allocation model itself. In the experimental application of the model described in the next two sections, prevalence is determined on the basis of separately estimated incidence and duration-of-episode parameters. Consequently, we will state prevalence in terms of these parameters in the model below. For a more suggestive notation, let $\overline{v}_j(t) \equiv \overline{TR}_j(t)$, the expected *transition rate* of the individual into state j over a period of length t; and let $\overline{\tau}_j \equiv \overline{D}_j$, the expected duration-of-stay per entry into j. Letting t be large, we now state the objective function and constraint set of the health resource allocation model:

$$\text{maximize } \Delta H(t) = \sum_{d=1}^{D} \sum_{m=1}^{M} \sum_{i=0}^{S_d} \left[\sum_{j=1}^{N} U_j \left(\overline{TR}_{jm}^{d_0}(t) \cdot \overline{D}_{jm}^{d_0} - \overline{TR}_{jm}^{d_i}(t) \cdot \overline{D}_{jm}^{d_i} \right) \right] P_m^{d_i} X_m^{d_i}$$

$$\text{subject to } \sum_{d=1}^{D} \sum_{m=1}^{M} \sum_{i=0}^{S_d} A_{mp}^{d_i}(t) X_m^{d_i} \leq R_p(t), \text{ for } p = 1, \ldots, Q;$$

$$\sum_{i=0}^{S_d} X_m^{d_i} = 1, \text{ for } m = 1, \ldots, M$$
$$d = 1, \ldots, D; \text{ and}$$

$$X_m^{d_i} \geq 0, \text{ for } i = 0, \ldots, S_d$$
$$d = 1, \ldots, D,$$
$$m = 1, \ldots, M \text{ where}$$

U_j = the consumer-provided preference, or utility weight for state j,

$\overline{TR}_{jm}^{d_i}(t)$ = the expected number of times a typical member of module m will enter (via a real transition) the stages of disease d associated with health state j over the interval t, given that intervention strategy i against disease d is implemented,

$\overline{TR}_{jm}^{d_0}(t)$ = the special case of $\overline{TR}_{jm}^{d_i}(t)$ when no special intervention strategy (i = 0) is implemented and the status quo is assumed.

t = the time duration over which the semi-Markov process is observed (and over which the strategies are being evaluated),

$\overline{D}_{jm}^{d_i}$ = the expected duration of stay per real transition to the disease d stage associated with state j for a typical member of module m, given that intervention strategy i against disease d is implemented,

$\overline{D}_{jm}^{d_o}$ = the special case of $\overline{D}_{jm}^{d_i}$ when the status quo (i = 0) is assumed,

P_m^d = the size of that population at risk to disease d in module m which, in addition, can *potentially* be affected by intervention strategy i,

$A_{mp}^{d_i}(t)$ = the total amount of resource p required to treat the expected prevalency of disease d, in its entirety, with strategy i over the period t in module m,

$R_p(t)$ = total amount of p available over t,

$X_m^{d_i}$ = that fraction of the population of module m, potentially treatable under strategy i against disease d, which should in fact be treated via that strategy if the optimal allocation of resources is to result,

N = the total number of health states,

S_d = the number of intervention strategies against disease d subject to allocative decisions,

M = the number of population modules,

D = the number of diseases in the decision problem, and

Q = the number of resources subject to allocation decisions.

The objective function, $\Delta H(t)$, may be interpreted as *expected improvement in the health status of the entire target population (all modules) over time period t*. To see this, note first that the expression within the inner parentheses represents the expected change in the total time of occupancy of state j over (t_o, t) for a typical individual in module m who is subject to strategy i instead of the status quo against diseased. While t may be set at any value it is desirable to choose t such that the transition rates and durations of stay are reasonably stable, so as to approximate the stationarity requirement. The parameter U_j represents the relative social utility of one fundamental time unit of state j. Therefore, the expression within square brackets can be defined as the expected change in health status *for an individual* in module m who receives treatment strategy i. Multiplication by $P_m^{d_i}$ yields the total expected change in health status if strategy i against disease d is administered to the *entire* population assumed to be at risk to d in module m. In solving the mathematical program, one is seeking values for $X_m^{d_i}$ on the closed interval [0, 1], each of which represents the fraction of a population at-risk which should receive a certain treatment strategy. While the model is specified here as a general linear program, one can convert it to a dichotomous (0–1) integer program by restricting the $X_m^{d_i}$ to lie on an endpoint of [0, 1]. Under this specification a treatment strategy—if it were administered within a module at all—would be made available to the entire at-risk population in the module. This permits one to acknowledge analytically the arguments of Chen et al. (1975) and Torrance et al (1973) that fractional funding of modules may be administratively and politically infeasible.

Consider now the Q inequality resource constraints. Each $A_{mp}^{d_i}(t)$ represents the total amount of resource p needed to administer strategy d_i to the entire population assumed to be at-risk to d in module m. Once the model is solved we can compute products of the form, $A_{mp}^{d_i}(t) \, X_m^{d_i}$, which are the key results from a policy perspective; each represents the optimal amount of resource p for treating disease d with intervention i in module m.

The second major group of constraints consists of equalities of the form $\sum_{i=0}^{S_d} X_m^{d_i} = 1$. Taken together, these insure that for each disease, each module member is subject to one and only one strategy. In a dichotomous integer programming model, each module will be allocated exactly one strategy for each disease.

Overall, the model may be viewed as a large production function, which indicates the maximum amount of output—defined as expected improvement in total population health status—obtainable from a given vector of inputs.[5] Another view, based on the typology of Donabedian [15], is that the model takes the *structure* of medical care (the $R_p(t)$) as given and chooses those *processes* (summarized in the $A_{mp}^{d_i}(t)$ (that maximize *outcome* (the objective function.)

As will be seen in the following section, the overall time interval (t) over which strategies will be evaluated is one year. All module members who survive that year are assumed to have the same expected time-flow of health status regardless of which active intervention strategies, if any, are introduced. This simplifying assumption is tenable because the two diseases studied here, infant gastroenteritis and infant respiratory infections, are acute problems that generally do not result in chronic organ impairment. Because of these assumptions—which are made for this particular application of the model only—introduction of a discount factor would have virtually no effect on the optimal pattern of resource allocations. We thus bypass for now the difficult task of validly converting expected future health status benefits to present value. In this application, t is assumed to be short enough that all health status gains and losses over that interval are regarded as objects of choice with virtually the same present value. Furthermore, the life expectancies at the end of t of all module members (i.e., all infants on the Papago Reservation) are assumed to be equal; the one long-term benefit of intervention—reduction in infant mortality—has the same time structure for all modules competing for resources.

III FURTHER SPECIFICATION AND THE ESTIMATION OF PARAMETERS FOR THE RESOURCE ALLOCATION MODEL

(a) Overview

The resource allocation model was presented in the last section in its most basic form. The purpose of this section is to examine each of the model's components in some detail and to describe how all of its parameters were estimated for this two-disease application on the Papago Reservation.[6] We will discuss sequentially the development of disease stages, health states, utility weights, modules, disease interventions, durations-of-stay in stages, transition rates between stages, resource requirements for intervention by module, and effective resource availabilities for the inputs in the analysis.

Subsections (b)–(d) and Appendices A and B deal interrelatedly with health states, disease stages, and consumer preferences (utility) weights. At this point it may be instructive to preview that part of the model.

We have defined health as a four-dimensional phenomenon, in that suboptimal health is characterized by varying degrees of physical dysfunction, social dysfunction, pain/anguish, and disease-induced disruption in the normal family environment. For each of these four dimensions we have developed a category scale which is nondisease-specific and whose end-points represent Good Health (or No Dysfunction) and Death; these scales are presented in subsection (d). At a point in time an individual can be regarded as being in one category along each of the four dimensions, so that the function status of an individual is uniquely described by a point in the corresponding four-dimensional space. It is to these generalized, nondisease-specific health states that a pilot sample of Papago Indian consumers have assigned utility weights. But the model requires utility numbers for the *disease stages* under study. Thus, in the manner of Bush et al. (1973), we have created linkages between disease stages and the generalized health states; the aim has been to map each stage into the most appropriate point in the four-dimensional health state space. In this way, each disease stage takes on the utility value of its associated health state.[7]

(b) Disease Stages

The two diseases that are the focus of this application are infant gastro-enteritis (GE) and infant respiratory infections (RI). Physician scientists at the Indian Health Service's Office of Research and Development (ORD) at Tucson have defined each disease in terms of mutually exclusive and exhaustive "stages" through which any patient may move during an episode. The presence of each stage is manifested in the patient's exhibiting specific objective and subjective clinical symptoms; a patient is assigned to a disease stage on the basis of the provider's objective and subjective assessment of the prevalence of these symptoms. Stages for both diseases are given descriptively in Figure 1.

The subjective and objective criteria for assigning infants to GE stages are contained in Figure 2. The decision rule adopted by Papago tribal outreach workers is to assign each infant to the most severe stage indicated in the responses to all questions. Thus, if there were blood found in the infant's diarrhea but all other clinical responses were at the Stage I level, the infant would be classified as Stage III. Likewise, Figure 3 contains the clinical criteria for staging RI. These definitions are arbitrary, but highly useful delineations; associated with each stage is a prescribed set of medical processes to be initiated by providers if the infant is to receive a "minimum acceptable" level of health care. There is one other characteristic of these stages to note for now: *by construction, if the infant moves through the stages at all, the movement must be in numerical (for GE) or alphabetical (for RI) sequence.* Thus, for example, for an infant to be in Stage III, he/she must have passed through Stage I and Stage II; conversely, to return to good health (Stage 0), the infant must move back eventually through Stage II and Stage I. This feature greatly reduces the number of possible (stage-contingent) parameters that must be estimated. But it does require a rather tedious expansion and restate-

Figure 1. Disease Stages

Gastroenterisits

0	Well Infant
I	Mild Gastroenteritis
II	Moderate Gastroenteritis
III	Severe Gastroenteritis with Minimal Dehydration
IV	Severe Gastroenteritis with Dehydration
V	Death

Respiratory Infection

A	Well Infant
B	Cold or Mild Influenza
C	Moderate Pneumonia
D	Severe Pneumonia
E	Death

Figure 2. Standards of Stage Assessment for Gastroenterisits
Age Category: Babies Up to 3 Years Old

	Information Gathering	Stage I	Stage II	Stage III	Stage IV
SUBJECTIVE	24-hour follow-up				
	5-day follow-up				
	Is the baby less than 3 months old?	No		Yes	
	What is the baby's risk level? ☐ Average ☐ High				
	Is the diarrhea mushy or liquid?				
	Mushy – For how many days?	1-4	5-7	Over 7	
	Mushy – How many in last 6 hours?	1-3	4-5	Over 5	
	Liquid – For how many days?	1	2	Over 2	
	Liquid – How many in last 6 hours?	1	2-3	Over 3	
	Is there blood in the diarrhea?	No		Yes	
	Is there mucus in the diarrhea?	No	Yes		
	Is the baby vomiting?	No	Yes		
	For how many days?	1	2	Over 2	
	How many times in last 6 hours?	1	2	Over 2	
	Can the baby keep down clear fluids?	Yes		No	
	Is the baby urinating a normal amount?	Yes		Deceased	
OBJECTIVE	Rectal temperature	98-102°	102-103°	Over 103°	
	Making tears when crying?	Yes		Deceased	No
	Soft spot (Fontanelle)?	Normal			Fallen
	Lining of Mouth	Moist			Dry or Sticky
	Eyes look sunken in?	No			Yes
	Skin tenting?	No			Yes

Figure 3. Community Health Representative Program

Problem: Respiratory Infections

Age Category: Infants and Children up to 4 Years

Information Gathering	Stage B	Stage C	Stage D
Subjective:			
How long has it been present	less than 5 da.	5-7 days	7 da. or more
Is there coughing?	Yes/No		
Does he/she cough so hard he passes out or turns blue?	No		Yes
Does he/she indicate that his ear hurts?	No		Yes
Is there pus in the ear?	No		Yes
Does he/she have a sore throat?	No	Yes	
Is he/she throwing up? — after coughing only?	No		Yes
after each feeding?	No		Yes
Objective:			
Temperature: age 0-6 months	less than 100°		100° or more
age 6 months to 2yrs.	less than 100^5	100^5-101^5	101^5 or more
age 2 yrs. to 4 yrs.	less than 101	101-102^5	102^5 or more
Respiratory Rate	less than 32/min.	32-40/min.	40/min. or more
Are there retractions present?	No		Yes
Is there flaring of the nostrils?	No		Yes
Is there grunting when he/she breathes out?	No		Yes
Is the baby lethargic?	No		Yes
Does he/she have a stiff neck?	No		Yes

Assessment	Treatment Plan	1st
Well child	Do Educational Task A	
Respiratory Infection	Treat as below; do educational Task A & follow-up in 5 days; Refer	
Stage B	to Clinic if not better	1
Respiratory Infection	Treat as below; do educational Task A & follow-up in 24 hours;	
Stage C	Refer to Clinic if not better	1
Respiratory Infection Stage D	Refer to Clinic right away	1
No sickness — medicine to be kept on hand		1

Treatment

1. Fever or headache (use acetaminophen Drops or baby aspirin tablets 75 mg.)

   0-6 months-acetaminophen drops 0.3cc every 4 hrs.
   6-12 months-acetaminophen dorps 0.6cc every 4 hrs.
   12-18 months-acetaminophen drops 0.9cc every 4 hrs.
   18 months-2 yrs. — baby aspirin 75mg — 1 tablet for each year of age, every 4 hrs.

2. Runny or stuffy nose: Saline nose drops 1 drop in ea. side/3-4 hrs.

3. Coughing: (Use /DO NOT GIVE TO BABIES LESS THAN 6 MONTHS OLD
   Glycerol
   Guaiacolate Cough 6 mos.-2 yrs. – ½ teaspoonful 3 times a day
   Syrup)   2 yrs.-4yrs. – ½ teaspoonful 4 times a day
4. Sore throat: Throat culture – label with name, date, number and village &
                   send to Disease Control Lab within 24 hrs.
5. Educational Task A
   Other: Encourage fluids

Identification

Name. . . . .
              Last   First   Middle
B-date . . . . Age: . . . . Sex: . . . . Signed: . . . . CHR(900)
ID-No. . . . .
Residence: . . . .
Location of Encounter: . . . .   Reviewed: . . . . . .
Date: . . . .   CHR Supervisor

ment of the transition rate and durations-of-stay expressions introduced in section II.

To accomplish the mapping of disease stages into health states, a panel of pediatricians was asked to assess each clinically defined stage with respect to its likely impact on the modal infant's well-being defined along four dimensions—physical, social, pain/anguish, and family environment. The pediatricians included ORD research scientist Paul Nutting and seven other physicians on the medical school faculties at Duke University and the University of North Carolina at Chapel Hill. Aided by the staging schemes summarized in Figures 2 and 3, each was asked to write a succinct narrative characterizing the impact of each stage on infant-functioning along each of the four dimensions. These initial descriptions were summarized and integrated by the principal author and then redistributed to each pediatrician for further comments, additions, or deletions. Based on the results of this second iteration of responses, the ORD staff agreed upon the narrative stage descriptions given in Appendix A.

(c) Health States

The health states given in Figure 4 were developed by the IHS Office of Research and Development in cooperation with a number of Papago Indian volunteers.[8] The use of physical and social dimensions as components in a definition of health is in keeping with the approach adopted by Fanshel and Bush (1970), Chen et al. (1975), Bush et al. (1973), and Torrance et al. (1976) for the construction of function status scales. The addition of the pain dimension allows us to index the perceived impact of the sharp, sudden discomfort that often accompanies acute health problems. With the "Family Dependence and Environmental Disruption" scale, we

Figure 4. Health State Dimension Scales

Physical Limitation

1.1 Being able to get around physically to where you usually go.
1.2 Small physical problem like some trouble walking on one foot.
1.3 Needing crutches to walk.
1.4 Needing a wheelchair to get around.
1.5 Unable to move any part of your body.
1.6 Death.

Social Limitation

2.1 Being with your family and friends.
2.2 Not being able to be with a few of your very close friends.
2.3 Not being able to be with most of your family or friends.
2.4 Only able to see one or two people you know for a few minutes a day.
2.5 Completely separated from all family and friends.
2.6 Death.

Pain/Anguish

3.1 Feeling well — no pain.
3.2 A small pain in one part of your body.
3.3 Moderate pain which would make it hard to do your regular work.
3.4 Sharp pain where you wouldn't be able to think about anything else.
3.5 Very intense pain that would make you pass out.
3.6 Dying.

Family Dependence and Environmental Disruption

4.1 Able to take care of yourself without any extra help from your family.
4.2 You would need a little more help than usual from someone in a small way.
4.3 You would need a lot of extra help from someone for several things like getting dressed and eating.
4.4 One person in your family would have to take care of you all the time.
4.5 Everybody in family would have to help take care of you or be very careful around you.
4.6 Death.

are attempting to capture in a simple fashion the complex effects which alterations in the family home environment may have on the sick person whose illness initiates the disruption. For instance, a sick adult may derive disutility from knowing that he is dependent upon other family members for care and that others in the household are inconvenienced in various ways because of his illness. Also, it might be argued that an infant can sense the alarm and anguish felt by his fearful parents.[9]

As a final step, we must establish the linkages between the GE and RI disease stages and these health state dimension scales. For the purpose of this study, the authors assumed the role of arbiter and associated each dimension-specific stage description—as developed by the pediatricians—with one particular category along that dimension's health state scale. These assignments are given in Figure 5.

Figure 5. Disease Stage-Health State Linkages

Gastroenteritis

	Physical	Social	Pain/Anguish	Family Dependence
Stage 0	1.1	2.1	3.1	4.1
Stage I	1.2	2.2	3.2	4.2
Stage II	1.2	2.2	3.3	4.3
Stage III	1.4	2.4	3.4	4.4
Stage IV	1.4	2.5	3.4	4.5
Stage V	1.6	2.6	3.6	4.6

Respiratory Infections

	Physical	Social	Pain/Anguish	Family Dependence
Stage A	1.1	2.1	3.1	4.1
Stage B	1.2	2.2	3.2	4.2
Stage C	1.3	2.3	3.3	4.3
Stage D	1.4	2.4	3.4	4.5
Stage E	1.6	2.6	3.6	4.6

(d)   Consumer Preference Weights for Health States

In this subsection we (1) discuss the implementation of a working instrument to measure Papago preferences for the health states; (2) derive utility weights based on responses to the instrument by a pilot sample of Papago Indians; and (3) link these health state dimension weights to their corresponding disease stage dimensions.

(1) The Instrument.   Based on the health state dimension descriptions presented above, the staff of the Office of Research and Development developed the preference instrument reproduced below in Figure 6. Papago Indian employees of ORD assisted directly both in the specification of individual scale items and in establishing the format of the instrument.[10] On Part I the 16 dimension scale items are arrayed in random order; the consumer is told nothing about the presumed duration of each state dimension, but is asked simply to associate each item with a point on the category scale of severity. This exercise serves as a preliminary to the completion of the primary component of the instrument, Part II. Its format differs from that of Part I in one crucial respect: each state dimension item to be evaluated now has an associated time of duration. Four alternative time durations for the state dimensions were selected: seven hours, three days, one month, and ten months.[11] These times are logarithmically related (approximately) and are designed to facilitate our inferring the relative disutility of state-dimension occupancies corresponding to both acute and more chronic problems. It has been suggested by Fanshel and

Bush (1970) and especially by Torrance et al. (1973) that the disutility of a health state may be no simple linear function of time of occupancy.

To anticipate the discussion, we will develop utility weights for those states corresponding to the morbid but nonfatal stages of GE and RI by employing a multidimensional scaling analysis of preferences for the dimension scale items whose associated duration is closest to the corresponding GE and RI stage durations. Based on these responses, utility weights for the states involving endpoints of the four dimensions will be assigned heuristically.[12]

As a whole, the instrument represents a first effort in developing a mechanism to measure Papago preferences for health states. It was submitted successfully to a pilot group of 42 Papago, who were predominantly female, under ago 40, and members of the ORD clerical staff.[13]

(2) Estimation of State Utility Weights. The preference instruments required consumers to rate dimension scale items (DSI) singly and sequentially. Without data reflecting preferences for alternative health states— i.e., four-element vectors of DSI's, with one DSI for each dimension—we could not proceed as Patrick et al. (1973) and compute health state utility weights as the simple means (or medians) of sample preferences for such states. Nor could we employ more sophisticated psychometric techniques, such as polynomial conjoint scaling [Luce et al. (1964)] and functional measurement [Anderson (1970)] to attempt to discriminate among functional rules for aggregating individual preferences into interval scale weights. Our psychometric analysis consequently will be based on two assumptions: (1) the functional rule for preference aggregation is additive and (2) the scale of perceived dysfunctions of the health states (whose values are to be estimated) can be represented as a vector in the "health state space" which lies at the same angle with respect to each of the component dimensions.[14] While additivity, in particular, should be properly regarded as an hypothesis to be tested in more sophisticated preference aggregation models, recent work by Kaplan et al. (1976) lends support to its reasonableness. For more discussion of some of the theoretical issues in the psychometric assessment of preferences, see Appendix B, section (1).

Utility weights for the dimension scale items were estimated here by Thurstone's "method of successive categories," employing a least squares approach developed by Diederich, et al. (1957). The model underlying this method assumes that judgments on the value of each DSI are drawn from a normal distribution with a mean equal to that DSI's perceived value and a variance also unique to that DSI. Recall that the scale for Part I contains 40 ordered and equally-spaced increments, which we now term scale "categories." Each scale in Part II has 12 ordered categories. Each category on a scale is assumed to have a normal distribu-

Figure 6. Preference Instrument

Part I

Listed below are some of the different kinds of problems people have when they are sick. The people who work in the health programs would like to know what is important to you. Please read each item and then show on the line that goes from Very Small Problem to Very Large Problem how you feel about the item. For example, if you feel that item 1, "One person in your family would have to take care of you all the time" is a very large problem, you put the "1" near the bottom of the line. If you feel that the item is somewhere between a very small problem and a very large problem, put "1" along the line where you feel it belongs. Please do the same for the rest of the items that are numbered 2 through 16. People have different feelings as to what is a problem and how serious it is. Your feelings are very important and are needed.   Thank you.

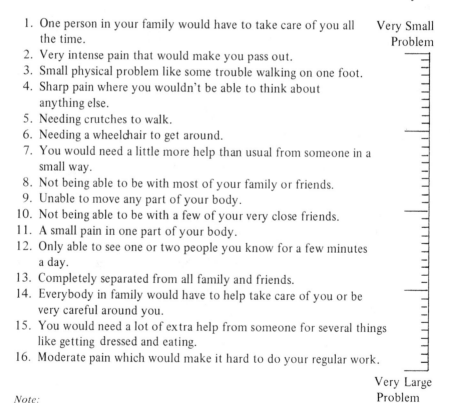

1. One person in your family would have to take care of you all the time.
2. Very intense pain that would make you pass out.
3. Small physical problem like some trouble walking on one foot.
4. Sharp pain where you wouldn't be able to think about anything else.
5. Needing crutches to walk.
6. Needing a wheelchair to get around.
7. You would need a little more help than usual from someone in a small way.
8. Not being able to be with most of your family or friends.
9. Unable to move any part of your body.
10. Not being able to be with a few of your very close friends.
11. A small pain in one part of your body.
12. Only able to see one or two people you know for a few minutes a day.
13. Completely separated from all family and friends.
14. Everybody in family would have to help take care of you or be very careful around you.
15. You would need a lot of extra help from someone for several things like getting dressed and eating.
16. Moderate pain which would make it hard to do your regular work.

Very Small Problem

Very Large Problem

Note:

When you are finished with this page, all 16 numbers will be located somewhere between "Very Small Problem" and "Very Large Problem."

Figure 6 (cont.)

Part II

Listed below are some of the different kinds of problems people have when they are sick. The people who work in the health programs would like to know what is important to you. Please read each item and then show on the line that goes from Very Small Problem to Very Large Problem how you feel about the item. For example, if you feel that item 1 "Needing crutches to walk for one month" is a Very Small Problem, you place a check mark (√) under Very Small Problem. If you feel it would be a very large problem, place a check mark under Very Large Problem. If you feel that it is something between a very small problem and a very large problem, put the check mark where you feel it belongs.

	Very Small Problem	Very Large Problem

1. Needing crutches to walk for one month.

2. Not being able to be with a few of your very close friends for ten months.

3. Needing crutches to walk for ten months.

4. Sharp pain where you wouldn't be able to think about anything else for three days.

5. Not being able to be with most of your family or friends for three days.

6. Not being able to be with a few of your very close friends for one month.

7. One person in your family would have to take care of you all the time for three days.

8. Unable to move any part of your body for three days.

9. Needing a wheelchair to get around for one month.

10. You would need a little more help than usual from someone in a small way for ten months.

11. Needing a wheelchair to get around for seven hours.

12. Small physical problem like some trouble walking on one foot for ten months.

13. Not being able to be with most of your family or friends for one month.

14. Not being able to be with most of your family or friends for seven hours.

15. You would need a lot of extra help from someone for several things like getting dressed and cutting for ten months.

Figure 6 (cont.)

Very Small Problem Very Large Problem

16. Very intense pain that would make you pass out for seven hours.

17. Moderate pain which would make it hard to do your regular work for three days.

18. Unable to move any part of your body for seven hours.

19. One person in your family would have to take care of you for all the time for ten months.

20. Only able to see one or two people you know for a few minutes a day for one month.

21. Only able to see one or two people you know for a few minutes a day for ten months.

22. Only able to see one or two people you know for a few minutes a day for three days.

23. You would need a lot of extra help from someone for several things like getting dressed and eating for one month.

24. Not being able to be with a few of your very close friends for three days.

25. Everybody in family would have to help take care of you or be very careful around you for three days.

26. Completely separated from all family and friends for ten months.

27. Everybody in family would have to help take care of you or be very careful around you for one month.

28. You would need a little more help than usual from someone in a small way for three days.

29. You would need a lot of extra help from someone for several things like getting dressed and eating for seven hours.

30. Needing crutches to walk for seven hours.

31. You would need a lot of extra help from someone for several things like getting dressed and eating for three days.

32. Not being able to be with most of your family or friends for ten months.

33. Moderate pain which would make it harder to do your regular work for one month.

34. You would need a little more help than usual from someone in a small way for one month.

35. A small pain in one part of your body for three days.

Figure 6 (cont.)

36. Completely separated from all family and friends for three days.

37. Sharp pain so that you wouldn't be able to think about anything else for seven hours.

38. Unable to move any part of your body for ten months.

39. Unable to move any part of your body for one month.

40. Very intense pain that would make you pass out for three days.

41. Moderate pain which would make it hard to do your regular work for ten months.

42. Everybody in family would have to help take care of you or be very careful around you for ten months.

43. Completely separated from all family and friends for one month.

44. Small physical problem like some trouble walking on one foot for one month.

45. You would need a little more help than usual from someone in a small way for seven hours.

46. Needing a wheelchair to get around for three days.

47. Not being able to to be with a few of your very close friends for seven hours.

48. A small pain in one part of your body for ten months.

49. Moderate pain which would make it hard to do your regular work for seven hours.

50. Completely separated from all family and friends for seven hours.

51. Sharp pain so that you wouldn't be able to think about anything else for one month.

52. Small physical problem like some trouble walking on one foot for three days.

53. Needing crutches to walk for three days.

54. Needing a wheelchair to get around for ten months.

55. A small pain in one part of your body for one month.

56. Sharp pain so that you wouldn't be able to think about anything else for ten months.

57. A small pain in one part of your body for seven hours.

58. Small physical problem like some trouble walking on one foot for seven hours.

59. One person in your family would have to take care of you all the time for one month.

tion of perceived values centered around its true perceived value, and a variance equal to that of all other categories. The proportion of times that a DSI is judged less than or equal to a category is proportional to the area left of zero of a bivariate normal distribution whose mean is the true value of the category minus the true value of the DSI and whose variance is the sum of the DSI's variance plus the constant variance associated with each category. The square root of this combined variance measure is called the "discriminal dispersion" of the dimension scale item.[15]

In the successive categories model, each subject's judgments carry the same "weight" as the judgments of other subjects. There is no extrinsic process that places added emphasis on the judgments of certain subjects, nor is there any intrinsic process—such as is present in the computation of a group mean—where emphasis is placed on the outliers. This method of preference aggregation is thus consistent with a "one man-one vote" decision rule.

From the successive categories analysis we derived the 16 basic preference numbers which are the raw input for constructing the utility weights. These estimates are based on the responses of 42 individuals to the 16 items from Part II pertaining to state dimensions of three-day duration; as will become evident from (h) below, the average duration of most GE and RI stages is closer to three days than to any of the other time horizons built into the DSI definitions of Part II. The preference weights are presented in Figure 7. A detailed discussion of their derivation and of the construction of dimension scale endpoint weights is contained in Part (2) (b) of Appendix B and footnote 16 below.

The final task is to construct the set of health state weights, U_j, from these dimension scale item values. For each intermediate state weight, we also want to compute a standard deviation, so that the sensitivity of model solutions to random variations in the utility weights can be checked. Unfortunately, the discriminal dispersion of an item value is the square root of the sum of the item variance and a positive constant. Consequently, the variance of a health state weight in the context of the additive model assumed here will always be less than the sum of the four associated discriminal dispersion estimates. The square root of this latter sum represents a conservative (over-) estimate of the standard deviation of the health state weight. For convenience, denote this statistic as "< S. D." Based on the disease stage-health state linkages presented at the end of subsection (c) above, the raw dimension state item weights estimated here, and the additive aggregation model assumed, the health state weights and < S.D. values associated with the GE and RI disease stages are presented in Figure 8. Since each dimension scale is on [0,1], the health state scale in this additive model is on [0,4].[16]

Figure 7. Dimension Scale Item (DSI) Means and Discriminal Dispersions

Physical Limitations				Social Limitations		
DSI	Mean	Discriminal Dispersion		DSI	Mean	Discriminal Dispersion
1.1	0	– –		2.1	0	– –
1.2	.413	.165		2.2	.255	.189
1.3	.386	.163		2.3	.365	.164
1.4	.406	.161		2.4	.316	1.89
1.5	.649	.208		2.5	.336	.159
1.6	1.0	– –		2.6	1.0	– –

Pain/Anguish				Family Dependence and Environmental Disruption		
DSI	Mean	Discriminal Dispersion		DSI	Mean	Discriminal Dispersion
3.1	0	– –		4.1	0	– –
3.2	.427	.173		4.2	.403	.129
3.3	.495	.142		4.3	.507	.153
3.4	.605	.162		4.4	.487	.150
3.5	.753	.271		4.5	.486	.190
3.6	1.0	– –		4.6	1.0	– –

Figure 8. Health State Utility
Weights and Relative
Dispersion Measures

Disease Stage	Mean Weight	< S.D.
O (and A)	0	– –
I	1.498	.810
II	1.670	.806
III	1.821	.814
IV	1.833	.820
B	1.498	.810
C	1.753	.790
D	1.820	.838
V (and E)	4.0	– – –

(e) Modules

The purpose of dividing a target population into modules is to secure a set of subpopulations, each relatively homogeneous with respect to (1) transition rates between disease states, (2) durations-of-stay in stages, and (3) per capita resource requirements for each treatment strategy. For this application of the model, 30 modules have been defined. This delineation is based on the fact that for the two diseases under study, there are a total of three separate, currently measurable disease "groups" into which the infant populations of each of the 10 Papago Reservation districts may be distributed. The three groups consist of disease-specific patient "risk" levels. Two risk levels—average risk and high risk—have been established for infant GE based on regression and Bayesian analysis of data gathered on the reservation since 1972.[17] Disease-stage specific data on respiratory infections were first analyzed in 1974, and the development of district risk levels is still in the formative stage. For this study each infant in each district has been assigned to the one RI category and, depending on his/her risk score, into one of two GE risk levels. Thus, each infant in fact occupies two modules, one for each disease for which he/she is at risk. The element of "double-counting" here is intentional, for each disease represents a competing risk in the infant's environment which should be acknowledged in the resource allocation solution.[18]

Modules are defined also with respect to geographic region because transition rates, durations-of-stay in states, and resource requirements for intervention strategies may vary systematically by location. The quality of housing, food, and other environmental factors, for instance, may be a function of geographic location; and these variables are likely to have an impact on transition rates and durations. Because the difficulty of physical access to outpatient clinics and hospitals is also a function of geography, resource requirements for patient triage will vary by district.[19] While current data limitations rule out distinct epidemiologic parameters for each district, we are able to calculate district-specific triage resource requirements for triage to outpatient and inpatient facilities. Thus, per infant resource requirements—as reflected in the constraint set—are a function here of both risk level and district of occupancy. This leads to $3 \times 10 = 30$ modules.

Total module populations (the P_m^{di} of section (ii)) have been estimated on the basis of a district-specific census of all infants (ages 0–1) whose records were in the IHS health information system as of March 1975. Because of the traditionally intensive concentration by the Papago Executive Health Staff, Community Health Representatives (CHR's) and Nutrition Aides (NA's) on infant health problems, these estimates closely approximate those that would be obtained from a complete census on the reservation. There was a total of 132 infants, 52 classified as being at high risk to GE; the remaining 80 were said to be at average risk to GE, and all 132 were placed in the single RI risk category. Total infant populations in the districts ranged from three to 42. The high-risk GE group varied from two infants, in three districts, to 13 in one district. Average-risk GE district populations varied significantly, from one infant to 32.

(f) Disease Intervention Strategies

As a prelude to the specification of alternative values for the transition rates and duration-of-stay parameters, intervention strategies must be specified. For each disease there are three active treatments, plus the status quo. The latter "strategy" consists of the sequence of health care encounters and treatments that a typical infant, suffering from either GE or RI, can expect to receive in the absence of active assistance and supervision by tribal community health workers. The status quo strategy does not imply that the infant fails to encounter the reservation health-care system; rather, it means that all preventive care and triage of diseased infants is initiated and conducted by the family without external guidance. Figure 9 contains general descriptions of the intervention strategies. Clearly, they focus on the use of community outreach workers in a variety of roles—from no intervention at all to almost complete management of the nonclinic and nonhospital treatment of the infant. The task content of these strategies will be specified in subsection (i) below.

(g) Transition Rates Between Stages

From section II, define $\bar{v}_{fj}(t) \equiv \overline{TR}_{fj}(t)$. Because disease stages here must be occupied sequentially by definition, $\overline{TR}_j(t) = \overline{TR}_{j-1,j}(t) + \overline{TR}_{j+1,j}(t)$. The model requires such transition rate estimates for all modules and disease interventions. However, because of a paucity of observations on the stage-specific incidence of GE and RI, we were not able to estimate transition rates at this point by standard statistical techniques. Rather, they are based on available point estimates of incidence, supplemented where necessary by expert judgment.

Indian Health Service researchers felt that the most representative stage- and risk-level-specific data available on the effects of certain GE interventions were generated during the October–December period of 1972 (see Nutting et al.). Likewise, the most adequate data from which to estimate RI transition rates were gathered in the January–February, 1974 study of the effects of patient education and provider problem-solving on stage occupancy [Nutting et al. (1974)].[20] Expert judgment—provided by IHS clinicians at Tucson—was used to supplement this transition rate data where necessary. Transition rates for GE rates are for a 92-day interval encompassing the October–December period, while RI rates are based on the 59-day, January–February period. Knowledge of the length

Figure 9. Disease Intervention Strategies

Gastroenteritis

SQ — Status Quo.

A/C — Individual education of the parents of the infant, to focus on causes, spread, prevention, danger, recognition, and treatment of diarrhea; assignment of the infant to a disease stage and initiation of a problem-solving algorithm; education of parents in the administration of electrolyte solution; giving solution during home visit, if necessary; *parents responsible for triage of ill infant to clinic or hospital;* physicians and nurses at clinic and/or hospital subsequently responsible for treatment and triage of infant.

C/T — Assignment of infant to a disease stage and initiation of a problem-solving algorithm; *community health worker responsible for triage of infant to clinic or hospital;* physicians and nurses at clinic and/or hospital subsequently responsible for treatment and triage of infant.

A/C/T— Strategies A/C and C/T combined.

Respiratory Infection

SQ — Status Quo.

A/C — Individual education of the parents of the infant, to focus on the nature, complications, danger signs, treatment, and prevention of respiratory infections; assignment of the infant to a disease stage and initiation of a problem-solving algorithm; *parent(s) principally responsible for triage of ill infant to clinic or hospital;* physicians and nurses at clinic and/or hospital responsible for treatment of infant (including triage) once he/she is registered at either type of facility.

C/T — Assignment of the infant to a disease stage and initiation of a problem-solving algorithm; *community health worker responsible for triage of infant to clinic or hospital;* physicians and nurses at clinic and/or hospital responsible subsequently for treatment and triage of infant.

A/C/T— Strategies of A/C and C/T combined.

and seasonal position of these intervals is mandatory for the proper adjustment of the rates for their use in the allocation models, it will be seen shortly. The rates are presented in Figure 10 and now take the general form $\overline{TR}^{di}_{fjm}(t)$, meaning the transition is from stage f to stage j. Since there is insufficient information at present to distinguish among transition rates

Figure 10. Transition Rates by Treatment Strategies and Stages
of Exit of Entry
Gastroenteritis, Average Risk (GEAR)
(t = 92 days)

Exit Stage f	Entry Stage j	SQ	A/C	C/T	A/C/T
0	I	.89*	.89*	.89	.89*
I	II	.68*	.63*	.68	.63*
II	III	.25*	.20*	.23	.20*
III	IV	.05*	.03*	.02	.02
IV	V	.002	.002	.002	.002
V	IV	0	0	0	0
IV	III	.048	.028	.018	.018
III	II	.248	.198	.228	.198
II	I	.678	.628	.678	.628
I	0	.888	.888	.888	.888

Gastroenteritis, High Risk (GEHR)
(t = 92 days)

Exit Stage f	Entry Stage j	SQ	A/C	C/T	A/C/T
0	I	1.27	.79*	1.27	.79*
I	II	1.20*	.74*	1.20	.74*
II	III	1.07*	.32*	.72	.25
III	IV	.93*	.16*	.43	.10
IV	V	.19	.03	.04	.02
V	IV	0	0	0	0
IV	III	.74	.13	.39	.08
III	II	.88	.29	.68	.23
II	I	1.01	.71	1.16	.72
I	0	1.08	.76	1.23	.77

Respiratory Infections, No Risk Differential (RINR)
(t = 59 days)

Exit Stage f	Entry Stage j	SQ	A/C	C/T	A/C/T
A	B	.270	.270	.270	.270
B	C	.180	.027	.180	.027
C	D	.170	.026	.080	.010
D	E	.050	.008	.020	.003
E	D	0	0	0	0
D	C	.120	.018	.060	.007
C	B	.130	.019	.160	.024
B	A	.220	.262	.250	.267

* Estimate based on observations from operation of programs on the Papago Reservation.

for districts, the subscript m refers only to a particular risk level of disease d. Rates based on quasi-experimental observation are denoted by asterisks.

The next task is to convert these raw transition rates into a form that can be used in the allocation model. As seen in section II, it is desirable to subdivide the entire time horizon of program analysis into a set of mutually exclusive and exhaustive subintervals so the underlying Markov transition matrix $[p_{ij}]$, can reasonably be assumed to be stationary over each subinterval. The resource allocations for each subinterval are influence by the transition rates appropriate to that subinterval. In this sense the allocations over the entire time horizon are derived from a model that is "piece-wise" stationary over the entire allocation time frame. Define this time horizon as one year. To determine the most appropriate subintervals, we examine (see Figure 11) the monthly patterns of total GE and RI incidence for Papago infants age 0–1 over the 12-month interval from September 1973 to September 1974. Based on these data, three subintervals were defined:

(1) May–September, when GE tends to be high incidence and RI low incidence;

(2) December–April, when GE tends to be low incidence and RI high incidence; and

(3) October–November, when both GE and RI are high incidence.

Figure 11. Monthly Incidence of
Gastroenteritis and Respiratory Infections
Among Papgo Infants
(Age 0-1)

	GE	RI
September (1973)	24	16
October	52	61
November	72	65
December	22	63
January	19	96
February	10	90
March	17	118
April	33	63
May	44	3
June	53	0
July	43	0
August (1974)	86	0

To compute the transition rates appropriate for each subinterval and disease, one multiplies the disease's raw transition rates by an adjustment factor equal to the ratio of the expected incidence during the given subinterval to the expected incidence during the interval over which the raw rates are computed. For example, the GE adjustment factor for subinterval (1) is calculated as:

$$\frac{\text{Incidence for May–September}}{\text{Incidence for October–December}} = \frac{44 + 53 + 43 + 86 + 24}{52 + 72 + 22} = 1.71.$$

That is, for use in the model appropriate to subinterval (1), each raw (1972) GE transition rate is multiplied by 1.71; the result is a seasonally adjusted *and* interval-length adjusted set of GE transition rates. For this procedure, the following adjustment factors have been calculated:

	GE	RI
(1) May–September	1.71	.10
(2) December–April	.69	2.31
(3) October–November	.85	.68

Clearly, these adjustment factors are only approximations to demonstrate how one can cope with seasonal variations in incidence over the time horizon. As will be seen, one actually implements three allocation models, each appropriate to one subinterval.

(h) Durations-of-Stay in Disease Stages

From clinical experience, IHS researchers were not able to provide estimates of D_j as such, but rather of stage durations contingent on the stage of next occupancy, i.e., of $\overline{\tau}_{je} \equiv \overline{D}_{je}$. Fortunately, this information suffices, since (by construction) a patient moves through the stages in a specific, ordered sequence. Thus, our prevalence expression $\overline{TR}_j(t) \cdot D_j$ assumes the operational form

$$\overline{TR}_{j,j+1}(t) \cdot \overline{D}_{j|j+1} + \overline{TR}_{j,j-1}(t) \cdot \overline{D}_{j|j-1}.$$

One other conceptual issue must be confronted in this stage duration analysis. It appears that there is nothing in the semi-Markovian theory itself to suggest the proper termination times for trapping states. Death is the ultimate trapping state, and we are forced to appeal to exogenous assumptions as a basis for assigning a duration to the death state. Let t be the subinterval over which optimization is to occur. Assume first that death, if it occurs at all in the interval, would occur on average at the midpoint; thus, the expected duration of death within t is t/2. The target population consists of all infants age 0–1; assume that the typical age at the beginning of the period t is six months. The number of days of life lost between the end of t and the infant's first birthday is, on average (assuming again that death does occur in that first year) equal to $(182.5 - t)$. Now the life expectancy *at age one* on the Papago Reservation has recently been calculated by the ORD staff as 76.1 years, or 27,776.5 days. Then the expected amount of life lost for an infant death, occurring in the first year, is $\frac{t}{2} + (182.5 - t) +$ 27,776.5 days. As a matter of notation, let $(182.5 - t) + 27,776.5 = \overline{T}^*$. Since death is a trapping state and assumed to occur either during t (in fact, at $\frac{1}{2}$ or at the end of $\overline{T}^*$, the transition rate into death during t can also be regarded as the probability of "enduring" death throughout $\overline{T}^*$. However, at this point in our analysis of Papago health problems, we do not have estimates of the expected prevalency of each of the $(N-1)$ nondeath states over $\overline{T}^*$. Consequently, we must approximate these crudely by defining U^* as the "average" expected health state utility experienced per day per surviving infant over the period $\overline{T}^*$. Then $U^*\overline{T}^*$ is the health status assumed for the infant over $\overline{T}^*$, and we may let $U^*\overline{T}^* \equiv \sum\limits_{\substack{j=1 \\ (j \neq \delta)}}^{N-1} U_j \overline{TR}_{jm}(\overline{T}^*) \cdot \overline{D}_{jm}$, where

δ represents the death state.[21]

Ignoring (for simplicity) the stage sequencing requirement for now, the health status of the modal infant in module m who is subject to intervention strategies denoted by d_i can be expressed in general form

$$\left(\sum\limits_{\substack{j=1 \\ (j \neq \delta)}}^{N-1} U_j \overline{TR}_{jm}^{d_i}(t) \cdot \overline{D}_{jm}^{d_i} \right) + \left(U_\delta \overline{TR}_{\delta,m}^{d_i}(t) \cdot \frac{(t)}{2} \right) + \left(U_\delta \ \overline{TR}_{\delta,m}^{d_i}(t) \cdot \overline{T}^* \right)$$

$$+ \left(U^* (1 - \overline{TR}_{\delta,m}^{d_i}(t)) \ \overline{T}^*{}_{\delta,m}^{d_i} \right)$$

When this expression is subtracted from the corresponding one for the status quo intervention, the U^*T^* terms cancel. Thus, the expected change in health status per person in module m, is

$$\sum\limits_{\substack{j=1 \\ (j \neq \delta)}}^{N-1} U_j(\overline{TR}_{jm}^{d_o}(t) \cdot \overline{D}_{jm}^{d_o} - \overline{TR}_{jm}^{d_i}(t) \cdot \overline{D}_{jm}^{d_i}) + U_\delta \ (\overline{TR}_{\delta,m}^{d_o}(t) - \overline{TR}_{\delta,m}^{d_i}(t)) \frac{(t)}{2}$$

$$+ (U_\delta - U^*) (\overline{TR}_{\delta,m}^{d_o}(t) - \overline{TR}_{\delta,m}^{d_i}(t)) \ \overline{T}^*.$$

As a practical matter, the longer the lengths-of-stay in stages, the easier it becomes to observe the $\overline{D}_j$ in a sample of patients. For acute diseases like infant gastroenteritis and infant respiratory infections, the length-of-stay in some stages may range from only a few hours to four or five days. Only those very ill infants who have been hospitalized are subject to the kind of continuous professional observation required to determine, in most cases, exactly when one clinical stage ends and another begins. The majority of Papago infants who contract either GE or RI do not reach that stage of either disease where hospitalization is required. Thus, it has been necessary to use clinical judgment in estimating the $\overline{D}_j$. With the fundamental time unit defined to be one day (24 hours), researchers at ORD, led by Paul Nutting, concluded that duration is a function of the risk level of the infant but is not systematically related to intervention strategy employed or district of residence. Consequently, while interventions are assumed to affect crucially the transition rates between stages, the stage durations are regarded as unaltered. This may not be a reasonable assumption generally, but for these two diseases and the intervention strategies designated the proposition may closely approximate reality. For the strategies all emphasize prevention, and there is little variation among them in treatment of the infant once contact is made with an outpatient clinic or hospital. The stage duration estimates are presented in Figure 12.

(i) Intervention Resource Requirements

As the basic production coefficient in the allocation model, $A_{mp}^{d_i}(t)$ has been defined as the *total* amount of resource p needed to implement intervention i against disease d in all of module m over t. In expanded form we may write $A_{mp}^{d_i}(t) = \sum\limits_{\substack{j=1 \\ j \neq f}}^{N} \sum\limits_{f=1}^{N} A_{fjmp}^{d_i}(t) + \tilde{Z}_{mp}^{d_i}(t) \cdot P_m^{d_i}$, where $A_{fjmp}^{d_i}(t)$ is the corresponding total quantity of p required for the curative treatment rendered to individuals in stage j who just came from stage f, and $\tilde{Z}_{mp}^{d_i}(t)$ is the *per infant* consumption of p for preventive activity in module m over period t according to strategy d_i. The purpose of this subsection, and of Appendix C, is to describe how the $A_{fjmp}^{d_i}(t)$ and $\tilde{Z}_{mp}^{d_i}(t)$ were calculated for the resources, diseases, and treatment programs in this application of the model. This is facilitated by noting further that $A_{fjmp}^{d_i}(t) = TR_{fjm}^{d_i}(t) \cdot W_{fjmp}^{d_i} \cdot Z_{fjmp}^{d_i} \cdot P_m^{d_i}$, where $Z_{fjmp}^{d_i}$ is the amount of resource p required to treat disease d *per patient episode* in module m, given intervention i and that contact is first made with p upon entry into j from f; and $W_{fjmp}^{d_i}$ is the frequency of triage to p, given d and i and that the patient, in module m, arrived at stage j from stage f. Note that $W_{fjmp}^{d_i}$ may equal zero either because the infant will not make contact with resource p in that episode or because contact is made with p at some other transition in the episode. The non-zero triage frequencies assumed for this study are presented in Figure 13; they were provided by IHS staff scientists and are thought to reflect current standards of care. These frequencies are assumed not to vary by module (i.e., by risk level and district of residence). Since the pattern of provider contacts for outpatient and inpatient treatment will be assumed below to vary only by the disease stage of the infant, the usual resource subscript p is used in Figure 13 only to denote whether triage is to an outpatient clinic (OP) or to the Papago Reservation hospital (IP) at Sells, Arizona.

Figure 12. Durations of Stay in Disease Stages

(in days)

Gastroenteritis, High Risk (GEHR)		Gastroenteritis, Average-Risk (GEAR)	Respiratory Infection, No Risk Differential (RINR)	
$\overline{D}_{I/II}$	$= 1$	1	$\overline{D}_{B/C}$	$= 5$
$\overline{D}_{II/III}$	$= 2$	1	$\overline{D}_{C/D}$	$= 2$
$\overline{D}_{III/IV}$	$= 3$	2	$\overline{D}_{D/E}$	$= 2$
$\overline{D}_{IV/V}$	$= 1$	1	$\overline{D}_{E/E}$	$= \dfrac{t + (182.5\text{-}t)}{2}$ $+ 27{,}776.5$
$\overline{D}_{V/V}$	$= \dfrac{t + (182.5\text{-}t)}{2}$ $+ 27{,}776.5$	$\dfrac{t + (182.5\text{-}t)}{2}$ $+ 27{,}776.5$	$\overline{D}_{D/C}$	$= 2$
$\overline{D}_{IV/III}$	$= 1$	1	$\overline{D}_{C/B}$	$= 3$
$\overline{D}_{III/II}$	$= 3$	2	$\overline{D}_{B/A}$	$= 1$
$\overline{D}_{II/I}$	$= 2$	2		
$\overline{D}_{I/0}$	$= 1$	1		

For both *outpatient* and *inpatient* care, we assume that the per episode resource requirements do not vary by (outreach) intervention or by module in this model application; thus Z^{di}_{tjmp} becomes Z^{d}_{tjp}. We further assume for GE that resource consumption is not significantly affected by stage of entry—not so heroic an assumption since only infants at or near the very worst nonfatal stage are hospitalized. For RI, we are able to distinguish two inpatient resource consumption patterns per episode, depending upon stage of entry into the hospital. Five resources will be contained explicitly in the constraint set of the model: physician outpatient time (DOCOP), physician inpatient time (DOCIP), nurse outpatient time (NUROP), nurse inpatient time (NURIP), and outreach worker time (OUTREACH). Generation of the type of detailed input-output information needed for statistical estimation of these parameters would ideally require time-motion studies of considerable magnitude. Such studies have not been conducted yet within the reservation health care system—nor perhaps within any system of similar size and diversity.[22] Consequently, task time estimates are based on the expert judgment of IHS researchers, led by staff scientist Paul Nutting. Most of these estimatés upon which all the $A_{mp}^{di}(t)$ are finally based are summarized in a narrative format in Figure 14. Times for triage to clinic or hospital are district-specific and are given only in general form in the figure. The derivations of all of these estimates are considered in more detail in Appendix C.

Note that the $A_{mp}^{di}(t)$ are clearly seasonally dependent, being explicit functions of seasonally dependent transition rates. Consequently, the five resource constraints of the allocation model must be adjusted for each subinterval over which the model is applied.

(j) Resource Availabilities

Estimation of the right-hand side resource availabilities, the $R_p(t)$, for $p = 1, \ldots, Q$, is particularly difficult in this first application of the model; GE and RI—while they have a relatively major impact on a portion of the population—still absorb only a fraction of the health care labor inputs on the Papago Reservations. Ideally, one would first determine the subset of all resources that should be devoted overall to GE and RI, then optimally allocate these quantities with the disease model. But this raises two problems, one conceptual and one practical. In the absence of a more encompassing allocation model, how can one rationally determine the fractions of all resources which are to be set aside exclusively for GE and RI? Clearly, as more diseases are brought into the model, one would sequentially increase the fraction of each resource category subject to the allocation algorithm. If the model were finally to include a sufficient number of problems to account for virtually all disease prevalence, the $R_p(t)$ would reflect the total availability of each resource. Secondly, there is the practical difficulty of determining those fractions of each input's total availability which are *effectively* devoted to patient care of each type. This is a special problem with labor inputs. Without detailed time-motion observations on the actual labor utilization in the treatment of each episode, how does one adjust the $R_p(t)$ for the downtime that is inevitable in the operation of a health care system? Studies on the production of dental services by Kilpatrick et al. (1972), and Lipscomb and Scheffler (1975) have employed direct estimates of various categories of downtime. Since such

Figure 13. Rules of Triage from Home to Outpatient
and Inpatient Care

Gastroenteritis

Status Quo (SQ)

0% of Stage II infants to outpatient clinic ($W_{I, II, OP}$ = 0.0)
40% of Stage III infants to clinic ($W_{II, III, OP}$= 0.40)
10% of Stage III infants to hospital at Sells ($W_{II,III, IP}$ = 0.10)
100% of Stage IV infants to hospital at Sells ($W_{III, IV, IP}$ = 1.00)

Education and Workup (A/C)

75% of Stage II to clinic ($W_{I, II, OP}$ = 0.75)
60% of Stage III to clinic ($W_{II, III, OP}$ = 0.60)
15% of Stage III to hospital ($W_{II, III, IP}$ = 0.15)
100% of Stage IV to hospital ($W_{III, IV, IP}$ = 1.00)

Workup and Triage (C/T)

100% of II to clinic ($W_{I, II, OP}$ = 1.00)
80% of III to clinic ($W_{II, III, OP}$ = 0.80)
20% of III to hospital ($W_{II, III, IP}$ = 0.20)
100% of IV to hospital ($W_{III, IV, IP}$ = 1.00)

Education, Workup, and Triage (A/C/T)

100% of II to clinic ($W_{I, II, OP}$ = 1.00)
80% of III to clinic ($W_{II, III, OP}$ = 0.80)
20% of III to hospital ($W_{II, III, IP}$ = 0.20)
100% of IV to hospital ($W_{III, IV, IP}$ = 1.00)

Respiratory Infections

Status Quo (SQ)

0% of Stage B to clinic ($W_{A, B. OP}$ = 0.0)
50% of Stage C to clinic ($W_{B, C, OP}$ = 0.50)
15% of Stage C to hospital ($W_{B, C, IP}$ = 0.15)
100% of Stage D to hospital ($W_{C, D, IP}$ = 1.00)

Education and Workup (A/C)

20% of Stage B to clinic ($W_{A, B, OP}$ = 0.20)
75% of Stage C to clinic ($W_{B, C, OP}$ = 0.75)
then 22.5% to hospital ($W_{B, C, IP}$ = 0.225)

Education and Workup (A/C) cont.

100% of Stage D to clinic ($W_{C, D, OP} = 1.00$)

then 100% to hospital ($W_{C, D, IP} = 1.00$)

Workup and Triage (C/T)

30% of Stage B to clinic ($W_{A, B, OP} = 0.30$)

100% of Stage C to clinic ($W_{B, C, OP} = 1.00$)

then 30% to hospital ($W_{B, C, IP} = 0.30$)

100% of Stage D to clinic ($W_{C, D, OP} = 1.00$)

then 100% to hospital ($W_{C, D, IP} = 1.00$)

Education, Workup, and Triage (A/C/T)

30% of Stage B to clinic ($W_{A, B, OP} = 0.30$)

100% of Stage C to clinic ($W_{B, C, OP} = 1.00$)

then 30% to hospital ($W_{B, C, IP} = 0.30$)

100% of Stage D to clinic ($W_{C, D, OP} = 1.00$)

then 100% to hospital ($W_{C, D, IP} = 1.00$)

Under all interventions, hospitalized infant is triaged home when, and only when, the asymptomatic stage (either 0 for GE or A for RI) is reached. Outpatient visits not resulting in hospitalization have an implicit triage-to-home probability of one.

time-motion studies have not been conducted yet within the reservation's health care system, we must turn to additional criteria in choosing the $R_p(t)$.

With regard to the four nonfield-based inputs—nurse outpatient time, nurse inpatient time, physician outpatient time, and physician inpatient time—it is assumed there will always be a sufficient supply of each to guarantee treatment of GE and RI in the clinic and/or hospital according to the minimum standards outlined in the previous subsection. Even without specific information on the other diseases competing for nurse and doctor time, this assumption is completely realistic; infant diseases have traditionally been given high priority by the medical staff and the Papago tribe.

Associated with any optimal solution is a certain disease-, module-, and intervention-specific pattern of utilization for each input. This information

Figure 14. Summary of Basic Task Times for Treatment and Prevention
of Infant Gastroenteritis and Infant Respiratiory Infections*

GE Outpatient Visit

$$Z_{DOCOP}^{GE} = .20 \qquad\qquad Z_{NUROP}^{GE} = .25 \; .$$

GE Inpatient Stay

$$Z_{DOCIP}^{GE} = 5.44 \qquad\qquad Z_{NURIP}^{GE} = 26.50$$

RI Outpatient Visit

$$Z_{DOCOP}^{RI} = .55 \qquad\qquad Z_{NUROP}^{RI} = .12$$

RI Inpatient Stay

$$Z_{B,C, DOCIP}^{RI} = 1.75 \qquad\qquad Z_{B,C,NURIP}^{RI} = 11.84$$

$$Z_{C,D,DOCIP}^{RI} = 2.25 \qquad\qquad Z_{C,D,NURIP}^{RI} = 17.52$$

Outreach Worker Activity

· Education and Workup (A/C)

$$Z_{OUTREACH}^{\sim GE} = Z_{OUTREACH}^{\sim RI} = 4.50$$

· Workup and Triage (C/T)

$$Z_{OUTREACH}^{GE} = 1.00 + TT_{fjm, OUTREACH}^{GE}$$

$$Z_{OUTREACH}^{RI} = 1.00 + TT_{fjm, OUTREACH, where,}^{RI}$$

Figure 14 (Cont.)

in general, TT^{d_i} = the triage time required of
$\qquad$ fjmp

input p from module (district) m, given intervention
strategy d_i and that the infant has just entered
stage j from stage f.**

Education, Workup, and Triage (A/C/T)

$$Z^{\sim GE}_{OUTREACH} + Z^{GE}_{A/C}{}_{OUTREACH} = 5.50 + TT^{GE}_{fjm, OUTREACH}$$

$$Z^{RI}_{A/C}{}_{OUTREACH} + Z^{RI}_{C/T}{}_{OUTREACH} = 5.50 + TT^{RI}_{fjm, OUTREACH}$$

* All times expressed in hours. See Appendix D for the derivation of estimates.
** As shown in Appendix D, the complicated expression for triage time arises because triage can be either to the clinic or hospitals and the rules of triage are disease-stage specific.

can be easily aggregated for each input, as will be seen in the next section, to obtain the total treatment time—for each module and for the system as a whole—corresponding to a given optimal solution. While nurse and physician time is not specifically subject to an allocation decision here, the amount of *treatment* time required of these inputs is readily computed.

The key input for allocation is the outreach worker. Again, the most appropriate specification of total resource availability is not obvious. Essentially, our strategy will be to solve the model sequentially for successively decremented values of outreach worker availability, noting how intervention strategy assignments respond to the shrinking constraint set.

EMPIRICAL RESULTS

The resource allocation results obtained by implementing the model of section II with the data developed in section III will be presented now. We focus on several issues, including: (1) the expected impact of outreach workers on infant health status; (2) variations in the optimal allocation of resources as the relative prevalencies of infant GE and RI fluctuate over a 12-month period; and (3) the pattern of optimal allocation solutions induced by successively reducing the supply of outreach worker time presumed to be available for GE and RI activities. We also look briefly at the sensitivity of optimal allocations to random variations in the estimated utility weights and the practicability of solving the model specified as a dichotomous integer program [Geoffrion and Nelson (1968)]. The latter issue is of some importance if one suspects that it may be politically or administratively infeasible to allocate fractionally to modules. In fact, Chen et al. (1975) have proposed an integer optimization model which can account for a number of such non-technological constraints.

Before proceeding it may be useful to collect the various strands of the refined model, as developed in subsections (g), (h), and (i) of Section II. Acknowledging explicitly our stage transition sequencing restrictions, we present the model in general form in Figure 15.

In section III we presented estimates of the utility weights, the durations of stay, and the transition rates, the latter based on 92 days of high prevalence GE and 59 days of high prevalence RI. The right-hand-side resource availabilities will be subject to parametric variation in the analysis and will not have preassigned values. The parameter $\overline{T}^*$ is equal to $[27,776.5 + (182.5 - t)]$ days and thus depends on the length of the optimization interval; recall that $\overline{T}^*$ assumes that the modal infant is six months old at the beginning of t.

The most troubling element in the model is $(U_\delta - U^*)$, the per person per day health status "opportunity cost" of death which occurs in the first year of life. Since at this point there is no substantive basis for calculating U^* for the Reservation, we let this opportunity cost measure assume the value of U_δ ($=4$). Clearly, this results in an overstatement of the health status impact of programs which avert infant death. But because the expected duration of death is overwhelmingly larger than the other GE and RI stage durations, marginal reductions in U_δ for the purpose of realistically reflecting this opportunity cost will have virtually no impact on allocation results.[23]

Finally, recall that the basic allocation interval is one year, divided into three mutually exclusive and exhaustive subintervals:

(1) May-September—High prevalence GE, low prevalence RI (t=153)
(2) October-November—High prevalence of both diseases (t=61)
(3) December-April—Low prevalence GE, high prevalence RI (t=151).

Results will be presented for models based on all three subintervals; these period-specific formulations will be designated, respectively, Model 1, Model 2, and Model 3. If we adjust the raw transition rates given in section II by the "prevalence adjustment factors" calculated there for each subinterval, we obtain the subinterval-specific transition rates required for optimization.

Figure 15. Final Form of the Resource
Allocation Model

$$\max \sum_{\substack{j=1 \\ (j \neq \delta)}}^{D} \sum_{m=1}^{M} \sum_{i=0}^{S} \sum_{j=1}^{N-2} U \left[\overline{TR}_{j,j+1,m}^{d_o}(t) \cdot \overline{D}_{j/j+1,m}^{d_o} - \overline{TR}_{j,j+1,m}^{d_i}(t) \cdot \overline{D}_{j/j+1,m}^{d_i} \right] +$$

$$\sum_{\substack{j=2 \\ (j \neq \delta)}}^{N-1} U_j \left[\overline{TR}_{j,j-1,m}^{d_o}(t) \cdot \overline{D}_{j/j-1,m}^{d_o} - \overline{TR}_{j,j-1,m}^{d_i}(t) \cdot \overline{D}_{j,j-1,m}^{d_i} \right] +$$

$$U_\delta \left[\overline{TR}_{\delta m}^{d_0}(t) - \overline{TR}_{\delta m}^{d_i}(t) \right] \frac{(t)}{2} + (U - U^*)_\delta \left[\overline{TR}_{\delta,n}^{d_0}(t) - \overline{TR}_{\delta m}^{d_i}(t) \right] T^* \right\} P_m^{d_i} X_m^{d_i},$$

$$\text{subject to } \sum_{j=1}^{D} \sum_{m=1}^{M} \sum_{i=0}^{S} \left\{ \sum_{\substack{j=1 \\ (j \neq \delta)}}^{N-2} TR_{j,j+1,mp}^{d_i}(t) \cdot W_{j,j+1,mp}^{d_i} \cdot Z_{m,j+1,mp}^{d_i} + \right.$$

$$\left. \sum_{\substack{j=2 \\ (j \neq \delta)}}^{N-1} \overline{TR}_{j,j-1,mp}^{d_i}(t) \cdot W_{j,j-1,mp}^{d_i} \cdot Z_{j,j-1,mp}^{d_i} + \tilde{Z}_{mp}^{d_i} \right\} P_m^{d_i} X_m^{d_i} \leqslant R_p(t),$$

$$\text{where } p = 1, \ldots, Q;$$

$$\sum_{i=0}^{S_d} X_m^{d_i} = 1 \qquad \text{for } d = 1, \ldots, D; \\ m = 1, \ldots, M; \text{ and}$$

$$X_m^{d_i} \geqslant 0 \qquad \begin{matrix} i = 0, \ldots, S_d \\ d = 1, \ldots, D \\ m = 1, \ldots, M. \end{matrix}$$

Employing both linear and integer programming methods, we solved
the model for all three subintervals and for a number of alternative values
of the effectively available outreach worker time. As noted, it is assumed
for now that sufficient doctor and nurse time is available for outpatient
and inpatient infant GE and RI cases. Thus, the four resource constraint
parameters DOCOP, NUROP, DOCIP, and NURIP were set at arbitrarily
large values. Whether the optimal solution is constrained or unconstrained depends upon the assumed value of OUTREACH; five alterna-

tive levels of this parameter were employed in each of the three seasonal models.

To illustrate the program management information that can be derived from Models 1–3, we present in Figures 16.1–16.9 the allocation results obtained when OUTREACH is specified at 150 hours/month for GE and RI. Appendix D contains additional reports summarizing how resources are reallocated over the May-September period (Model 1) as OUT-REACH assumes successive monthly values of 300, 200, 100, and 50 hours.

Based on these reports, and similar ones available from the authors upon request, the following conclusions emerged:

The availability and effective utilization of outreach workers can significantly reduce the morbidity and mortality impacts of gastroenteritis and respiratory infection in infants.

Outreach workers are most actively employed and have their greatest influence on health status in Model 2, that is, in October and November when GE and RI are both at high prevalence. The next most active season is May-September, when GE alone is high prevalence.

As OUTREACH is reduced and hard choices have to be made about the allocation of workers, several trends are apparent:

(a) allocations to high risk GE infants consistently took precedence over those for average risk infants, who were assigned the "Status Quo," after a point, in virtually all districts;

(b) high risk GE interventions generally received a higher priority than respiratory infection tasks—the major exception being in Model 3 (high RE–low GE) when OUTREACH was restricted to be 50 hours per month;

(c) as OUTREACH became binding, the general pattern of retrenchment within a given risk category was a shift from A/C/T allocations, to C/T to A/C, and finally to SQ.

Regardless of the psychometric model of consumer preferences adopted, the U_j employed in practice can properly be viewed as random because of sampling and measurement error. The question arises as to the stability of "optimal" resource allocations to random variations in these preference weights.[24] To explore this we undertook a small Monte Carlo analysis by drawing randomly from the estimated distributions of the U_j and solving Model 1 sequentially. The results reported in Figure 17 are based on five drawings and suggest (though very tentatively) that allocation solutions are reasonably stable.

Integer programming solutions most closely approximated the linear ones when the constraints were not severely binding; when none were binding, the linear and integer solutions were identical. As the value of OUTREACH was decremented, a number of equality constraints were not met often, particularly in the average risk GE modules.[25]

Figure 16.1.

Model 1 – High Gastroenteritis, Low Respiratory Infection Prevalence
(May - September)

District - Specific Allocation of Providers for Delivering Care
to Infants at "Average Risk" to Gastroenteritis
(in hours)

Providers Districts	DOCOP	DOCIP	NUROP	NURIP	OUTREACH Education & Workup	Workup & Triage	Education, Workup & Triage	Total
0	1.78	5.54	2.22	27.29	0.0	12.52	0.0	12.52
1	0.53	1.23	0.67	5.98	0.0	0.0	19.02	19.02
2	2.39	5.54	2.99	26.93	0.0	0.0	83.91	83.91
3	0.80	1.85	0.99	8.98	0.0	0.0	29.22	29.22
4	2.07	6.46	2.58	31.84	0.0	17.92	0.0	17.92
5	0.26	0.62	0.33	2.99	0.0	0.0	9.37	9.37
6	0.53	1.23	0.67	5.98	0.0	0.0	19.34	19.34
7	9.28	27.65	11.59	135.97	0.0	57.26	57.27	114.52
8	3.56	11.08	4.43	54.58	0.0	30.25	0.0	30.25
9	1.78	5.54	2.22	27.29	0.0	13.27	0.0	13.27
Total Allocation to Average Risk Gastroenteritis	22.99	66.74	28.69	327.84	0.0	131.22	218.13	349.34
Maximum Resources Available ($R_p(t)$)	1533.6	728.0	656.6	1640.0	—	—	—	750.0

Figure 16.2.

Model 1 — High Gastroenteritis, Low Respiratory Infection Prevalence
(May - September)

District - Specific Allocation of Providers for Delivering Care
to Infants at "High Risk" to Gastroenteritis
(in hours)

Providers Districts	DOCOP	DOCIP	NUROP	NURIP	OUTREACH			
					Education & Workup	Workup & Triage	Education, Workup & Triage	Total
0	3.39	18.09	4.22	88.48	0.0	0.0	90.49	90.49
1	0.51	2.79	0.65	13.61	0.0	0.0	15.10	15.10
2	2.34	12.53	2.92	61.25	0.0	0.0	64.66	64.66
3	1.04	5.57	1.30	27.22	0.0	0.0	31.19	31.19
4	0.79	4.17	0.97	20.42	0.0	0.0	23.27	23.27
5	0.51	2.79	0.65	13.61	0.0	0.0	14.60	14.60
6	0.51	2.79	0.65	13.61	0.0	0.0	15.10	15.10
7	2.60	13.92	3.25	68.06	0.0	0.0	71.19	71.19
8	1.04	5.57	1.30	27.22	0.0	0.0	30.80	30.80
9	0.79	4.17	0.97	20.42	0.0	0.0	22.11	22.11
Total Allocation to High Risk Gastroenteritis	13.53	72.40	16.89	353.90	0.0	0.0	378.51	378.51
Maximum Resources Available ($R_p(t)$)	1533.6	728.0	656.5	1640.0	—	—	—	750.0

Figure 16.3.

Model 1 – High Gastroenteritis Low, Respiratory Infection Prevalence
(May-September)

District - Specific Allocation of Providers for Delivering Care
to Infants at Risk to Respiratory Infections
(in hours)

Providers Districts	DOCOP	DOCIP	NUROP	NURIP	OUTREACH			Total
					Education & Workup	Workup & Triage	Education, Workup & Triage	
0	0.12	0.07	0.03	0.51	0.0	0.0	3.14	3.14
1	0.02	0.01	0.01	0.11	0.0	0.0	0.68	0.68
2	0.11	0.07	0.02	0.49	0.0	0.0	3.01	3.01
3	0.04	0.03	0.01	0.19	0.0	0.0	1.20	1.20
4	0.06	0.04	0.01	0.27	0.0	0.0	1.71	1.71
5	0.02	0.01	0.00	0.08	0.0	0.0	0.50	0.50
6	0.02	0.01	0.01	0.11	0.0	0.0	0.68	0.68
7	0.26	0.15	0.06	1.13	0.0	0.0	6.99	6.99
8	0.10	0.06	0.02	0.43	0.0	0.0	2.73	2.73
9	0.05	0.03	0.01	0.24	0.0	0.0	1.51	1.51
Total Allocation to Respiratory Infections	0.80	0.49	0.19	3.56	0.0	0.0	22.16	22.16
Maximum Resources Available ($R_p(t)$)	1533.6	728.0	´656.6	1640.0	—	—	—	750.0

Figure 16.4.

Model 2 – High Respiratory Infection, Low Gastroenteritis Prevalence
(December - May)

District - Specific Allocation of Providers for Delivering Care
to Infants at "Average Risk" to Gastroenteritis
(in hours)

Providers Districts	DOCOP	DOCIP	NUROP	NURIP	OUTREACH			
					Education & Workup	Workup & Triage	Education, Workup & Triage	Total
0	0.08·	1.70	0.10	8.24	0.0	0.0	0.0	0.0
1	0.03	0.57	0.03	2.75	0.0	0.0	0.0	0.0
2	0.12	2.55	0.16	12.36	0.0	0.0	0.0	0.0
3	0.04	0.85	0.05	4.12	0.0	0.0	0.0	0.0
4	0.10	1.98	0.12	9.61	0.0	0.0	0.0	0.0
5	0.01	0.28	0.02	1.37	0.0	0.0	0.0	0.0
6	0.03	0.57	0.03	2.75	0.0	0.0	0.0	0.0
7	0.44	9.05	0.55	43.94	0.0	0.0	0.0	0.0
8	0.17	3.39	0.21	16.48	0.0	0.0	0.0	0.0
9	0.08	1.70	0.10	8.24	0.0	0.0	0.0	0.0
Total Allocation to Aveage Risk Gastroenteritis	1.10	22.63	1.38	109.85	0.0	0.0	0.0	0.0
Maximum Resources Availabe ($R_p(t)$)	1533.6	728.0	656.6	1640.0	—	—	0.0	300.0

Figure 16.5.

Model 2 – High Respiratory Infection, Low Gastroenteritis Prevalence
(December - May)

District - Specific Allocation of Providers for Delivering Care
to Infants at "High Risk" to Gastroenteritis
(in hours)

Providers / Districts	DOCOP	DOCIP	NUROP	NURIP	OUTREACH			
					Education & Workup	Workup & Triage	Education, Workup & Triage	Total
0	1.37	7.30	1.70	35.70	0.0	0.0	36.51	36.51
1	0.21	1.12	0.26	5.49	0.0	0.0	6.09	6.09
2	0.95	5.06	1.18	24.72	0.0	0.0	26.09	26.09
3	0.42	2.25	0.52	10.98	0.0	0.0	12.59	12.59
4	0.32	1.68	0.39	8.24	0.0	0.0	9.39	9.39
5	0.21	1.12	0.26	5.49	0.0	0.0	5.89	5.89
6	0.21	1.12	0.26	5.49	0.0	0.0	6.09	6.09
7	1.05	5.62	1.31	27.46	0.0	0.0	28.72	28.72
8	0.42	2.25	0.52	10.98	0.0	0.0	12.43	12.43
9	0.32	1.68	0.39	8.24	0.0	0.0	8.92	8.92
Total Allocation to High Risk Gastroenteritis	5.46	29.21	6.82	142.80	0.0	0.0	152.73	152.73
Maximum Resources Available ($R_p(t)$)	1533.6	728.0	656.6	1640.0	—	—	152.73	300.0

Figure 16.6.

Model 2 – High Respiratory Infection, Low Gastroenteritis Prevalence
(December - May)

District - Specific Allocation of Providers for Delivering Care
to Infants at Risk to Respiratory Infections
(in hours)

Providers / Districts	DOCOP	DOCIP	NUROP	NURIP	OUTREACH			Total
					Education & Workup	Workup & Triage	Education, Workup & Triage	
0	7.90	12.31	2.19	89.54	0.0	20.58	0.0	20.58
1	1.66	2.49	0.46	18.85	0.0	5.71	0.0	5.71
2	7.48	11.23	2.08	84.82	0.0	22.52	0.0	22.52
3	2.33	6.95	0.49	53.36	0.0	0.0	0.0	0.0
4	3.35	9.84	0.70	75.48	0.0	0.43	0.0	0.43
5	1.25	1.87	0.35	14.14	0.0	4.16	0.0	4.16
6	1.66	2.49	0.46	18.85	0.0	5.82	0.0	5.82
7	17.46	26.20	4.85	197.92	0.0	49.18	0.0	49.18
8	6.65	9.98	1.85	75.40	0.0	25.62	0.0	25.62
9	3.74	5.61	1.04	42.41	0.0	13.26	0.0	13.26
Total Allocation to Respiratory Infections	53.50	88.98	14.47	670.77	0.0	147.28	0.0	147.28
Maximum Resources Available ($R_p(t)$)	1533.6	728.0	656.6	1640.0	–	–	–	300.0

Figure 16.7.

Model 3 — High Gastroenteritis, High Respiratory Infection Prevalence
(October - November)

District - Specific Allocation of Providers for Delivering Care
to Infants at "Average Risk" to Gastroenteritis
(in hours)

Providers / Districts	DOCOP	DOCIP	NUROP	NURIP	OUTREACH			
					Education & Workup	Workup & Triage	Education, Workup & Triage	Total
0	0.79	1.84	0.99	8.92	0.0	0.0	27.38	27.38
1	0.26	0.61	0.33	2.97	0.0	0.0	9.45	9.45
2	1.19	2.75	1.49	13.39	0.0	0.0	41.71	41.71
3	0.40	0.92	0.49	4.46	0.0	0.0	14.53	14.53
4	0.93	2.14	1.16	10.41	0.0	0.0	33.83	33.83
5	0.10	0.28	0.10	1.35	5.86	0.0	0.0	5.86
6	0.26	0.61	0.33	2.97	0.0	0.0	9.61	9.61
7	4.22	9.79	5.28	47.60	0.0	0.0	147.81	147.81
8	1.58	3.67	1.98	17.85	0.0	0.0	57.84	57.84
9	0.79	1.84	0.99	8.92	0.0	0.0	28.07	28.07
Total Allocation to Average Risk Gastroenteritis	10.52	24.45	13.13	118.86	5.86	0.0	370.24	376.10
Maximum Resources Available ($R_p(t)$)	1533.6	728.0	656.6	1640.0	—	—	—	750.0

Figure 16.8.

Model 3 – High Gastroenteritis, High Respiratory Infection Prevalence
(October - November)

District - Specific Allocation of Providers for Delivering Care
to Infants at "High Risk" to Gastroenteritis
(in hours)

Providers					OUTREACH			
Districts	DOCOP	DOCIP	NUROP	NURIP	Education & Workup	Workup & Triage	Education, Workup & Triage	Total
0	1.68	8.99	2.10	43.98	0.0	0.0	44.98	44.98
1	0.25	1.39	0.32	6.77	0.0	0.0	7.51	7.51
2	1.16	6.23	1.45	30.45	0.0	0.0	32.14	32.14
3	0.52	2.77	0.65	13.53	0.0	0.0	15.50	15.50
4	0.39	2.07	0.48	10.15	0.0	0.0	11.57	11.57
5	0.25	1.39	0.32	6.77	0.0	0.0	7.26	7.26
6	0.25	1.39	0.32	6.77	0.0	0.0	7.51	7.51
7	1.29	6.92	1.61	33.83	0.0	0.0	35.39	35.39
8	0.52	2.77	0.65	13.53	0.0	0.0	15.31	15.31
9	0.39	2.07	0.48	10.15	0.0	0.0	10.99	10.99
Total Allocation to High Risk Gastroenteritis	6.72	35.99	8.40	175.92	0.0	0.0	188.15	188.15
Maximum Resources Available ($R_p(t)$)	1533.6	728.0	656.6	1640.0	—	—	188.15	750.0

Figure 16.9.

Model 3 – High Gastroenteritis, High Respiratory Infection Prevalence
(October - November)

District - Specific Allocation of Providers for Delivering Care
to Infants at Risk to Respiratory Infections
(in hours)

Providers					OUTREACH			
Districts	DOCOP	DOCIP	NUROP	NURIP	Education & Workup	Workup & Triage	Education, Workup & Triage	Total
0	0.79	0.48	0.18	3.49	0.0	0.0	21.38	21.38
1	0.16	0.10	0.04	0.73	0.0	0.0	4.62	4.62
2	0.75	0.46	0.17	3.30	0.0	0.0	20.44	20.44
3	0.29	0.18	0.07	1.29	0.0	0.0	8.16	8.16
4	0.41	0.25	0.10	1.84	0.0	0.0	11.63	11.63
5	0.12	0.07	0.03	0.55	0.0	0.0	3.42	3.42
6	0.16	0.10	0.04	0.73	0.0	0.0	4.62	4.62
7	1.74	1.05	0.40	7.71	0.0	0.0	47.56	47.56
8	0.67	0.40	0.15	2.94	0.0	0.0	18.57	18.57
9	0.37	0.22	0.09	1.65	0.0	0.0	10.30	10.30
Total Allocation to Respiratory Infection	5.47	3.32	1.26	24.24	0.0	0.0	150.71	150.71
Maximum Resources Available ($R_p(t)$)	1533.6	728.0	656.6	1640.0	—	—	—	750.0

Figure 17. Variations in the "Optimal" Model 1 Allocation of Outreach
Worker Time Among Papago Reservation Districts, As Generated
by (Five) Random Drawings on the Estimated Distributions of
Consumer Preference Weights

District	Mean*	Standard Deviation*	Coefficient of Variation
0	164.43	0.0 **	0.0 **
1	38.46	2.05	.05
2	169.39	9.96	.06
3	64.08	3.38	.05
4	96.00	6.50	.07
5	25.45	1.33	.05
6	36.82	2.33	.06
7	423.67	43.93	.10
8	159.98	13.82	.09
9	91.55	6.41	.07

*   Time in hours.
** All district 0 allocations were identical.

DISCUSSION

Based on earlier research by Indian Health Service scientists showing the effectiveness of certain GE and RI treatment programs Nutting et al. (1974), Torrance et al. (1975), the trends in the allocation results of section IV are to be expected. That they did emerge supports the internal validity of the model.

But beyond these trends, what the model does purport to provide are specific resource allocation prescriptions; over a particular time period, *how many* workers are required to implement the *most* effective intervention against GE and RI for *each* district, given *supply constraints*. However, just because this is a practical allocation question—perhaps even the most obvious—does not mean that it is always the one the planner will ask. Almost by definition, a manpower reallocation involves organizational change and the reordering of some group and individual priorities. Administrative considerations may limit the planner's range of decision making and permit the institution of only marginal and sporadic resource reallocations. Nonetheless, we adopt the view that it is valuable for the planner to have precise decision guidelines. For when the policy choice set is found to be restricted, such guidelines do indicate the desired *direc-*

tion of change. And when the policy maker has a freer hand, the allocation can reflect all of the available epidemiological, consumer preference, technological, and supply side information relevant to the problem. Practically, the planner's ability to implement a model is strengthened whenever provider groups are directly involved both in its development and subsequent improvement. While this approach to resource allocation has just recently been introduced and is not now a basis for decision making in the Indian Health Service, the aim is to develop an iterative planning process involving both IHS clinicians and consumer representatives in the refinement of the model.

All things being equal, an allocation model becomes more meaningful to policy makers as (1) the validity and reliability of its components are borne out (logically and statistically) by experience and (2) the allocation problem considered in the model approaches in scope the corresponding real-world problem that must be solved. Regarding the latter point, we hope to expand the model to include additional high-prevalence chronic and acute problems affecting the Papago tribe. As the focus extends to chronic disease, we should be able to utilize the wealth of information contained in the reservation's health information system to estimate statistically many of the transition rates and duration-of-stay parameters. But to consider chronic disease is also to complicate matters significantly from a theoretical standpoint. Program effects will often be delayed in time. Different age groups will be found to be in direct competition for scarce resources. The result is that one must squarely face the problem of converting to present value a potentially diverse set of expected program benefits.

In subsequent applications we hope to attack important validity and reliability issues with more precision; guidelines for such analyses have been suggested in recent work by Kaplan et al (1976), Bergner et al (1976), Pollard et al. (1976), and Reynolds et al. (1974). However, the focus of much of this paper throughout has been on conceptual problems in health program evaluation, and we conclude with several theoretical topics deserving further study:

Measuring the Quality of Health Care

Let $I = [i]$ be the entire set of intervention strategies *currently* being implemented against all diseases in the analysis. There will be a corresponding set of transition rate forecasts, $[\overline{TR}_{jm}^{d_i}(t)]$, and of duration-of-stay forecasts, $[\overline{D}_{jm}^{d_i}]$. Given these epidemiological estimates, the consumer preference weights $[U_j]$ and module populations $[P_m^{d_i}]$, there will be an associated value of the objective function of the allocation model, $\Delta H(t)$, calculated simply by direct substitution. But given the prevailing technology and the supplies of allocable resources, $[R_p(t), p = 1, \ldots, Q]$, maximization of the model leads to an intervention set $I^* = [i^*]$, which generates an expected total change in health status of $\Delta H^*(t)$. On the other hand, the assignment of status quo strategies ($I° = [i°]$) throughout the system leads to an objective function maximum of $\Delta H°(t) = 0$. We define the resource "constrained" quality of care associated with I as

$$X = \frac{\Delta H(t) - \Delta H°(t)}{\Delta H^*(t) - \Delta H°(t)} = \frac{\Delta H(t)}{\Delta H^*(t)}.$$

The index is bounded from above at one (defined as optimal quality) and may assume negative values. A value of zero indicates that implementing the set of strategies, I, is expected to induce a health state occupancy pattern in the population over period t which is *value-equivalent* to the pattern that would likely prevail were no interventions undertaken at all. In fact, χ must be non-negative for the given intervention set I to be of net benefit to a population.

The index represents a logical extension of a quality-of-care measure proposed by Bush et al. (1975) and illustrated by them in the context of emergency medical services evaluation. Like that quality index, χ reflects the crucial point that medical care outcomes are inherently stochastic. The implication is that the quality of care associated with the implementation of intervention set I is *not* to be measured in relation to actual set of outcomes which happens to emerge over the single period t. Rather, the intervention set should be judged in accordance with the pattern of outcomes that would emerge were the set implemented identically over many periods of length t. This information on expected outcome is captured in the transition rate and duration forecasts. Also like the model of Bush et al., the indexes here assume implicitly that certain minimum process standards of care are met in the performance of tasks. In future work we hope to implement χ on the reservation.[26]

Resource Allocation and Consumer Demand

Recent cost-effectiveness models have implicitly assumed that once the optimal distribution of manpower and facilities has been effected, the desired consumption of resources by the target population would follow. Consumer demand considerations have been given little attention. This omission may not be serious in analyses of screening programs, for instance, and it may not have been crucial in this study. All of the intervention strategies here involved direct home provision of care by outreach workers. Further, there are no money prices, as such, for care rendered on the reservation. However, "time prices" faced by consumers [see Acton (1975)] may be significant on the reservation and are likely to vary across districts. In future applications, the possibility should be acknowledged that these prices might potentially be altered to lower access barriers to care.

Competing Risks

The disease d transition rates (and perhaps durations-of-stay) applicable to the individuals in a module may, in general, be viewed as conditional on the prevalence patterns of other diseases to which they are at risk. Chiang (1968) has analyzed this problem of "competing risks" theoretically in a continuous-time Markov model of disease. The most straightforward way to handle competing risks in our model would be to respecify the transition rate (and possibly stage duration) parameters so that they are stochastically dependent upon a vector of relevant (competing) disease prevalencies. These parameters would then, in principle, reflect the indirect impact of other health problems on the apparent effectiveness of interventions aimed at disease d. (For a regression strategy to facilitate such an analysis, see [Lipscomb (1976)].)

Evaluation of Intertemporal Benefits

With chronic problems such as hypertension in the resource allocation model, one must directly confront the problems of estimating and then comparing at the margin, the benefits of health programs whose time flow of (health status) payoffs will differ markedly. For instance, Stage III of diabetes may endure, on average, for ten years and be characterized by relatively small transition rates to fatal and near fatal stages. On the other hand, Stage III of gastroenteritis may last on average about two days—but if an infant is not treated properly at that point, the likelihood of death is high. Such examples suggest that modules would need to be made age-specific and that the model would have to explicitly consider tradeoffs in securing health status benefits for individuals at different points in the life cycle. Related to this is the problem of converting future expected health status benefits to present value. The approach adopted by Torrance et al (1972), Bush et al. (1973), and Feldstein (1970) was to use a "social rate of discount."

What has not been emphasized sufficiently, we think, is that (1) arriving at a "social" rate of discount involves all of the conceptual problems of deriving a "social" value for a health state as such; (2) there is no obvious operational scheme for eliciting individual preferences for rates-of-discount for social goods, nor for aggregating these preferences even if they were known; and (3) the time-flow-mix of health care programs will, in general, be a function of the rate-of-discount adopted, so that particular population sub-groups should not, in fact, be indifferent about the social rate adopted.

We have no easy response to the first two assertions. However, regarding the third, one could solve resource allocation models employing a wide range of discount rates and then study the sensitivity of solutions to rate changes.

FOOTNOTES

*An earlier version of this paper was presented at the Annual Meeting of the American Public Health Association, Miami Beach, October 1976.

1. For a somewhat more detailed discussion of the model—particularly regarding its potential use in the measurement of the quality of care and its relationship to social indicator and social policy models of program evaluation—the reader is referred to Lipscomb (1976).

2. A number of health status indexes have been introduced in the literature, but only a few are readily adaptable for use in mathematical programming models, we have argued at some length in U.S. Department of Health, Education, and Welfare, Indian Health Service (1975). This does not imply that one cannot attempt to use such indexes, for example Chen's $-T$ Index (1975), to compare the health (defined in some fashion) of two or more populations. What it does imply is that these indexes are of little direct help to the policy maker who poses the question, "What's the likely health status improvement differential from putting health workers of type Z into population B versus C?" In principle, optimization models can address such a query because the expenditure of dollars (or physical resources) can be linked structurally to population health status change. One can then perform parametric analysis with crucial cost and resource parameters in the constraint set to trace out a loci of optimal solutions—one for each particular parameter set specification.

Torrance (1976) has argued that all of the major health indexes proposed in recent years can be classified into one of a handful of basic structural categories, and he reformulates several models to bring out that point. But it seems clear that certain indexes—particularly those of Bush et al. (1972, 1973, 1975) and Torrance—do contain considerably more information about population preferences for and movements among *levels* of human function. These models are potentially more sensitive instruments for resource allocation.

3. A similar result can be derived for the asymptotic expected prevalence of j, given that the interval of analysis at the random moment of entry. One can write:

$$_r\overline{pp}_j(t) = \sum_{i=1}^{N} \phi_i \sum_{k=1}^{N} \sum_{m=0}^{t} {}_rp_{ik}\, {}_rh_{ik}(m) \left[\delta_{ij} \cdot m + \right.$$

$$\left. \sum_{s=0}^{t-m} e_{kj}(s) \sum_{n=0}^{t-m-s} {}^{>}w_j(n) \right].$$

If $t = \infty$,

$$_r\overline{pp}_j(\infty) = \sum_{i=1}^{N} \phi_i \sum_{k=1}^{N} \sum_{m=0}^{\infty} {}_rp_{ik}\, {}_rh_{ik}(m)\, \delta_{ij} \cdot m$$

$$+ \sum_{i=1}^{N} \phi_i \sum_{k=1}^{N} \sum_{m=0}^{\infty} {}_rp_{ik}\, {}_rh_{ik}(m) \left[\sum_{s=0}^{\infty} e_{kj}(s) \sum_{n=0}^{\infty} {}^{>}w_j(n) \right]$$

$$= {}_r^m\overline{pp}_j + {}_r^m\nu_j(\infty) - \overline{\tau}_j, \text{ where}$$

$$_r^m\overline{pp}_j \equiv \sum_{i=1}^{N} \phi_i \sum_{k=1}^{N} \sum_{m=0}^{\infty} {}_rp_{ik}\, {}_rh_{ik}(m)\, \delta_{ij} \cdot m$$

is the expected prevalence of j from the random entry point to the first observable transition after the random entry;

$$^m\bar{p}_j(\infty) \equiv \sum_{i=1}^{N} \phi_i \sum_{k=1}^{N} \sum_{m=0}^{\infty} {}_rp_{ik} \, {}_rh_{ik}(m) \sum_{s=0}^{\infty} e_{kj}(s) \ ,$$

the expected number of entries (incidence) into j over an unbounded horizon which begins at the moment of the first transition after the random entry; and

$$\sum_{n=0}^{\infty} {}^>w_j(n) = \bar{\tau}_j.$$

4. Since the objective function is structured, in fact, to represent a *minimization* of value-weighted disability, the U_j are better thought of here as disutility weights whose numerical values are inversely related to state desirability. This interpretation of the weights is equally as valid as the usual "positive health" conceptualization, since the U_j are assumed to be no more than interval-scale numbers and thus unique up to any desired linear transformation.

5. However, since this production function is structured basically as a linear program, there is a concomitant assumption that the care rendered with inputs explicitly in the constraint set is subject to constant returns-to-scale. This may seem unduly restrictive, but several steps can be taken to weaken its practical impact. First, for any *particular* application one must determine the nature of the shortrun within which production is proceeding.

Then for that application the constraint set should include only the factors assumed variable. The cost of fixed factors can be calculated for long-run planning purposes. Second, if it is believed the constant returns assumption is violated within the relevant output range, one can divide the range into regions such that over each the assumption is more reasonable. One then would adjust the $A_{mp}^{di}(t)$ where needed to reflect the particular input proportion characteristics relevant to each output region. Third, from a modeling viewpoint one can "un-fix" fixed factors and calculate the maximum obtainable output from all relevant short-run configurations of medical care structure. This also implies that one can calculate the optimal long-run input configuration for the system. Of course, the ability of a decisionmaker to move to that *optimum optimorum* may be limited by an external dollar funding constraint or an absolute shortage of one or more productive factors. With all of these complexities, one might be tempted to opt for a simpler neoclassical production function approach to the allocation problem; indeed, such a Cobb-Douglas specification has been introduced by Auster et al. (1969), albeit for a somewhat different purpose. But in cases where there exists information on the task structure of medical care, to adopt that aggregate production function methodology is to preclude the opportunity for studying the effects of alternative treatments on patient outcomes. Adopting that methodology in some cases may lead to ignoring prior information on the task structure of medical care and thus precluding the opportunity to study the way in which alternative processes of care affect outcomes. As the work of Smith et al. (1972) and Lipscomb and Scheffler (1975) suggest, it is possible to construct activity analysis models which capture the diverse processes of medical care, yet yield readily interpretable solutions.

6. There are approximately 13,700 Papago living in and around three contiguous reservations in southern Arizona whose total land area is about 400,000 square miles, about the size of the state of Connecticut. About 49 percent of the population is male and about 64 percent under the age of 30. The average family size is 4.8. The health-care delivery and research activity of the Indian Health Service's Office of Research and Development is focused within the nine districts of the main (Sells) reservation and the single-district San Xavier reservation. There are about 150 villages and settlements and 9,000 Papago in these ten districts. Health services are rendered at a 50-bed hostital and an outpatient clinic at Sells; at

outpatient clinics in Pisinimo, Santa Rosa, and San Xavier; and in the field by Community Health Representatives (CHR's) and Nutrition Aides (NA's).

The estimated annual per capita income is less than $1,000; among adults the median highest grade of school completed is 7.2. The occupational distribution is farming (25.1 percent), unskilled labor (25 percent), skilled labor (9.5 percent), clerical and professional (9.4 percent), and unemployed (31 percent).

7. If an allocation model is focused on only a few (one, two, or three, perhaps) diseases, it may be convenient to define the set of all possible clinical disease stages as the set of health states. This is precisely how Torrance et al. (1972) have proceeded thus far, and they have been reasonably successful in assigning utility weights to these states. But as the domain of an allocation model is generalized to include an increasing number of diseases, the policy of christening each new stage as a new health state soon leads to a proliferation of states and a probable administration burden. Bush et al. (1972, 1973, 1975) have worked to develop a generalized set of function levels, supplemented by a comprehensive list of "symptom-problem complexes." The hope is that such a set is sufficiently dense with health state alternatives to permit one-to-one associations with disease stages if need be, yet not so dense with states as to preclude a successful assignment of utility weights by consumers.

8. The initial strategy had been to use scales for our four dimensions patterned after those employed by Chen et al (1975). We introduced a modified and expanded version of these scales to a small pilot sample of Papago and found that the item descriptions apparently did not adequately express the behavioral implications of suboptimal health as perceived by the Papago. Thus, a new set of dimension scales was developed which are believed to be more closely related, both in language and in functional description, to the Papago experience.

9. A somewhat different interpretation of the family dependence scale is that it may be used to measure the physical and emotional burden borne by family members in caring for the sick individual; the assumption is that this immediate spillover impact of ill health should be accounted for somehow in the allocation decision process. Now, it is not realistic, nor perhaps meaningful, to assume that the infant registers disutility from the empathetic knowledge that the family environment has been disrupted because of his sickness. Thus, in this particular model application it is probably more defensible to interpret the family dependence weights as measures of inconvenience, fear, or anguish inflicted upon those most closely involved with providing and caring for the infant.

10. The original instrument was in three parts, only two of which were employed in the analysis of preferences. A third, "force choice" part yielded responses which were not useful for the utility estimation model later adopted for the study.

11. There are only 59 separate scale items on Part II, because the ORD eliminated five possible items as illogical or highly unlikely.

12. The decision for now to exclude the death state from explicit consideration on the instrument was made by the ORD staff after consulting with Papago advisers; it was felt that, at this point, the focus should be on developing a preference elicitation format which would serve as an indicator of the consumer's willingness to render judgments about the relative utility of function levels. The view was, and is, that if this initial effort achieved significant consumer acceptance, modified instruments might then be introduced which would permit a closer examination of several empirical and methodological issues. The ORD staff excluded dimension levels corresponding to no dysfunction (i.e., good health) from Parts I and II to minimize the length of the instrument; it was felt that the utility weight for this most desirable state could be inferred from the other responses.

Bush and his colleagues have also had to cope with the problem of estimating a death-state preference, given data only on preferences for non-death states. A recent paper by Blischke, Bush, and Kaplan (1976) presents a multivariate analysis approach to determine scale end-points.

13. There is encouraging evidence that the instrument was acceptable and understandable. Of the 45 individuals originally approached, 42 volunteered to participate; and of these, 39 successfully completed all parts of the form. More than 70 percent of the respondents thought the item questions were "clear." For over 53 percent, both the questions and the instruments were "clear." The average completion time for the instrument was 20 minutes, and about 90 percent of the respondents were finished within 35 minutes. As we proceed in this planning effort with the advice and cooperation of the Papago tribe, an expansion toward a larger and more representative sampling framework will be of primary importance.

14. If we designate this angle as θ, then the perceived dysfunction of a DSI on dimension j, denoted by x_j, can be related to its utility scale value, s_j, by the formula $x_j = ms_j + b$, where $m = \cos \theta$ and b is some additive constant. The values of m and b are not affected by the value of j. We can then symbolically represent the perceived dysfunction of state i as

$$U_i = \sum_{j=1}^{r} x_{ij},$$ where x_{ij} is the particular DSI on dimension j associated with state i and r is the

number of dimensions. Substitution yields $U_i = \sum_{j=1}^{r} (ms_{ij} + b) = m\left(\sum_{j=1}^{r} s_{ij}\right) + rb$, which im-

plies that the perceived dysfunction of a state is being measured on an interval scale and can be expressed as the sum of perceived dysfunctions of the associated health state dimension scale items. A more complete discussion of utility estimation procedures is given in Appendix B, section (2).

15. Consider the expression $\nu_{jk} = (\tau_k - \mu_j)/\sigma_j$, where μ_j is the mean value of DSI j, τ_k is the mean value of category k, σ_j is the discriminal dispersion associated with DSI j, and ν_{jk} is a unit normal deviate. The area under the unit normal curve between $-\infty$ and ν_{jk} represents the model's prediction of the proportion of times that DSI j is judged less than or equal to category k. The computational procedure involves finding values for the μ's, τ's, and the σ's such that the best fit between the μ's and the observed proportions is obtained. It should be noted that there is no direct relationship between μ_j and the average category assigned to DSI j. We refer to μ_j as a "mean" in the sense that it is the center of an hypothesized normal distribution of the perceived dysfunctions that subjects attach to DSI j. While the value of μ_j certainly affects the subjects' responses, that relationship is indirect. It should also be noted that the τ's and μ's lie on the same interval scale; i.e., subjecting the τ's and μ's to the same linear transformation, does not alter the model's predictions concerning the proportions. If $\tau'_k = m\tau_k + b$ and $\mu'_j = m\mu_j + b$, then $\sigma'_j = m\sigma_j$ and $\nu'_{jk} = \dfrac{\tau'_k - \mu^{\circ}_j}{\sigma'_j} = \dfrac{m\tau_k - m\mu_j + b - b}{m\sigma_j}$

$\dfrac{\tau_k - \mu_j}{\sigma_j} = \nu_{jk}.$

The input to the successive categories procedure is a DSI's-by-categories matrix, where each cell represents the proportion of subjects responding to the DSI who judged its value as being less than or equal to the value of the category.

16. Derivation of a single set of state utility weights from the dimension weights given above involves at this point three tasks: (1) estimation (or assignment) of weights for the states corresponding to Good Health and Death; (2) transforming the dimension weights so that all are nonnegative; and (3) summing the four dimension weights corresponding to each state to arrive at state weights in accordance with the basic additive model assumed for now.

Recall that consumers were not directly asked in this initial application of the instrument to value Good Health and Death; but the basic model requires these utility weights nonetheless, so a somewhat arbitrary estimation procedure was devised. First, notice from the raw weights given above that "social limitation" appears to be the dimension which has the *least* undesirable consequences; that is, relative to the other three dimensions, scale items for social limitation are rather more negative. Notice also from Figure B.1 of Appendix B, that as the time of duration decrements logarithmically from 10 months, the disutility of item (2.2)—the *least* undesirable item on the social scale—decreases from −.75 to −1.20 to −1.86 to −2.58. If one linearly extrapolates these utility weights through two further logarithmic decrements, one finds that the disutility of 4.2 minutes of (2.2) (i.e., "Not being able to be with a few of your very close friends.") is about −3.80. This we designated as the utility weight for the Good Health category along each of the four dimensions. Proceeding similarly for the Death state, notice that the Pain/Anguish dimension was valued, overall, as a relatively undesirable dimension of health. Along this dimension, item 3.5 (i.e., "Very intense pain that would make you pass out") was assigned a value 1.32 at the seven-hour duration level and 1.949 at the three-day level. Extrapolating this utility difference forward for four successive logarithmic duration increments, one finds that the disutility of 8.33 years of intense pain is 3.836. This we designate as the utility weight for the death item along each of the four dimensions. *We emphasize that these are crude estimates not derived from the Thurstone scaling procedures used to determine the intermediate state weights; in particular, the death disutility weight should be viewed as a perhaps reasonable, but finally arbitrary estimate.* It should be the aim of future preference elicitation efforts to secure information for a more direct estimate of this important parameter.

Finally, given the values assigned to the end-point items, Good Health and Death, each raw scale item value s_{ij} given in Part (2) (b) of Appendix B was mapped onto the 0–1 interval by the linear transformation, $x_{ij} = .498 + .131 \, s_{ij}$. The discriminal dispersion of each transformed item value is the product of the discriminal dispersion of the untransformed value and the multiplicative constant in the linear transformation, .131. The transformed data are given in Figure 7 in the text.

The weight for each intermediate (non-Good Health and non-Death) dimension item indexes the relative disutility associated with three days of occupancy in the condition depicted by the item. To be internally consistent, we arbitrarily let 0 and 1.0 represent the disutilities associated with *three* days of Good Health and *three* days of Death, respectively, along each dimension. Now since the duration-of-stay parameters, $\overline{D}_j$, in the basic model will be expressed in terms of days, the U_j in the objective function must, in fact, represent utility *per day* of occupancy in state j. Note, however, that no distortion occurs if we redefine each of the above dimension scale item weights as the "utility *per day* of occupancy if the occupancy is three days." The *relative* positions of all weights are maintained under this interpretation, which is all that matters.

17. Infants were assigned to GE risk levels on the basis of a Bayesian analysis of factors thought to affect both the probability of incurring the disease and its severity once Stage I has been entered. The analysis, Sanders (see Department of Health, Education, and Welfare, Indian Health Service (1975) focuses on the production of a posterior odds ratio which indicates the ratio of the probability that the infant is at high risk to the probability that he/she is at average risk to GE. To develop a general expression for this ratio, first let us assume conditional independence of the data. Then we can write:

$$\ln \text{POR (HR:AR)} = \sum_{i=1}^{R} \ln \text{LR}(x_i) + \ln \text{PROR (HR:AR)}$$

where ln = the natural logarithm function,

POR(HR:AR) = posterior odds ratio of high-risk to average-risk level,

PROR(HR:AR) = prior odds ratio or high-risk to average-risk infants,

LR(x_i) = the likelihood ratio associated with the ith potential risk factor, given the observation x_i on that factor, and

R = the number of potential risk factors.

If POR(HR:AR) > 1, the infant is assigned to the high-risk group; if POR(HR:AR) < 1, the infant is designated average risk. In the absence of prior information, PROR(HR:AR) is assumed to be unity, so that ln PROR(HR:AR) is zero.

Another way to express the likelihood ratio is:

$$\frac{\text{Prob (factor i present, given that infant is at high-risk)}}{\text{Prob (factor i is present, given that infant is at average risk)}}.$$

In practice, this ratio is estimated as the percent of the observed population possessing characteristic i who are at high-risk, divided by the percent possessing the characteristic who are at average risk. Clearly, calculation of this likelihood ratio requires some prior definition of the extent of GE morbidity associated with high risk and average risk infants. Researchers at ORD developed in 1972 a simple morbidity scoring system, which assigns an infant one point for each episode of GE and four points for each hospital day due to GE. In an earlier analysis by Nutting et al. (1974), an infant with more than five points accumulated over the three-month period from October through December, 1972, was assumed to have excessive GE morbidity and was assigned to the high-risk category; those who had fewer than five morbidity points over that period were placed in the average-risk category. For each of these infants, the presence or absence of a number of potential risk factors was noted, and it is on this basis that the LR(x_i) can be calculated.

Sanders began by examining the impacts of the following factors under the assumption that there were no significant factor interactions:

Birth weight less than six pounds
Principal guardian under 20 or over 40
Residence in a traditionally high prevalence village
More than five siblings
Family tendency to child neglect
Alcoholism in parent or guardian
Mental problems in parent or guardian
Overcrowded home

The first four factors can be measured objectively, while the final four must be estimated subjectively for each infant by health care personnel. Further experimentation revealed that the predictive power of the Bayesian model could be increased considerably by dropping the independence assumption and including among the x_i interaction terms involving two or more factors. In general, an interaction factor, consisting of n separate factors, was considered to be present for an infant if the infant possessed all of the n individual factors comprising the composite factors. Research to determine the most predictive set of individual and interaction risk factors for infant GE is continuing, so we will postpone further discussion of the choice of factors until the results of a more definitive analysis are available. It can be noted encouragingly that this initial Bayesian scheme yields a risk level classification that correlates well with the results of an earlier linear regression analysis performed on the same data by Englander and Strotz (1972).

18. However, it should be noted that we make no allowance in this application for the possibility that the transition rates and durations in certain modules may be statistically dependent with those of other modules. That is, the fact that an infant has had, or is highly susceptible to GE is not assumed here to affect the transition rates and durations-of-stay for RI, and vice versa. Thus, the problem of competing risks is not fully dealt with, in the sense that transition rates and durations for one indicator disease are not made conditional on those for other diseases. We view this as an important topic for further research.

19. These are, in no particular order, Pisinimo, Gu Vo, Gu Achi, Sells, Chukut Kuk, Baboquivari, Schuk Toak, Sid Oidak, Hickiwan, and San Xavier.

20. Because of a scarcity of health-care manpower during each of these periods, ORD

researchers were able to observe the outreach component of the health care system operating implicitly within a loose quasi-experimental design in which parent education and infant problem-solving algorithms could be administered to only a subset of the infant target population. Specifically, over the October-December GE observation period, 38 infants high-risk and 30 average-risk infants (age 0–2) received intervention, and their function status was monitored by the system. Over the two-month observation period for respiratory infection, 32 individuals (age 0–4) were subject to intervention A, 31 others were administered task C, and 110 others received no preventive intervention. Unlike the GE data, these observations were derived from a study of several major villages on the reservations and therefore do not represent anything like a complete enumeration of the children at risk during the period. Certain inherent weaknesses in these data for our purposes are evident: (1) the number of observations is relatively small and would be smaller still if only the subset of children age 0–1 were included; (2) the impact of outreach worker triage, especially transportation provision, is not gauged, and (3) there is but one observation interval specified for each disease, so that it is not feasible to estimate the $\overline{TR}_{jm}^{d_i}$ by the usual statistical methods.

21. By varying U* appropriately, one can cause U*T̄* to take on all possible values that the right-hand side expression could, in fact, assume. Consequently, one could test the sensitivity of solutions to variations in U*—and thus to variations in the individual's health status over T̄*.

22. Task-specific estimates of resource requirements for patient care have been employed in the production studies of Smith et al. (1972), Kilpatrick et al. (1972), and Lipscomb and Scheffler (1975), among others. But data for these estimates were generated in a few private practice and experimental settings. The accuracy of our model will doubtlessly be strengthened as estimates from subsequent production studies on the reservation are incorporated.

23. Similarly, we would expect the allocation results in this application of the model to be robust with respect to the choice of the death state weight itself—a welcomed possibility given our ad hoc procedure (described in Appendix B) for obtaining a value for U_δ.

24. Clearly, the same issue rises regarding the effects of randomness in the transition rate and duration-of-stay variables. In this model application there is insufficient data to estimate the relevant distributions, and we thus postpone consideration of this point.

25. We are continuing to investigate this problem in light of the computational algorithm employed here, a modified Balasian procedure developed at the Rand Corporation [Geoffrion and Nelson (1968)].

26. For a more thorough discussion of this "systems" approach to quality measurement and for a regression strategy for obtaining intervention-specific forecasts of transition rate and duration-of-stay parameters, see Lipscomb (1976).

APPENDIX A
Narrative Stage Descriptions

Infant Gastroenteritis

Stage I

Physical Dysfunction—The baby's activity is curtailed; he may vomit once or twice a day, but eats and drinks fairly well. The infant is alert and physically active, but suffers 6–10 loose stools/24 hours period. Possibly has a low-grade fever. There is a minimal effect on physical status at this stage. Appetite and play activity are not impaired.

Social Dysfunction—Frequent trips to toilet and need for diaper change mean infant must stay close to home. The infant remains mentally alert and can enjoy a generally normal family life in the home. The infant plays, eats, and sleeps in a relatively normal fashion.

Pain-Anguish-Discomfort—Little pain except possibly diaper rash; would be apparent to child when diaper was changed. Infant may have the discomfort associated with low-grade fever. Infant suffers minimal pain. Child is comfortable between episodes of diarrhea.

Family Dependence-Disruption—At least one parent (probably mother) is forced to stay at home. Family life is not disrupted, but the infant's caretaker has to be constantly on alert to change diapers, treat diaper rash, and give the child plenty of liquids. Very little family disruption except for frequent diaper change.

Stage II

Physical Dysfunction—The infant remains physically active, but physical mobility is limited by the 6–10 watery stools likely per 24-hour period and by vomiting. The infant is likely to be hindered by a low-grade fever.

Social Dysfunction—Infant is fussy; often hungry and frustrated because he cannot understand reason for restrictions on food intake. Infant tends to be irritable at times, prompted by loose stools and diaper rash. Sleep may be disturbed.

Pain-Anguish-Discomfort—Diaper rash causes persistent discomfort, which worsens during stools, which are frequent. Infant feels quite ill from nausea. Child is quite uncomfortable even when not having diarrhea.

Family Dependence-Disruption—Normal household functions of mother disrupted; constant care of infant needed and frequent diaper change may necessitate extra laundry burden. Child may have to be separated from rest of family to avoid spread of disease. The caretaker spends increased time in observing infant fluid intake. The infant's diarrhea and irritability are becoming a source of frustration to the parents.

Stage III

Physical Dysfunction—Infant is plagued by frequent mushy stools. Fever is present and there is difficulty in keeping down even clear fluids. Infant must stay confined to sleeping quarters of house.

Social Dysfunction—Infant is very ill. Little social interaction except with mother or nurse. May require hospitalization, which would involve adjustment to new surroundings. Infant is very fretful and irritable. Will generally be severed from normal social relationships, including those involving outside day care. Child cries frequently, sleeps poorly or excessively, and can engage in no play activity. Infant's overall appearance is unhappy. He may be anxious and demanding.

Pain-Anguish-Discomfort—Child is anguished, irritable most of the time. Infant's buttocks and perianal skin are red and very tender. Nausea and fever are persistent and cause the child to be very fussy. Specific abdominal discomfort may be observed, especially in association with bowel movements. Infant may engage in continuous crying and will be in a general state of discomfort.

Family Dependence-Disruption—Hospitalization will likely cause one or both parents to give up normal activity, resulting in some family members being left alone at home or to be cared for by neighbors or other members of extended family. Wage earner in family is likely to miss some work and thus reduce family income. There may also be considerable parental fear of implications of medical therapy, such as blood drawing. Parents may fear for child's life and thus feel continual anguish. Child's caretaker is generally frustrated by the inconvenience of caring for patient constantly. Mother is required to forego most normal activities to care for child. Great disruption of family life. Infant requires nearly constant attention because of diaper changes, efforts aimed at getting child to drink, and general comforting that is required for an unhappy child.

Stage IV

Physical Dysfunction—Rapid deterioration of infant's strength. Mobility quite limited. Eyes sunken. The infant is listless and weak, with minimal physical activity. Infant's skin color is poor, tears are minimal, little or no urine output. Infant exhibits marked lethargy.

Social Dysfunction—Infant is very ill. No social interaction except with mother or nurse. Will require hospitalization, which would involve adjustment to new surroundings. Infant can no longer stay in home and must be hospitalized. He will tend to be sleepy and will have little personal involvement or interaction with other members of the family. Infant is listless, cries weakly, is unable to play, and has little interest in activities around him.

Pain-Anguish-Discomfort—Infant experiences considerable pain and anguish when dehydration is mild, and discomfort becomes intense as dehydration becomes severe. However, anguish subsides if severe comatose condition develops.

Family Dependence-Disruption—Infant will require transportation to and care in hospital, which may cause some family members to be neglected at home and others to miss work and forego income. Infant requires the constant attention of one or more persons (if not in hospital, then likely caretakers are mother and father). Parents no longer able to work normally. Infant is totally dependent on fluids that are administered by parents, if he is not hospitalized.

Infant (Lower) Respiratory Infections

Stage B

Physical Dysfunction—Infant is physically active, but there is possibility that difficulty in sleeping can lead to daytime fatigue. Infant has runny nose, sneezes, has a cough and scratchy throat; physical activities may be somewhat curtailed. Infant probably does *not* have earache or sore throat; slight fever could dampen desire for physical activity.

Social Dysfunction—Infant engages in normal social activity; eating habits are unchanged. Infant may have a decreased attention span. The child is alert and relates in the usual way with family, but may be a bit fussy.

Pain-Anguish-Discomfort—Infant suffers the discomfort associated with a runny nose, sneezing, coughing, a scratchy throat, and a mild fever. Unless his nose becomes tender from continual wiping, infant will probably feel nearly normal most of the time. The primary discomfort may derive from the necessity of mouth breathing, particularly at night, and the resulting sore throat.

Family Dependence-Disruption—Except for efforts to keep child out of inclement weather, there is little alteration in family behavior or activity. Infant tends to want to spend extra time with mother, forcing her to curtail some normal household activities. Infant's difficulty in sleeping will likely disrupt family sleeping patterns. Family needs to provide slightly increased attention and care, but unusual assistance is not needed. Except for periods of irritability and except for help in nose wiping, family behavior is hardly altered.

Stage C

Physical Dysfunction—Infant's mobility is not greatly impaired, but extent of activity may be limited by fever and other symptoms of severe cold. Child is not as active as usual and there is a decreased tolerance for activity. Patient may take many long naps. Activity may be further restrained because of vomiting accompanying cough.

Social Dysfunction—Child will not play as much as usual, and play will be less vigorous. Eating and sleeping patterns become disturbed. Infant will be confined to home; will have a decreased attention span. Social interaction is decreased at all levels, but child is not obviously lethargic. May want to spend much of day in quiet activity. Socialization outside home is greatly reduced, or nonexistent. Infant may be irritable, fretful, and is likely to cry frequently.

Pain-Anguish-Discomfort—Infant has persistent fever and discomfort from heavy congestion. Also may be pained by inflamed pharynx. There will be intermittent physical discomfort from coughing and wheezing, but the child may be comfortable when resting. There may be additional discomfort from vomiting, but this is most likely to occur when infant is coughing heavily. Infant feels generally ill and complains a great deal.

Family Dependence-Disruption—The child will need constant attention at home; special effort will be required to deal with his irritability. Mother's normal activities will be considerably disrupted. The infant is cranky, demanding, and disrupts family sleeping patterns with persistent coughing and crying.

Stage D

Physical Dysfunction—Child will appear to be quite ill, with breathing difficulties, wheezing, grunting, noises, or retractions, and stiff neck. Mobility greatly impaired. Infant will be less active than usual; he may appear extremely anxious and devote his total energies to the work of breathing. He will probably alter his feeding. Fatigue results from fever and efforts to breathe.

Social Dysfunction—The infant is quite irritable. There is little social interaction with family members; child tends either to sleep or demand continual attention of parents (particularly mother). Infant feels considerable anxiety, and this mood is transmitted throughout home environment. Infant has little or no interaction with anyone other than mother or nurse. Child will virtually cease all play activity.

Pain-Anguish-Discomfort—The child will experience considerable discomfort. Extreme lower tract congestion will be painful. The child may be uncomfortable, even at rest. Infant experiences the anguish of a high, persistent fever. The infant's face will swell, neck will be stiff; there will be flaring of the nostrils and considerable wheezing.

Family Dependence-Disruption—Family members are constantly involved in treatment of child. If infant is hospitalized, normal daily function of one or both parents is impaired, resulting possibly in neglect of other children or possible earnings loss because of missed work. All social engagements will be cancelled. Family is also worried that infant may need continual treatment and formal medical care. In severe cases, parents and brothers and sisters may fear for the life of the ill infant. Family sleeping patterns will be disrupted considerably, thus worsening fatigue and irritability among family members.

APPENDIX B
Health State Utility Estimation

(1) *Theoretical Comments*

The four health state dimensions constitute a taxonomy by which disease stages can be classified. We have made the assumption that this taxonomy is present not only at the overt level—so that we can map disease stages into health states—but is also present at the cognitive level; we have assumed that when a subject perceives the dysfunction of a disease stage, he is attaching some value with respect to each of the dimensions of that stage. On the basis of these four values, the subject applies some sort of judgmental model and arrives at the value for the perceived dysfunction of the disease stage. It is assumed that we have developed a matrix of health states from these four health state dimensions and that each disease stage can be validly mapped into one element of this matrix. Thus, if utility weights can be estimated for each element of the health state matrix, the weights for the disease stages themselves are known.

In order to measure the perceived dysfunctions attached to a set of health states, the most straightforward procedure is to have subjects assess these states—each one considered as a complete entity—on rating scales and input these ratings to some model of perceptual processes; the output of this model would be the perceived values of the dysfunctions, assuming that the subjects behave in a manner analogous to the model. This approach has a limitation. Should we wish to expand the set of possible states, every element of the set must be rated to insure that all the perceived values lie on the same scale. An alternative to this is to develop a function taxonomy where each health state can be characterized according to the levels of the various attributes it possesses. The attributes, in the terminology we are using, are the health state dimensions. If we can then measure the perceived dysfunctions for all the dimensions and if we can assume that the taxonomy contains all the relevant dimensions that might enter into the perception of the state, then it is reasonable to suppose, as researchers such as Bush have suggested, that a functional rule can be found which relates the various perceptions of the separate dimensions to the overall perceived dysfunction associated with each state. Should the state set be expanded, perceived dysfunctions for the new elements can be computed by locating the new states in the taxonomy and inputting the dimension values into the functional rule.

The search for functional rules has been given two different labels in the literature. The first of these is polynomial conjoint measurement; it has been developed by Luce and Tukey (1964) and has been implemented as a computational procedure. The other is functional measurement, which has been developed by Anderson (1970), who has tended to use the standard analysis of variance for the computational implementation of his procedure. In both of these methods, the objective is the same: given a set of observations which are assumed to be the result of some underlying components that lie on one or more dimensions, find the rule which combines the components and then assign values to the components such that the predictions of the model using these values fit the data as closely as possible.

For our purposes, such a procedure would involve using as our observed data the perceived dysfunctions attached to various states and their dimensions. With these values and a knowledge of the components (i.e., health state dimension levels) that each disease possesses, we could then apply functional measurement analysis in an effort to determine if the functional rule for the aggregation of dimension effects is additive, multiplicative, etc. Having decided on the nature of the rule, values for the levels could then be computed by regression techniques. Since our input data had been measured on an interval scale, in all likelihood the levels would also lie on an interval scale. Validation of the model and validation of the values assigned to the levels are intrinsically linked, since one is the direct consequence of the other. Should poor fits to the data be obtained, we have no way of knowing if this is the result of errors in the computation of the values or the model being inappropriate. Since we must assume that the model is at fault, it is clear that a model's robustness is limited by its computational implementation.

Validation of our perceived dysfunction model could take several forms. The most straightforward would be to expand the disease set and get perceived dysfunction values for the new members. If the model is valid, then we should be able to predict these values from knowing the positions in the health state taxonomy of the new members.

(2) *Implementation of the Thurstone Successive Interval Estimation Procedure*

(a) Two sets of ratings for the health state dimension scale items were analyzed. Recall regarding Part I that subjects placed the sixteen DSI's on a single 40 point scale. For Part II recall also that a set of four time periods (seven hours, three days, one month, ten months) was attached to each of the DSI's; 59 of 64 time-DSI combinations were then judged on separate 12-point preferability scales. Both sets were judged by the 42 subjects and the ratings were input to the successive categories analysis program. The resulting perceived values for each DSI are plotted in Figure B.1. Dotted lines have been drawn to connect the perceived values of the four DSI's of each health state dimension as derived from the Part I responses; solid lines connect the values of the four DSI's of each time-dimension scale combination. Visual inspection of these plots reveals, first, that perceived dysfunction was a monotonic function of duration for all four DSI's of all four dimensions. Second, while individual fluctuations did exist, in general the ordering of the DSI's for a dimension was the same for all time periods as well as for when no time period was specified.

While the two sets of rating differed with respect to the existence of a time specification and the nature of the rating instrument, the results seem quite comparable. To investigate this further, we computed correlation coefficients between the values from the first (Part I) set and the values for each of the time periods from the second set. These correlations were:

	Second Set (Part II)			
	Seven hours	Three days	One month	10 months
First Set (Part I)	.280	.519	.741	.651

Since the category scaling model, by definition, produces as interval scale of level and category values, these results indicate that the ratings in both sets are based on the same interval scale and that subjects tended to impose a duration of close to one month on a state dimension when asked to judge it in the absence of a time specificat on.

(b) The 16 preference numbers used for computing the health state utility weights were derived on the basis of the 42 responses to the 16 items from Part II of the preference solicitation instruments pertaining to dimension items of three-day duration. These numbers are first presented on the normalized interval scale produced by the computer algorithm which implements the Thurstone successive categories method. Dimension scale items are denoted by the numerical nomenclature introduced in the text above; thus item 3.2 corresponds to the pain/anguish dimension level, "A small pain in one part of your body." The raw weights and associated discriminal dispersions are:

Physical Limitation			Social Limitation		
Dimension Scale Item	Weight	Discriminal Dispersion	Dimension Scale Item	Weight	Discriminal Dispersion
1.2	-.652	1.261	2.2	-.1855	1.446
1.3	-.858	1.245	2.3	-1.012	1.255
1.4	-.699	1.228	2.4	-1.338	1.444
1.5	1.151	1.585	2.5	-1.237	1.213

Pain/Anguish			Family Dependence and Environmental Disruption		
Dimension Scale Item	Weight	Discriminal Dispersion	Dimension Scale Item	Weight	Discriminal Dispersion
3.2	-.542	1.321	4.2	-.742	.981
3.3	-.026	1.081	4.3	.065	1.166
3.4	.813	1.236	4.4	-.081	1.145
3.5	1.949	2.067	4.5	-.092	1.449

See footnote 16 for a discussion of how these values were transformed into preference weights for the health states employed in the analysis.

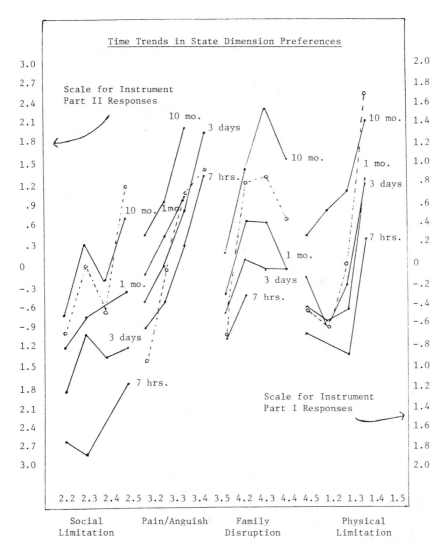

Figure B.1

APPENDIX C

Derivation of Task Times for Treatment and Prevention of Infant Gastroenteritis and Infant Respiratory Infections

As a preliminary, it is useful to note that there may be more than one outpatient or outreach worker contact per episode of GE or RI. Thus let z^{di}_{fjmp} be the amount (in hours) of resource p required *per patient contact* in module m to treat disease d according to intervention i, given that the patient has arrived at stage j from f. The following discussion summarizes the logic and the assumptions employed by the IHS scientists in arriving at the task time estimates given in Figure 14.

GE Outpatient Visit. Infant's history is read from outreach worker charts and certain items may be rechecked, including perhaps rectal temperature, tears, existence of soft spot, appearance of eyes and skin. Additional diagnostic tasks include stool culture, stool smear, total white blood count, and urine examination. Electrolyte solution and other medications administered as needed. Presence of leukocytes on stool smear > 5/hpf is strongly indicative of a bacterial etiology; use of ampicillin or Neomycin may be indicated prior to obtaining culture results. Parents/guardians are counseled in proper care of infant with GE at the stage indicated. Physician time per infant and nurse time per infant are estimated, respectively, at .20 hours and .25 hours. Let DOCOP and NUROP represent, respectively, the physician and nurse inputs in an outpatient seting. Then we could write $z^{GE}_{DOCOP} = .20$ and $z^{GE}_{NUROP} = .25$. Although there will obviously be some exceptions, one clinic visit per episode is assumed, so that $Z^{GE}_{DOCOP} = .20$ hours and $Z^{GE}_{NUROP} = .25$ hours.

GE Inpatient Visit. On the day of admission, a physician will spend .75 hours on initial work-up plus an estimated .84 hours on additional care activities. The physician will expend .41 hours/days during the remaining days of the infant's hospital stay. Assuming an average length-of-stay of ten days, that amounts to 3.19 hours of care after the first day. Additionally, about 20 percent of all infants will suffer a relapse, requiring the physician to put in about one-half of the time required on the day of admission. If we let DOCIP represent the physician inpatient input, $Z^{GE}_{DOCIP} = 5.44$ hours.

On the day of admission, the nurse will spend about .50 hours initially settling the patient and .33 hours carrying out initial physician orders. A diaper change and temperature check requiring a total of about .16 hours is required hourly throughout the remainder of the first day. There will be .33 hours worth of additional physician-generated tasks on that day.

Starting with the second day and continuing through the tenth, there will be about .33 hours of physician-generated tasks per day, plus about .08 hours of care required per hour around-the-clock. Assuming again a relapse in 20 percent of all admissions (so that one-half of the first day's tasks are repeated) and letting NURIP be the nurse inpatient input, Z^{GE}_{NURIP} = 26.50 hours.

RI Outpatient Visit. Physician will spend .20 hours in information gathering, .04 hours for throat culture, .12 hours for treatment planning, and about .01 hours for blood count per infant visit; the throat culture and blood count estimates reflect the assumptions that only 85 per cent and 20 per cent, respectively, of all infants receive these tasks. Thus, z^{RI}_{DOCOP} = .37 hours. Now about 50 percent of all infants will make a follow-up visit, regardless of stage at which initial visit occurred. Thus, the physician outpatient time required per episode can be expressed as Z^{RI}_{DOCOP} = .55 hours.

To be consistent with current delivery practices at the clinics, it is assumed that the physician plays the major role here and that the nurse will only be absorbed about .08 hours per visit (for information gathering). Then, z^{RI}_{NUROP} = .08 hours and Z^{RI}_{NUROP} = .12 hours.

RI Inpatient Visit. On the day of admission, physician will spend .75 hours at intake and .25 hours during the day monitoring patient progress. Physician monitoring on the second day requires .25 hours and about .125 per day for all succeeding days of stay. On the day of admission, nurse will be used .50 hours at intake and will spend .33 hours immediately thereafter carrying out physician instructions. Nurse will allocate 5 minutes per hour around the clock checking on infant, will be involved another .25 hours in response to physician orders, and will devote .25 additional hours on the first day to related care activity. On the second day, nurse spends a total of about .58 hours responding to physician orders, a total of about two hours on routine condition checks, and about .25 hours in related care activity. From the third day to the day of release, nurse will devote about 1.42 hours/day to the patient. For patients admitted at Stage C, the average length-of-stay is 6 days; for patients admitted at Stage D, it is 10 days. Thus, $Z^{RI}_{B,C,DOCIP}$ = 1.75; $Z^{RI}_{C,D,DOCIP}$ = 2.25; $Z^{RI}_{B,C,NURIP}$ = 11.84; and $Z^{RI}_{C,D,NURIP}$ = 17.52 hours.

Outreach Worker Effort. The principal input being allocated in this application of the model is the outreach worker. For both GE and RI, outreach worker time required per infant over period t is intervention-specific. The worker's activities related to GE and RI may involve preventive and curative educational tasks, information gathering, treatment planning, some treatment, and triage if appropriate. While the field-based care and treatment of GE and RI are generically similar, the precise contents of the tasks vary, of course, between the two diseases.

Figure C.1 is an outline of the activities involved in GE tasks A, individual education. The GE task C defined in this study calls for the outreach worker to complete the Task C contained in Figure C.2, plus the information gathering and disease staging routine as summarized in Figure C.3. The respiratory infection Task A is also designed as a patient education routine, and its contents are summarized in Figure C.4. The information gathering, treatment planning, and treatment algorithm, which is defined as RI Task C, is depicted in Figure C.5.

In developing time estimates for these outreach worker activities, a number of assumptions and operational decision rules were employed. For each educational and for each treatment-rendering task, summary estimates of the total amount of worker time required per episode were made by the IHS staff. These times are assumed not to vary by district nor by disease stage at which the tasks are first administered. This invariance by district assumes, in particular, that workers can be sufficiently dispersed about the reservation that the expected time required for a house call for a given purpose does not vary systematically by district. This condition clearly can be approximated in principle, and is not grossly violated by the current distribution of workers among districts.

A recent estimate of the distribution among the districts of Community Health Representatives is as follows: Baboquivari, 4; Gu Vo, 3; Hickiwan, 2; Gu Achi, 2; Sif Oidak, 2; Chukut Kuk, 2; and Schuk Toak, 3. Nutrition Aides were located as follows (fractions indicate NA-equivalents): Baboquivari, 1.5; Gu Vo, 1; Hickiwan, 1; Gu Achi, .5; Sif Oidak, 1; Chukut Kuk, .5; and Schuk Toak, .5.

On the other hand, it is explicitly assumed that the amount of outreach worker time required for triage to a clinic or to the hospital at Sells is a function of the district of occupancy. For each district, estimates were developed for the average triage time from a typical home in the district to the closest clinic and also from the typical home to Sells. The heavy dots on the Reservation map in Figure C.6 designate four clinics—at Pisinimo, at San Xavier, at Santa Rosa in Gu Achi, and at the Sells hospital. The most reliable published information on distance and travel times within the reservation is based on a 1967 study, part of whose results are summarized in Figure C.7. To choose a travel time from a typical home in each district to Sells, we computed a weighted average of the travel times from each village listed in the district, with each weight being the fraction that village population is of the total of all village populations in the district. If we assume that the relative dispersion of infants across villages in a district is proportionally related to the relative dispersion of the general populations across villages in a district, our approach can be viewed as a crude attempt to weight each village travel time by its probability of occurrence, given that a triage *from the district* is to occur.

For districts whose appropriate clinic is also at Sells, no further calculation is required. But estimating triage time to Santa Rosa and Pisinimo involves new problems, since information or travel times comparable to that contained in Figure C.7 is not available. Thus, a second, cruder approach was taken in which triage occurring *within* either the Pisinimo or Gu Achi districts was assumed to require the same outreach worker time as triage to Sells from within the Sells district. Also, triage to either of the two clinics from an adjacent district (the only other possibility) was assumed to require the same worker time as triage from the Chukut Kuk district to the Sells Clinic.

Finally, triage times from San Xavier, Santa Rosa, and Pisinimo to the hospital at Sells are, respectively, 1.17, .67, and 1.0 hours, as indicated in Figure C.7.

We turn finally to the outreach worker task times. These estimates are clearly approximations. In particular, for lack of more discriminating information we are forced to assume that field-based tasks which are generically similar, e.g. Task A for GE and Task A for RI, require approximately the same amount of worker time. The estimates are:

Task A (GE and RI)—1.5 hours per infant, administered once (if at all) during the optimization interval t. This estimate incorporates travel time and some allowance for normal "downtime" during the visit. It is convenient to view this resource usage as being independent of the various transition rates and rules of triage that govern the more curative resource consuming processes. Recall from section iii that $Z_{mp}^{d_i}$ represents the per infant consumption of resource p in module m from this one-shot, non-probabilistic prevention component. Here we have $Z_{OUTREACH}^{GE_A C} = 1.5$ hours $= Z_{OUTREACH}^{RI_A C}$, with the same estimate applying as well within intervention strategy A/C/T for each disease. The estimate thus is assumed not to vary across modules (i.e., districts and risk levels).

Task C (for GE and RI)—When performed as part of strategy A/C, it is assumed to require two home visits per episode (see Figure C.2), each requiring 1.5 hours of outreach worker time. Again, this per visit estimate includes travel to and from the infant's home and allowance for normal nontreatment activity at the home. When Task C is performed as part of Task T (triage), it is assumed to require 1.0 hours, encompassing the trip to the infant's home and delivery of care in the home prior to triage.

Task T (for GE and RI)—As noted, this time estimate will be a function of the infant's district and stage of occupancy (for the latter governs the rules of triage). Let OT_{mp} and IT_{mp} be the average outpatient and inpatient triage time requirements for input p from module (district) m. Then $OT_{mp} \cdot W_{fjm,OP}^{d_i} + IT_{mp} \cdot W_{fjm,IP}^{d_i} = TT_{fjmp}^{d_i} =$ expected triage time required of input p from district m, given intervention d_i and that the infant has just entered stage j and from stage f. The subscripts OP and IP in the triage probability expressions refer, respectively, to triage to outpatient and inpatient settings. In general, TT^{di}_{fjmp} is a component of Z^{di}_{fjmp}. For the present study, p = OUTREACH only, and triage time is added to Task C time (to get the time for C/T) or to Task C and Task A time (to get the time for A/C/T). Unlike for outpatient and inpatient care, the consumption of field-based resources varies by module.

Figure C.1.

TASK A   Individual Education (30 min.)

If Task A Has Been Done Within 2 Weeks, Then Do Task B

1. Causes of Diarrhea
    a. Virus
    b. Bacteria — most severe — need stool culture for diagnosis
    c. Parasites

2. Spread of Diarrhea
    a. Feces — human or animal — source of germs
    b. Food — spoiled or not refrigerated
    c. Flies — carry germs
    d. Water — stagnant or contaminated
    e. Garbage — germs and flies multiply

3. Prevention of Diarrhea
    a. Wash hands with soap after going to the bathroom
    b. Keep flies off of food and baby
    c. Use screens for fly control
    d. Make privy flyproof
    e. Boil baby's water
    f. Do not give baby milk that is left over from last feeding
    g. Keep baby's bottle nipple clean
    h. Avoid contact between baby and people with diarrhea

4. Danger of Diarrhea
    a. Dehydration — an emergency
        loss of water from blood
        loss of water from brain
    b. Spread to other people

5. Recognition of Dehydration — (Dehydration is an emergency)
    a. Sunken eyes
    b. Sunken soft spot
    c. Dry or sticky lining of mouth
    d. Few or no tears when crying
    e. Skin "tents"

6. Treatment of Diarrhea
    a. If dehydrated — to hospital immediately
    b. If no signs of dehydration present:
        (1) Give nothing by mouth for three (3) hours
        (2) Give clear fluids for 24 hours (small amounts given often)
        (3) Half strength milk or formula for 24 hours
    c. Give aspirin for fever
    d. If the cause is a bacteria — Doctor will prescribe antibiotic

Figure C.2.

TASK C   Education in the Use of
Electrolyte Solution (30 min.)

For Use only in Babies up to Two Years Old

1. Explain how to use it.
    a. Nothing by mouth for three (3) hours.
    b. Give electrolyte solution for 24 hours. (Small amounts given very often)
    c. Give half strength milk or formula for 24 hours.
    d. Instruct patient to watch for:
        (1) Signs of dehydration
        (2) If baby vomits and can't keep electrolyte solution down, must be seen at the clinic.

2. Explain why it is used.
    a. "Rests" the intestines
    b. Supplies water to replace losses in diarrhea
    c. Supplies electrolytes to replace losses in diarrhea
    d. Supplies calories

3. *Re-evalute the baby tomorrow – (go through history and physical examination and determine the stage in 24 hours).*

Figure C.3.

Standards of Stage Assessment for Gastroenteritis

Age Category: Babies up to Three Years Old

INFORMATION GATHERING	STAGE I	STAGE II	STAGE III	STAGE IV
24-hour follow-up				
5-day follow-up				
Is the baby less than three months old	No		Yes	
What is the baby's risk level? ☐ Average ☐ High				
Is the diarrhea mushy or liquid?				
Mushy – for how many days?	1-4	5-7	Over 7	
Mushy – how many in last 6 hours?	1-3	4-5	Over 5	
Liquid – for how many days?	1	2	Over 2	
Liquid – how many in last 6 hours?	1	2-3	Over 3	
Is there blood in the diarrhea?	No		Yes	
SUBJECTIVE				
Is there mucous in the diarrhea?	No	Yes		
Is the baby vomiting?	No	Yes		
For how many days?	1	2	Over 2	
How many times in last 6 hours?	1	2	Over 2	
Can the baby keep down clear fluids?	Yes		No	
Is the baby urinating a normal amount?	Yes		Deceased	
OBJECTIVE				
Rectal temperature	98-102°	102-103°	Over 103°	
Making tears when crying?	Yes		Deceased	No
Soft spot (fontanelle)?	Normal			Fallen
Lining of mouth	Moist			Dry or Sticky
Eyes look sunken in?	No			Yes
Skin tenting?	No			Yes

Figure C.4.

Community Health Representative Program

Respiratory Infection Educational Task A   30 Minutes

1. Colds are usually not serious
   a. No medicine or "shots" will cure a cold
   b. Cold will go away by itself

2. Babies with colds must be watched carefully, because they might develop a "complication" of the cold — pnemonia is main complication — also see infectious meningitis.

3. Danger signs in a baby with a cold
   a. High fever 0 - 3 months — 100
                   3 - 12 months — 100^5
                   1 - 4 years — 102^5
   b. Breathing fast — more than 40 times/minute
   c. Retractions — explain
   d. Flaring — explain
   e. Grunting — explain
   f. Wheezing — explain difference between wheezing and nasopharyngeal congestion

   — If any danger sign appears, should take to CHR or clinic right away.

4. Treatment
   a. Encourage baby to drink a lot of fluids — fruit juices are ideal.
   b. Liquid aspirin every 4 hours for fever
      1) 0 - 6 months   .3 cc
      2) 6 - 12 months   .6 cc

5. Prevention of Respiratory Infections
   a. Keep baby warm, but not too hot
   b. Baby's bed should be in a part of the room that has nearly constant temperature — avoid draft
   c. If baby gets a cold, watch for danger signs
   d. If danger signs appear, report this to CHR or clinic right away.
   e. Change baby's diapers when they are wet
   f. Encourage children to wear warm clothing and socks during cold weather.

Figure C.5.

Community Health Representative Program

Problem: Respiratory Infections

Age Category: Infants and Children up to 4 years

Information Gathering	Stage B	Stage C	Stage D
Subjective:			
How long has it been present?	less than 5 da.	5-7 days	7 da. or more
Is there coughing?	Yes/no		
Does he/she cough so hard he/she passes out or turns blue?	No		Yes
Does he/she indicate that the ear hurts?	No		Yes
Is there pus in the ear?	No		Yes
Does he/she have a sore throat?	No	Yes	
Is he/she throwing up?—after coughing only?	No		Yes
after each feeding?	No		Yes
Objective:			
Temperature: age 0-6 months	less than 100^{0}		100^{0} or more
age 6 months to 2 yrs.	less than 100^{5}	100^{5}-101^{5}	101^{5} or more
age 2 yrs. to 4 yrs.	less than 101	101-102^{5}	102^{5} or more
Respiratory rate	less than 32/min.	32-40/min.	40/min. or more
Are there retractions present?	no		Yes
Is there flaring of the nostrils?	No		Yes
Is there grunting when he breathes out?	No		Yes
Is there wheezing present when he/she breathes out?	No		Yes
Is the baby lethargic?	No		Yes
Does he/she have a stiff neck?	No		Yes

Assessment	Treatment Plan	1st
Well child	Do educational Task A	
Respiratory infection	Treat as below: do educational Task A & follow-up	1
Stage B	in 5 days; Refer to Clinic if not better	
Respiratory infection	Treat as below; do educational Task A & follow-up	1
Stage C	in 24 hrs.; Refer to Clinic if not better	
Respiratory Infection	Refer to Clinic right away	1
Stage D		

No sickness — medicine given to be kept on hand

Treatment

1. Fever or Headache   0-6 months-Acetaminophen drops 0.3cc every 4 hrs.
   (Use Acetaminophen   6-12 months-Acetaminophen drops 0.6cc every 4 hrs.
   Drops or Baby   12-18 months-Acetaminophen drops 0.9cc every 4 hrs.
   Aspirin tablets   18 mos.-2 yrs. — Baby Aspirin 75 mg. - 1 tablet for each
   75 mg.)   year of age, every 4 hrs.
2. Runny or stuffy nose: Saline nose drops 1 drop in ea. side / 3-4 hrs.

3. Coughing: (Use   /DO NOT GIVE TO BABIES LESS THAN 6 MOS. OLD
   Glycerol
   Guaiacolate Cough   6 mos. - 2 yrs. – ½ teaspoonful 3 times a day
   Syrup–   2 yrs. - 4 yrs. – ½ teaspoonful 4 times a day
4. Sore throat: Throat culture – label with name, date, number and village &
                        send to Disease Control Lab within 24 hrs.

5. Educational Task A
   Other: Encourage fluids
Identification   Last   First   Middle
Name: . . . .
B-date . . . . Age: . . . . Sex: . . . .   Signed: . . . .
                                                                              CHR (900)
ID - No.: . . . .
Residence: . . . .   Reviewed: . . . .
Location of Encounter: . . . .   CHR Supervisor
Date: . . . .

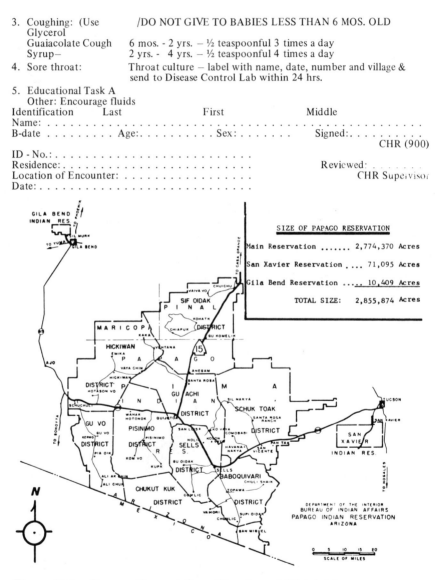

Figure C.6.   Papago Reservations (Roads and Districts)

Figure C.7.

Estimated Travel Time from Sells Hospital
to Principal Villages on Papago Reservation
(Distances, Direction, Population and Districts Indicated)

	Minutes to Sells	Miles	Average Speed	Direction	Population	District
Ali Chuckson	10	7.4	44	E	124	Baboquivari
Topawa	12	7.9	39	SE	252	Baboquivari
Gu Oidak	18	10.0	33	W	198	Sells
Havana Nakya	20	15.4	46	NE	71	Schuk Toak
Nolia	20	11.6	35	NW	25	Sells
Quijotoa	25	22.6	54	NW	97	Gu Achi
Cowlic	25	13.8	33	SW	91	Sells
Supi Oidak	25	17.6	42	SE	28	Baboquivari
San Luis	30	12.5	25	N	26	Sells
Choulic	30	19.2	38	SE	64	Baboquivari
Chiuli Shalik	30	20.5	41	SE	56	Baboquivari
San Miguel	35	22.8	39	SE	93	Chukut Kuj
Pan Tak	35	24.4	42	NE	45	Schuk Toak
Ko Vaya	35	15.1	26	N	38	Gu Achi
Vamori	35	19.1	33	S	63	Chukut Kuk
Comobabi	35	22.7	39	NE	76	Schuk Toak
Santa Rosa	40	33.7	51	NW	309	Gu Achi
Anegam	40	41.4	62	NW	146	Sif Oidak
Chuwut Murk	60	19.1	19	W	44	Pisinimo
Sil Nakya	60	37.5	38	Ne	58	Schuk Toak
Pisinimo	60	43.0	43	NW	170	Pisinimo
San Xavier	70	62.5	54	NE	563	San Xavier
Ventana	70	47.2	40	NW	71	Hickiwan
Kohatk	70	62.6	54	N	57	Sif Oidak
Schuchuli	75	56.6	45	NW	32	Hickiwan
Hotason Vo	75	56.3	45	NW	42	Hickiwan
Kom Vo	75	50.2	40	W	48	Pisinimo
Chuichu	80	71.4	54	N	268	Sif Oidak
Gu Vo	80	58.8	44	NW	154	Gu Vo
Kaka	90	53.2	35	NW	88	Hickiwan
Vaiva Vo	90	66.2	44	N	59	Sif Oidak
Hickiwan	90	60.2	40	NW	130	Hickiwan
Ali Chuk	120	73.8	37	SW	78	Gu Vo

APPENDIX D

Allocation Results Under Alternative Assumptions about Outreach Worker Availability

Figure D.1.

Model 1 – High Gastroenteritis, Low Respiratory Infection Prevalence
(May - September)

District - Specific Allocation of Providers for Delivering Care
to Infants at "Average Risk" to Gastroenteritis
(in hours)

Providers					OUTREACH			
Districts	DOCOP	DOCIP	NUROP	NURIP	Education & Workup	Workup & Triage	Education, Workup & Triage	Total
0	1.59	3.69	1.98	17.98	0.0	0.0	55.03	55.08
1	0.53	1.23	0.67	5.98	0.0	0.0	19.02	19.02
2	2.39	5.54	2.99	26.93	0.0	0.0	83.91	83.91
3	0.80	1.85	0.99	8.98	0.0	0.0	29.22	29.22
4	1.86	4.31	2.33	20.95	0.0	0.0	68.06	68.06
5	0.26	0.62	0.33	2.99	0.0	0.0	9.37	9.37
6	0.53	1.23	0.67	5.98	0.0	0.0	19.34	19.34
7	8.48	19.70	10.62	95.76	0.0	0.0	297.37	297.37
8	3.18	7.39	3.98	35.91	0.0	0.0	116.37	116.37
9	1.59	3.69	1.98	17.95	0.0	0.0	56.46	56.46
Total Allocation to Average Risk Gastroenteritis	21.23	49.25	26.55	239.40	0.0	0.0	754.19	754.19
Maximum Resources Available ($R_p(t)$)	1533.6	728.0	656.6	1640.0	–	–	–	1500.0

Figure D.2.

Model 1 — High Gastroenteritis, Low Respiratory Infection Prevalence
(May - September)

District - Specific Allocation of Providers for Delivering Care
to Infants at "High Risk" to Gastroenteritis
(in hours)

| Providers | | | | | OUTREACH | | | |
Districts	DOCOP	DOCIP	NUROP	NURIP	Education & Workup	Workup & Triage	Education, Workup & Triage	Total
0	3.39	18.09	4.22	88.48	0.0	0.0	90.49	90.49
1	0.51	2.79	0.65	13.61	0.0	0.0	15.10	15.10
2	2.34	12.53	2.92	61.25	0.0	0.0	64.66	64.66
3	1.04	5.57	1.30	27.22	0.0	0.0	31.19	31.19
4	0.79	4.17	0.97	20.42	0.0	0.0	23.27	23.27
5	0.51	2.79	0.65	13.61	0.0	0.0	14.60	14.60
6	0.51	2.79	0.65	13.61	0.0	0.0	15.10	15.10
7	2.60	13.92	3.25	68.06	0.0	0.0	71.19	71.19
8	1.04	5.57	1.30	27.22	0.0	0.0	30.80	30.80
9	0.79	4.17	0.97	20.42	0.0	0.0	22.11	22.11
Total Allocation to High Risk Gastroenteritis	13.51	72.40	16.89	353.90	0.0	0.0	378.51	378.51
Maximum Resources Available ($R_p(t)$)	1533.6	728.0	656.6	1640.0	—	—	—	1500.0

Figure D.3.

Model 1 – High Gastroenteritis, Low Respiratory Infection Prevalence
(May - September)

District - Specific Allocation of Providers for Delivering Care
to Infants at Risk at Respiratory Infections
(in hours)

Providers / Districts	DOCOP	DOCIP	NUROP	NURIP	OUTREACH			Total
					Education & Workup	Workup & Triage	Education, Workup & Triage	
0	0.12	0.07	0.03	0.51	0.0	0.0	3.14	3.14
1	0.02	0.01	0.01	0.11	0.0	0.0	0.68	0.68
2	0.11	0.07	0.02	0.49	0.0	0.0	3.01	3.01
3	0.04	0.03	0.01	0.19	0.0	0.0	1.20	1.20
4	0.06	0.04	0.01	0.27	0.0	0.0	1.71	1.71
5	0.02	0.01	0.00	0.08	0.0	0.0	0.50	0.50
6	0.02	0.01	0.01	0.11	0.0	0.0	0.68	0.68
7	0.26	0.05	0.06	1.13	0.0	0.0	6.99	6.99
8	0.10	0.06	0.02	0.43	0.0	0.0	2.73	2.73
9	0.05	0.03	0.01	0.24	0.0	0.0	1.51	1.51
Total Allocation to Respiratory Infection	0.80	0.49	0.19	3.56	0.0	0.0	22.16	22.16
Maximum Resources Available ($R_p(t)$)	1533.6	728.0	656.6	1640.0	—	—	—	1500.0

Figure D.4.

Model 1 – High Gastroenteritis, Low Respiratory Infection Prevalence
(May - September)

District - Specific Allocation of Providers for Delivering Care
to Infants at "Average Risk" to Gastroenteritis
(in hours)

Districts	DOCOP	DOCIP	NUROP	NURIP	OUTREACH			Total
Providers					Education & Workup	Workup & Triage	Education, Workup & Triage	
0	1.67	4.49	2.09	21.98	0.0	5.40	31.33	36.73
1	0.53	1.23	0.67	5.98	0.0	0.0	19.02	19.02
2	2.39	5.54	2.99	26.93	0.0	0.0	83.91	83.91
3	0.80	1.85	0.99	8.98	0.0	0.0	29.22	29.22
4	1.86	4.31	2.33	20.95	0.0	0.0	68.06	68.06
5	030	0.92	0.37	4.55	0.0	0.0	0.0	2.17
6	0.53	1.23	0.67	5.98	0.0	2.17	0.0	19.34
7	8.48	19.70	10.62	95.76	0.0	0.0	19.34	297.37
8	3.56	11.08	4.43	54.58	0.0	0.0	297.37	30.25
9	1.78	5.54	2.22	27.29	0.0	30.25	0.0	13.27
						13.27	0.0	
Total Allocation to Average Risk Gastroenteritis	21.91	55.89	27.37	272.99	0.0	51.09	548.25	599.33
Maximum Resources Available ($R_p(t)$)	1533.6	728.0	656.6	1640.0	—	—	—	1000.0

Figure D.5.

Model 1 — High Gastroenteritis, Low Respiratory Infection Prevalence
(May - September)

District - Specific Allocation of Providers for Delivering Care
to Infants at "High Risk" To Gastroenteritis
(in hours)

Providers / Districts	DOCOP	DOCIP	NUROP	NURIP	OUTREACH		Education, Workup & Triage	Total
					Education & Workup	Workup & Triage		
0	3.39	18.09	4.22	88.48	0.0	0.0	90.49	90.49
1	0.51	2.79	0.65	13.61	0.0	0.0	15.10	15.10
2	2.34	12.53	2.92	61.25	0.0	0.0	64.66	64.66
3	1.04	5.57	1.30	27.22	0.0	0.0	31.19	31.19
4	0.79	4.17	0.97	20.42	0.0	0.0	23.27	23.27
5	0.51	2.79	0.65	13.61	0.0	0.0	14.60	14.60
6	0.51	2.79	.065	13.61	0.0	0.0	15.10	15.10
7	2.60	13.92	3.25	68.06	0.0	0.0	71.19	71.19
8	1.04	5.57	1.30	27.22	0.0	0.0	30.80	30.80
9	0.79	4.17	0.97	20.42	0.0	0.0	22.11	22.11
Total Allocation to High Risk Gastroenteritis	13.53	72.40	16.89	353.90	0.0	0.0	378.51	378.51
Maximum Resources Available ($R_p(t)$)	1533.6	728.0	656.6	1640.0	—	—	—	1000.0

Figure D.6.

Model 1 – High Gastroenteritis, Low Respiratory Infection Prevalence (May - September)

District - Specific Allocation of Providers for Delivering Care to Infants at Risk to Respiratory Infections
(in hours)

Providers Districts	DOCOP	DOCIP	NUROP	NURIP	OUTREACH			Total
					Education & Workup	Workup & Triage	Education, Workup & Triage	
0	0.12	0.07	0.03	0.51	0.0	0.0	3.14	3.14
1	0.02	0.01	0.01	0.11	0.0	0.0	0.68	0.68
2	0.11	0.07	0.02	0.49	0.0	0.0	3.01	3.01
3	0.04	0.03	0.01	0.19	0.0	0.0	1.20	1.20
4	0.06	0.04	0.01	0.27	0.0	0.0	1.71	1.71
5	0.02	0.01	0.00	0.08	0.0	0.0	0.50	0.50
6	0.02	0.01	0.01	0.11	0.0	0.0	0.68	0.68
7	0.26	0.15	0.06	1.13	0.0	0.0	6.99	6.99
8	0.10	0.06	0.02	0.43	0.0	0.0	2.73	2.73
9	0.05	0.03	0.01	0.24	0.0	0.0	1.51	1.51
Total Allocation to Respiratory Infection	0.80	0.49	0.19	3.56	0.0	0.0	22.16	22.16
Maximum Resources Available ($R_p(t)$)	1533.6	728.0	656.6	1640.0	—	—	—	1000.0

Figure D.7.

Model 1 — High Gastroenteritis, Low Respiratory Infection Prevalence
(May - September)

District - Specific Allocation of Providers for Delivering Care
to Infants at "Average Risk" to Gastroenteritis
(in hours)

Providers / Districts	DOCOP	DOCIP	NUROP	NURIP	OUTREACH			
					Education & Workup	Workup & Triage	Education, Workup & Triage	Total
0	1.78	5.54	2.22	27.29	0.0	12.52	0.0	12.52
1	0.07	1.40	0.09	6.81	0.0	0.0	0.0	0.0
2	0.36	6.36	0.45	30.86	0.0	0.47	0.0	0.47
3	0.10	2.10	0.13	10.21	0.0	0.0	0.0	0.0
4	0.24	4.91	0.30	23.82	0.0	0.0	0.0	0.0
5	0.30	0.92	0.37	4.55	0.0	2.17	0.0	2.17
6	0.07	1.40	0.09	6.81	0.0	0.0	0.0	0.0
7	9.47	29.55	11.82	145.56	0.0	70.91	0.0	70.91
8	0.41	8.41	0.51	40.83	0.0	0.0	0.0	0.0
9	1.78	5.54	2.22	27.29	0.0	13.27	0.0	13.27
Total Allocation to Average Risk Gastroenteritis	14.58	66.14	18.20	324.03	0.0	99.34	0.0	99.34
Maximum Resources Available ($R_p(t)$)	1533.6	728.0	656.6	1640.0	—	—	—	500.0

Figure D.8.

Model 1 — High Gastroenteritis, Low Respiratory Infection Prevalence
(May - September)

District - Specific Allocation of Providers for Delivering Care
to Infants at "High Risk" to Gastroenteritis
(in hours)

| Providers | | | | | OUTREACH | | | |
Districts	DOCOP	DOCIP	NUROP	NURIP	Education & Workup	Workup & Triage	Education, Workup & Triage	Total
0	3.39	18.09	4.22	88.48	0.0	0.0	90.49	90.49
1	0.51	2.79	0.65	13.61	0.0	0.0	15.10	15.10
2	2.34	12.53	2.92	61.25	0.0	0.0	64.66	64.66
3	1.04	5.57	1.30	27.22	0.0	0.0	31.19	31.19
4	0.79	4.17	0.97	20.42	0.0	0.0	23.27	23.27
5	0.51	2.79	0.65	13.61	0.0	0.0	14.60	14.60
6	0.51	2.79	0.65	13.61	0.0	0.0	15.10	15.10
7	2.60	13.92	3.25	68.06	0.0	0.0	71.19	71.19
8	1.04	5.57	1.30	27.22	0.0	0.0	30.80	30.80
9	0.79	4.17	0.97	20.42	0.0	0.0	22.11	22.11
Total Allocation to High Risk Gastroenteritis	13.53	72.40	16.89	353.90	0.0	0.0	378.51	378.51
Maximum Resources Available ($R_p(t)$)	1533.6	728.0	656.6	1640.0	—	—	—	500.0

Figure D.9.

Model 1 – High Gastroenteritis, Low Respiratory Infection Prevalence
(May - September)

District - Specific Allocation of Providers for Delivering Care
to Infants at Risk to Respiratory Infections
(in hours)

Providers Districts	DOCOP	DOCIP	NUROP	NURIP	OUTREACH			Total
					Education & Workup	Workup & Triage	Education, Workup & Triage	
0	0.12	0.07	0.03	0.51	0.0	0.0	3.14	3.14
1	0.02	0.01	0.01	0.11	0.0	0.0	0.68	0.68
2	0.11	0.07	0.02	0.49	0.0	0.0	3.01	3.01
3	0.04	0.03	0.01	0.19	0.0	0.0	1.20	1.20
4	0.06	0.04	0.01	0.27	0.0	0.0	1.71	1.71
5	0.02	0.01	0.00	0.08	0.0	0.0	0.50	0.50
6	0.02	0.01	0.01	0.11	0.0	0.0	0.68	0.68
7	0.26	0.15	0.06	1.13	0.0	0.0	6.99	6.99
8	0.10	0.06	0.02	0.43	0.0	0.0	2.73	2.73
9	0.05	0.03	0.01	0.24	0.0	0.0	1.51	1.51
Total Allocation to Respiratory Infection	0.80	0.49	0.19	3.56	0.0	0.0	22.16	22.16
Maximum Resources Available ($R_p(t)$)	1533.6	728.0	656.0	1640.0	—		—	500.0

Figure D. 10.

Model 1 – High Gastroenteritis, Low Respiratory Infection Prevalence
(May - September)

District - Specific Allocation of Providers for Delivering Care
to Infants at "Average Risk" to Gastroenteritis
(in hours)

Providers Districts	DOCOP	DOCIP	NUROP	NURIP	OUTREACH			Total
					Education & Workup	Workup & Triage	Education, Workup & Triage	
0	0.21	4.21	0.26	20.42	0.0	0.0	0.0	0.0
1	0.07	1.40	0.09	6.81	0.0	0.0	0.0	0.0
2	0.31	6.31	0.38	30.63	0.0	0.0	0.0	0.0
3	0.10	2.10	0.13	10.21	0.0	0.0	0.0	0.0
4	0.24	4.91	0.30	23.82	0.0	0.0	0.0	0.0
5	0.03	0.70	0.04	3.40	0.0	0.0	0.0	0.0
6	0.07	1.40	0.09	6.81	0.0	0.0	0.0	0.0
7	1.09	22.44	1.37	108.89	0.0	0.0	0.0	0.0
8	0.41	8.41	0.51	40.83	0.0	0.0	0.0	0.0
9	0.21	4.21	0.26	20.42	0.0	0.0	0.0	0.0
Total Allocation to Average Risk Gastroenteritis	2.74	56.09	3.42	272.23	0.0	0.0	0.0	0.0
Maximum Resources Available ($R_p(t)$)	1533.6	728.0	656.6	1640.0	–	–	0.0	250.0

Figure D. 11.

Model 1 – High Gastroenteritis, Low Respiratory Infection Prevalence
(May - September)

District - Specific Allocation of Providers for Delivering Care
to Infants at "High Risk" to Gastroenteritis
(in hours)

Providers / Districts	DOCOP	DOCIP	NUROP	NURIP	OUTREACH			
					Education & Workup	Workup & Triage	Education, Workup & Triage	Total
0	8.00	69.14	9.87	337.01	0.0	66.33	0.0	66.33
1	0.51	2.79	0.65	13.61	0.0	0.0	15.10	15.10
2	4.32	34.37	5.34	167.59	0.0	31.56	24.70	56.25
3	0.58	38.58	0.74	188.03	0.0	0.0	0.0	0.0
4	0.44	28.93	0.55	141.02	0.0	0.0	0.0	0.0
5	0.51	2.79	0.65	13.61	0.0	0.0	14.60	14.60
6	0.51	2.79	0.65	13.61	0.0	0.0	15.10	15.10
7	6.16	56.60	7.59	259.24	0.0	54.21	0.0	54.21
8	0.60	37.45	0.75	182.52	0.0	0.0	1.06	1.06
9	0.79	4.17	0.97	20.42	0.0	0.0	22.11	22.11
Total Allocation to High Risk Gastroenteritis	22.43	277.60	27.76	1336.66	0.0	152.10	92.67	244.76
Maximum Resources Available ($R_p(t)$)	1533.6	728.0	656.6	1640.0	—	—	—	250.0

Figure D. 12.

Model 1 — High Gastroenteritis, Low Respiratory Infection Prevalence
(May - September)

District - Specific Allocation of Providers for Delivering Care
to Infants at Risk to Respiratory Infections
(in hours)

Providers / Districts	DOCOP	DOCIP	NUROP	NURIP	OUTREACH			
					Education & Workup	Workup & Triage	Education, Workup & Triage	Total
0	0.34	0.53	0.09	3.88	0.0	0.89	0.0	0.89
1	0.07	0.11	0.02	0.82	0.0	0.25	0.0	0.25
2	0.32	0.49	0.09	3.67	0.0	0.97	0.0	0.97
3	0.10	0.30	0.02	2.31	0.0	0.0	0.0	0.0
4	0.14	0.43	0.03	3.30	0.0	0.0	0.0	0.0
5	0.05	0.08	0.01	0.61	0.0	0.18	0.0	0.18
6	0.07	0.11	0.02	0.82	0.0	0.25	0.0	0.25
7	0.76	1.13	0.21	8.57	0.0	2.13	0.0	2.13
8	0.23	0.69	0.05	5.28	0.0	0.0	0.0	0.0
9	0.16	0.24	0.04	1.84	0.0	0.57	0.0	0.57
Total Allocation to Respiratory Infections	2.26	4.11	0.59	31.09	0.0	5.25	0.0	5.25
Maximum Resources Available ($R_p(t)$)	1533.6	728.0	656.6	1640.0	—	—	0.0	250.0

REFERENCES

Acton, Jan Paul (June 1975), "Nonmonetary Factors in the Demand for Medical Services: Some Empirical Evidence," *Journal of Political Economy* 83, No. 3: 595–614.

Anderson, N. H. (1970), "Functional Measurement and Psychophysical Judgment," *Psychological Review* 77: 153–170.

Auster, Richard; Leveson, Irving; and Sarachek, Deborah (Fall 1969), "The Production of Health, an Exploratory Study," *Journal of Human Resources* 4: 412–436.

Bergner, Marilyn; Bobbitt, Ruth A.; Pollard, William E.; Martin, Diane P.; and Gilson, Betty S. (January 1976), "The Sickness Impact Profile: Validation of a Health Status Measure," *Medical Care* 41, No. 1: 57–67.

Blischke, W. R.; Bush, J. W.; and Kaplan, R. M. (Summer 1975), "A Successive Intervals Analysis of Social Preference Measures in a Health Status Index," *Health Services Research* 10: 181–198.

Bush, J. W.; Blischke, W. R.; and Berry, C. C. (1975), "Health Indices, Outcomes, and the Quality of Medical Care," *Evaluation in Health Services Delivery;* Proceedings of an Engineering Foundation Conference, South Berwick, Me., August 19–24, 1973, edited by R. Yaffe and D. Zalkind. New York: Engineering Foundation Conferences.

———; Chen, M. M.; Patrick, D. L. (1973), "Health Status Index in Cost Effectiveness: Analysis of PKU Program," *Health Status Indexes,* edited by Robert E. Berg, Chicago: Hospital Research and Educational Trust.

———; Fanshel, S.; and Chen, M. M. (1972), "Analysis of a Tuberculin Testing Program Using a Health Status Index," *Socio-Economics Planning Sciences* 6: 49–68.

Chen, Martin K. (1975), "Aggregated Physiological Measures of Individual and Group Health Status," *International Journal of Epidemiology* 4, No. 2: 87–92.

Chen, Milton M.; Bush, J. W.; and Patrick, Donald L. (March 1975), "Social Indicators for Health Planning and Policy Analysis," *Policy Sciences* 6, No. 1: 71–89.

———; Bush, J. W.; and Zaremba, J. (1975), "A Critical Analysis of Effectiveness Measures for Operations Research in Health Services." *Operations Research in Health—A Critical Analysis.* Baltimore: Johns Hopkins University Press, 1975.

Chiang, Chin Long (1968), *Introduction to Stochastic Processes in Biostatistics.* New York: John Wiley and Sons, Inc.

Diederich, G. W.; Marsick, S. J.; and Tucker, L. R. (1957), "A General Least Squares Solution for Successive Intervals," *Psychometrics* 22: 159–173.

Donabedian, Avedis (1974), "Models for Organizing the Delivery of Personal Health Services and Criteria for Evaluating Them," *Organizational Issues in the Delivery of Health Services,* edited by Irving K. Zola and John B. McKinlay, New York: PRODIST.

——— (1967), "Evaluating the Quality of Medical Care," *Health Services Research,* edited by Donald Mainland, New York: Milband Memorial Fund.

Dunlop, David W. (1972), "The Development of an Output Concept for Analysis of Curative Health Services," *Social Science and Medicine* 6: 373–385.

Englander, Steven J., and Strotz, Charles R. (1972), "Correlation Between Risk Factors and Subsequent Infant Morbidity," unpublished paper, Tucson, Ariz.: Indian Health Service.

Fanshel, S., and Bush, J. W. (November–December 1970), "A Health Status Index and Its Application to Health Service Outcomes." *Operations Research* 18, No. 6: 1021–1066.

Fieldstein, Martin S. (May 1970), "Health Sector Planning in Developing Countries," *Economica* 37: 139–162.

Feldstein, Paul J. (1973), *Financing Dental Care: An Economic Analysis.* Lexington, Mass.: Lexington Books (D. C. Heath).

Feller, William (1968), *An Introduction to Probability Theory and Its Applications*, Vol. I, New York: John Wiley and Sons, Inc.

Geoffrion, Arthur M., and Nelson, A. B. (May 1968), *User's Instructions for 0–1 Integer Linear Programming, Code RIP30C*, Santa Monica, Calif.: Rand Corporation Memorandum RM-5627-PR.

———— (April 1967), "Integer Programming by Implicit Enumeration and 'Balas' Method," *SIAM Review* 9, No. 2: 178–190.

Grossman, Michael (March–April 1972), "On the Concept of Health Capital and the Demand for Health," *Journal of Political Economy*, 80, No. 2: 223–255.

Howard, Ronald A. (1971), "Dynamic Probabilistic Systems," *Semi-Markov and Decision Processes*, Vol. II, New York: John Wiley and Sons, Inc.

Kao, Edward P. C. (Fall 1972), "A Semi-Markov Model to Predict Recovery Progress of Coronary Patients," *Health Services Research:* 191–208.

Kaplan, Robert M.; Bush, J. W.; and Berry, Charles C. (February 1976), "Health Status: Validity of an Index of Well-Being," invited paper, symposium on "Health Status Indexes—Their Role in Tomorrow," at the Annual Meeting of the American Association for the Advancement of Sciences, Boston.

Kilpatrick, Kerry E.; MacKenzie, Richard S.; and Delaney, Allen G. (Winter 1972), "Expanded Function Auxiliaries in General Dentistry," *Health Services Research:* 288–300.

Lancaster, Kelvin (April 1966), "A New Approach to Consumer Theory," *Journal of Political Economy* 74: 132–157.

Lipscomb, Joseph (1978), "Health Resource Allocation and Quality of Care Measurement in a Social Policy Framework," *Policy Sciences* 9: 19–43.

———— and Scheffler, Richard M. (Spring 1975), "The Impact of the Expanded Duty Assistant on Cost and Productivity in Dental Care Delivery," *Health Services Research* 10, No. 1: 14–35.

Luce, R. D., and Tukey, J. W. (1964), "Simultaneous Conjoint Measurement: A New Type of Fundamental Measurement," *Journal of Mathematical Psychology* 1: 1–27.

Musgrave, Richard A. (1959) *The Theory of Public Finance*, New York: McGraw-Hill.

Nutting, Paul A.; Shorr, Gregory I.; London, Virginia L.; and Berg, Lawrence E. (September 1974), "Reduction of Respiratory Infection Morbidity by Community Health Representatives," unpublished paper, Tucson, Ariz.: Office of Research and Development, Indian Health Service.

Patrick, Donald L.; Bush, J. W.; and Chen, Milton M. (Fall 1973), "Methods for Measuring Levels of Well-Being for a Health Status Index," *Health Services Research:* 228–245.

Pollard, William E.; Bobbitt, Ruth A.; Bergner, Marilyn; Martin, Diane P.; and Gilson, Betty S. (February 1976), "The Sickness Impact Profile: Reliability of a Health Status Measure," *Medical Care* 14, No. 2: 146–155.

Reinhardt, Uwe E. (1975), "Health Manpower Planning in a Market Context: The Case of Physician Manpower," *Systems Aspects of Health Planning*, edited by Norman T. J. Bailey and Mark Thompson, Amsterdam: North-Holland Publishing Co.

Reynolds, W. Jeff; Rushing, William A.; and Miles, David L. (December 1974), "The Validation of a Function Status Index," *Journal of Health and Social Behavior* 15, No. 4: 271–288.

Scheffler, Richard M., and Lipscomb, Joseph (September 1974), "Alternative Estimations of Population Health Status: An Empirical Example," *Inquiry* 9: 220–228.

————, and ———— (July 1974), "The Consumption and Investment Benefits of Disease Programs," *Growth and Change* 5, No. 3: 8–16.

Smith, Kenneth R,; Miller, Marianne; and Golladay, Frederick L. (Spring 1972), "An Analysis of the Optimal Use of Inputs in the Production of Medical Services," *Journal of Human Resources* 7: 208–225.

Torrance, George W. (May 1976), "Health Status Models: A Unified Mathematical View," *Management Sciences* 22, No. 9: 990–1001.

———; Sackett, David L.; and Thomas, Warren H. (1973), "Utility Maximization Model for Program Evaluation: A Demonstration Application." *Health Status Indexes,* edited by Robert E. Berg, Chicago: Hospital Research and Education Trust.

———; Thomas, Warren H.; and Sackett, David L. (Summer 1972), "A Utility Maximization Model for Evaluation of Health Care Programs." *Health Services Research:* 118–133.

U.S. Department of Health, Education, and Welfare, Indian Health Service (November 1975), *Health Status Maximization and Resource Allocation: A Report to the National Center for Health Services Research,* prepared by Joseph Lipscomb, Lawrence E. Berg, Virginia L. London, and Paul A. Nutting.

Research in Health Economics

A Research Annual

Series Editor: **Richard M. Scheffler, Department of Economics George Washington University.**

The contributions to each volume are based on original research by recognized scholars within the fields of their specialization. Each volume will have a central theme within the framework of health economics. The level of treatment will be comparable to that found in leading journals in the fields of economics and medicine.

Volume 2.   **Spring 1980**   **Cloth**   **375 pages**   **Institutions: $ 28.50**
ISBN 0-89232-100-8   **Individuals: $ 14.50**

CONTENTS: Demand for Dental Care, *Teh-Wei Hu, Pennsylvania State University.* **Physician Reimbursement,** *Martha Blaxall and John Gabel, Health Care Financing Administration.* **H.E.W. Demand for Medical Care in a Rural Area,** *Larry Miners, State University of New York, Stony Brook.* **Economic Incentives in Health Maintenance Organizations,** *David Wipple, U.S. Navy Post Graduate School.* **A Theoretical and Empirical Investigation into Hospital Output Measures,** *Mark Hornbrook and John Rafferty, Division of Intramural Research, National Center for Health Services Research.* **H.E.W. Economics of Community Pharmacies,** *Lou Rossiter, Division of Intramural Research, National Center for Health Services Research.* **H.E.W. Current Issues in the Economics of Dentistry,** *John Cushman, University of California - Davis and Richard M. Scheffler, George Washington University.* **The American Hospital Industry Since 1900: A Short History,** *William D. White, University of Illinois - Chicago Circle.* **Health Manpower Credit Subsidies,** *Richard C. McKibbin, Wichita State University.* **Permanently Disabling Injuries: A General Model to Florida Work Injuries,** *Wayne Vroman, The Urban Institute.* **Determinants of Work Loss Days by Illness,** *Lynn Parringer, The Urban Institute.* **The Distribution of Health Services and the Effect on Health Status,** *Charles Stewart, George Washington University.* **Bibliography.**

A 10 percent discount will be granted on all institutional standing orders placed directly with the publisher. Standing orders will be filled automatically upon publication and will continue until cancelled. Please indicate which volume Standing Order is to begin with.

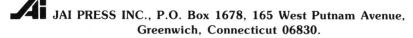 **JAI PRESS INC., P.O. Box 1678, 165 West Putnam Avenue, Greenwich, Connecticut 06830.**

Telephone: 203-661-7602   **Cable Address: JAIPUBL**

OTHER SERIES OF INTEREST FROM JAI PRESS INC.

Consulting Editor for Economics: Paul Uselding, University of Illinois

ADVANCES IN ACCOUNTING
Series Editor: George H. Sorter, New York University

ADVANCES IN APPLIED MICRO-ECONOMICS
Series Editor: V. Kerry Smith, Resources for the Future, Washington, D. C.

ADVANCES IN ECONOMETRICS
Series Editors: R. L. Basmann, Texas A & M University, and George F. Rhodes, Jr., Colorado State University

ADVANCES IN ECONOMIC THEORY
Series Editor: David Levhari, The Hebrew University

ADVANCES IN THE ECONOMICS OF ENERGY AND RESOURCES
Series Editor: Robert S. Pindyck, Sloan School of Management, Massachusetts Institute of Technology

APPLICATIONS OF MANAGEMENT SCIENCE
Series Editor: Randall L. Schultz, Krannert Graduate School of Management, Purdue University

RESEARCH IN AGRICULTURAL ECONOMICS
Series Editor: Earl O. Heady, The Center for Agricultural and Rural Development, Iowa State University

RESEARCH IN CORPORATE SOCIAL PERFORMANCE AND POLICY
Series Editor: Lee E. Preston, School of Management and Center for Policy Studies, State University of New York — Buffalo

RESEARCH IN ECONOMIC ANTHROPOLOGY
Series Editor: George Dalton, Northwestern University

RESEARCH IN ECONOMIC HISTORY
Series Editor: Paul Uselding, University of Illinois

RESEARCH IN EXPERIMENTAL ECONOMICS
Series Editor: Vernon L. Smith, College of Business and Public Administration, University of Arizona

RESEARCH IN FINANCE
Series Editor: Haim Levy, School of Business, The Hebrew University

RESEARCH IN HEALTH ECONOMICS
Series Editor: Richard M. Scheffler, George Washington University

RESEARCH IN HUMAN CAPITAL AND DEVELOPMENT
Series Editor: Ismail Sirageldin, The Johns Hopkins University

RESEARCH IN INTERNATIONAL BUSINESS AND FINANCE
Series Editor: Robert G. Hawkins, Graduate School of Business Administration, New York University

RESEARCH IN LABOR ECONOMICS
Series Editor: Ronald G. Ehrenberg, School of Industrial and Labor Relations, Cornell University

RESEARCH IN LAW AND ECONOMICS
Series Editor: Richard O. Zerbe, Jr., SMT Program, University of Washington

RESEARCH IN MARKETING
Series Editor: Jagdish N. Sheth, University of Illinois

RESEARCH IN ORGANIZATIONAL BEHAVIOR
Series Editors: Barry M. Staw, Graduate School of Management, Northwestern
University, and L. L. Cummings, Graduate School of Business, University of
Wisconsin

RESEARCH IN PHILOSOPHY AND TECHNOLOGY
Series Editor: Paul T. Durbin, Center for Science and Culture, University of
Delaware

RESEARCH IN POLITICAL ECONOMY
Series Editor: Paul Zarembka, State University of New York—Buffalo

RESEARCH IN POPULATION ECONOMICS
Series Editors: Julian L. Simoin, University of Illinois, and Julie DaVanzo, The
Rand Corporation

RESEARCH IN PUBLIC POLICY AND MANAGEMENT
Series Editor: Colin Blaydon, Institute of Policy Studies and Public Affairs,
Duke University

RESEARCH IN URBAN ECONOMICS
Series Editor: J. Vernon Henderson, Brown University

*ALL VOLUMES IN THESE ANNUAL SERIES ARE AVAILABLE AT
INSTITUTIONAL AND INDIVIDUAL SUBSCRIPTION RATES.
PLEASE ASK FOR DETAILED BROCHURE ON EACH SERIES.*

A 10 percent discount will be granted on all institutional standing orders
placed directly with the publisher. Standing orders will be filled automatically upon publication and will continue until cancelled. Please indicate
with which volume Standing Order is to begin.

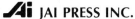 **JAI PRESS INC.**
P.O. Box 1678
165 West Putnam Avenue
Greenwich, Connecticut 06830

(203) 661-7602   Cable Address: JAIPUBL

Research in Human Capital and Development

A Research Annual

Series Editor: **Ismail Sirageldin, Departments of Population Dynamics and Political Economy The Johns Hopkins University.**

The purpose of this annual series is to bring together theoretical and empirical developments in the field of human capital formation that are relevant to the developmental issues including education and manpower training, fertility behavior, health and the important triangle of equity, efficiency and development. This series will serve as a vehicle to present a synthesis of recent developments in the field that is not only rigorous and interdisciplinary in nature, but will also bridge the gap between recent developments in theory and methodology and their applications to current developmental policy questions. Under the broad area of human capital formation, topics covered will include education and manpower development, health economics, population economics, social demography and developmental planning.

Volume 1.   **August 1979**   **Cloth**   **295 pages**   **Institutions: $ 27.50**
ISBN 0-89232-019-2   **Individuals: $ 14.00**

CONTENTS: Introduction, *Ismail Sirageldin.* **Health and Fertility. Relevance of Recent Development in the Theory of Human Capital Fertility Research,** *M. Ali Khan, The Johns Hopkins University.* **Health and Economic Development: A Theoretical and Empirical Review,** *Robin Barlow , University of Michigan.* **Health and Fertility in Bangladesh,** *W. H. Mosley, Cholera Research Laboratory, Dacca, with discussion by Ismail Sirageldin.* **Education and Manpower. College Quality and Earnings,** *J. N. Morgan and Greg Duncan, University of Michigan.* **Some Theoretical Issues in Manpower and Education Planning,** *M. Alamgir, Bangladesh Institute of Developmental Studies.* **Manpower Planning: With Special Reference to Latin America,** *Samuel Kelley, Center for Human Resources, University of Ohio.* **Barriers to Educational Development in Underdeveloped Societies: With Special Reference to Venezuela,** *Kristin Tornes, University of Bergen.* **The Growth of Professional Occupations in U.S. Manufacturing: 1900-1963,** *Carmel Ullman Chiswick, The World Bank, Washington, D.C., with discussion by Alan Sorkin, University of Maryland - Baltimore.* **Distribution and Equity. Equity, Social Mobility and Fertility,** *I. Sirageldin and J. F. Kantner, The Johns Hopkins University.* **Index.**

Guest Editor: **M. Ali Kahn, Department of Political Economy The Johns Hopkins University.**

Volume 2.   **Fall 1980**   **Cloth**   **Ca. 325 pages**   **Institutions: $ 28.50**
ISBN 0-89232-098-2   **Individuals: $ 14.50**

CONTENTS: Measures of Poverty and their Policy Implications, *K. Hamada and N. Takayama, University of Tokyo.* **Intergenerational Transfers and Distribution of Earnings,** *G. Loury, Northwestern University.* **Investment in Human Capital and Two-Sector Growth Models,** *R. K. Findlay and C. Rodriguez, Columbia University.* **The Effects on Income Maintenance on School Performance and Educational Attainment,** *C. R. Mallar and R. A. Maynard, Mathematica.* **An Analysis of Education, Employment and Income Distribution Using an Economic Demographic Model of the Phillipines,** *G. Rogers, International Labour Organization.* **Work and Consumption in the Twenty-First Century: Some Paradoxes of Late Twentieth Century Trends,** *N. Keyfitz, Harvard University.* **Relative Price Distortions and Inflation: An Application to the Case of Argentina,** *K. Chu and A. Feltenstein, International Monetary Fund.* **Theoretical Notes on Lactation and Fertility Behavior,** *W. Butz, The Rand Corporation.* **Index.**

Supplement 1 to Research in Human Capital and Development

Manpower Planning in the Oil Countries

Editor: **Naiem A. Sherbiny, International Bank for Reconstruction and Development, Washington, D.C.**

Fall 1980   Cloth   Ca. 350 pages   Institutions: $ 31.50
ISBN 0-89232-129-6   Individuals: $ 16.00

Editor's Introduction, I. Sirageldin. Introduction, Jan Tingergen.

CONTENTS: The Issues, Naiem A. Sherbiny, International Bank for Reconstruction and Development, Washington, D.C. **Structural Changes in Output and Employment in the Arab Countries,** Maurice Girgis, Indiana University, Ball State University and Kuwait Institute for Scientific Research. **Modeling and Methodology of Manpower Planning in the Arab Countries,** Ismail Serageldin, The World Bank. **An Econometric/Input-Output Approach for Projecting Sectoral Manpower Requirements: The Case of Kuwait,** M. Shokri Marzouk, Kuwait Institute for Scientific Research. **A Macroeconomic Simulation Model of High Level Manpower Requirements in Iraq,** Atif Kubursi, McMaster University and George T. Abed, International Monetary Fund, Washington, D.C. **Sectoral Employment Projections with Minimum Data Base: The Case of Saudi Arabia,** Naiem A. Sherbiny, International Bank for Reconstruction and Development, Washington, D.C. **Vocational and Technical Education and Development Needs in the Arab World,** Atif Kubursi, McMaster University. **The Complementarity of Labor and Capital Flows in the Arab World: Issues in Policy Planning,** Naiem A. Sherbiny, International Bank for Reconstruction and Development, Washington, D.C. **Index.**

A 10 percent discount will be granted on all institutional standing orders placed directly with the publisher. Standing orders will be filled automatically upon publication and will continue until cancelled. Please indicate which volume Standing Order is to begin with.

JAI PRESS INC., P.O. Box 1678, 165 West Putnam Avenue, Greenwich, Connecticut 06830.

Telephone: 203-661-7602   **Cable Address: JAIPUBL**

Research in Labor Economics

A Research Annual

Series Editor: **Ronald G. Ehrenberg, School of Industrial and Labor Relations, Cornell University.**

Volume 1. Published 1977 Cloth 384 pages Institutions: $ 27.50
ISBN 0-89232-017-6 Individuals: $ 14.00

REVIEWS: "...This volume, the first in a projected annual series, resembles a journal both in the diversity of subjects covered and the presence of advertisements at the back of the issue, but resembles a collection of essays in that the pieces are longer than the usual journal articles....If the editor can continue to find papers as high in quality as those published in this volume, the need for a publication like RLE will have demonstrated itself."— *Industrial and Labor Relations Review*

"Overall, the book should be very useful. The collection of papers presented in the volume is good and presents potentially new directions for future research in labor market phenomena." — *Southern Economic Journal*

CONTENTS: Human Capital: A Survey of Empirical Research, *Sherwin Rosen, University of Rochester.* **The Incentive Effects of the U.S. Unemployment Insurance Tax,** *Frank Brechling, Northwestern University.* **A Life Cycle Approach to Migration: Analysis of the Perspicacious Peregrinator,** *Solomon W. Polachek and Francis W. Horvath, University of North Carolina.* **Manpower Requirements and Substitution Analysis of Labor Skills: A Synthesis,** *Richard B. Freeman, Harvard University.* **Models of Labor Market Turnover: A Theoretical and Empirical Survey,** *Donald O. Parsons, Ohio State University.* **Work Effort, On-the-Job Screening and Alternative Methods of Remuneration,** *John H. Pencavel, Stanford University.* **A Simulation Model of the Demographic Composition of Employment, Unemployment and Labor Force Participation,** *Ralph E. Smith, The Urban Institute.* **Extensions of a Structural Model of the Demographic Labor Market,** *Richard S. Toikka, William J. Scanlon and Charles C. Holt, The Urban Institute.* **The Institutionalist Analysis of Wage Inflation: A Critical Appraisal,** *John Burton, Kingston Polytechnical and John Addison, Aberdeen University.*

Volume 2. Published 1978 Cloth 381 pages Institutions: $ 27.50
ISBN 0-89232-097-4 Individuals: $ 14.00

CONTENTS: Introduction, *Ronald Ehrenberg, Cornell University.* **The United Mine Workers and the Demand for Coal: An Econometric Analysis of Union Behavior,** *Henry S. Farber, Massachusetts Institute of Technology.* **Quelling for Union Jobs and the Social Returns to Schooling,** *John Bishop, University of Wisconsin.* **Labor Supply Under Uncertainty,** *Kenneth Burdett, University of Wisconsin and Dale T. Mortensen, Northwestern University.* **Governmentally Imposed Standards: Some Normative Aspects,** *Russell F. Settle, University of Delaware and Burton Weisbrod, University of Wisconsin.* **Cyclical Earnings Changes of Low Wage Workers,** *Wayne Vroman, National Bureau of Economic Research, Washington, D.C.* **Earnings, Transfers, and Poverty Reduction,** *Peter T. Gottschalk, Mount Holyoke College.* **The Influence of Fertility on Labor Supply of Married Women: Simultaneous Equation Estimates,** *T. Paul Schultz, Yale University.* **The Labor Market Adjustments of Trade Displaced Workers: The Evidence from the Trade Adjustment Assistance Program,** *George R. Newmann, University of Chicago.*

Supplement 1 to Research in Labor Economics

Evaluating Manpower Training Programs

(Revisions of papers originally presented at the Conference on Evaluating Manpower Training Programs, Princeton University, May1976)

Editor: **Farrell Bloch, Princeton University.**

June 1979   Cloth   375 pages   Institutions: $ 29.50
ISBN 0-89232-046-X   Individuals: $ 15.00

CONTENTS: Series Editor's Introduction. Editor's Introduction. **A Decision Theoretic Approach to the Evaluation of Training Programs,** Frank P. Stafford, U.S. Department of Labor and University of Michigan. **A Sensitivity Analysis to Determine Sample Sizes for Performing Impact Evaluation of the CETA Programs,** Hugh M. Pitcher, U.S. Department of Labor: (Discussant: John Conlisk, University of California - San Diego). **Estimating the Effect of Training Programs on Earnings with Longitudinal Data,** Orley Ashenfelter, Princeton University. **Earnings and Employment Dynamics of Manpower Trainees: An Explanatory Econometric Analysis,** Thomas F. Cooley, Tufts University and National Bureau of Economic Research, Timothy W. McGuire and Edward C. Prescott, Carnegie-Mellon University: (Discussant: Ronald G. Ehrenberg, Cornell University).**The Economic Benefits from Four Government Training Programs,** Nicholas M. Kiefer, Princeton University. **Estimates of the Benefits of Training for Four Manpower Training Programs,** Gordon P. Goodfellow, U.S. Department of Health, Education and Welfare:(Discussant: Daniel S. Hamermesh, Michigan State University). **The Labor Market Displacement Effect in the Analysis of the Net Impact of Manpower Training Programs,** George E. Johnson, University of Michigan: (Discussant: Robert E. Hall, Massachusetts Institute of Technology). **Potential Use of Markov Process Models to Determine Program Impact,** Hyman B. Kaitz, Westat, Inc: (Discussant: Michael L. Wachter, University of Pennsylvania). **Theoretical Issues in the Estimation of Production Functions in Manpower Programs,** Burt S. Barnow, U.S. Department of Labor. **Information Issues in Department of Labor Program Evaluation,** Ernst W. Stromsdorfer, U.S. Department of Labor: (Discussants: Michael E. Borus, Michigan State University and Robert S. Gay, Brooklyn College).

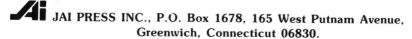 JAI PRESS INC., P.O. Box 1678, 165 West Putnam Avenue, Greenwich, Connecticut 06830.

Telephone: 203-661-7602   Cable Address: JAIPUBL